$\mathscr{C}$LIENT $\mathscr{E}$DUCAT

THEORY & PRACTICE

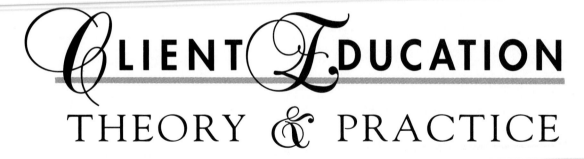

CLIENT EDUCATION

THEORY & PRACTICE

DOROTHY E. BABCOCK, RN, MS, C

Professor, Nursing and Health Care Management
Department of Nursing and Health Care Management
Metropolitan State College of Denver
Denver, Colorado

MARY A. MILLER, RN, GNP, PhD

Professor, Nursing and Health Care Management
Department of Nursing and Health Care Management
and
Associate Dean
School of Professional Studies
Metropolitan State College of Denver
Denver, Colorado

Illustrated

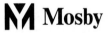 Mosby

St. Louis Baltimore Boston Chicago London Madrid Philadelphia Sydney Toronto

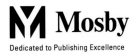

Mosby

Dedicated to Publishing Excellence

Executive Editor: N. Darlene Como
Associate Developmental Editor: Brigitte Wilke
Project Manager: Mark Spann
Production Editor: Amy Wastalu
Designers: Elise Lansdon, David Zielinski
Illustrator: Bob Rich

Copyright © 1994 by Mosby–Year Book, Inc.

Printed in the United States of America

Mosby-Year Book, Inc.
11830 Westline Industrial Drive
St. Louis, Missouri 63146

Library of Congress Cataloging in Publication Data
Babcock, Dorothy E.
   Client education: theory and practice / Dorothy E. Babcock, Mary A. Miller—
1st ed.
      p. cm.
   Includes bibliographical references and index.
   ISBN 0–8016–6942–1
   1. Patient education. I. Miller, Mary A. (Mary Alice)
II. Title.
   [DNLM: 1. Teaching—methods—nurses' instruction. 2. Learning—nurses' instruction. WA 18 B112c 1993]
   RT90.B3   1993
   610.73—dc20
   DNLM/DLC
   for Library of Congress   93-12114
                                                              CIP

93 94 95 96 97 WCB/WCB 9 8 7 6 5 4 3 2 1

To our students,
our clients,
our colleagues:
Our teachers.

This book is written for nursing students and nurses who are interested in learning more about effective health education and client teaching. Academic prerequisites to using this text include introductory courses in psychology, growth and development, and sociology. Clinical prerequisites include knowledge of nursing process application in a variety of settings. One should be advanced enough in education and practice to be comfortable with routine procedures and meeting the physiologic needs of clients. This allows for the psychic energy needed to identify client and family teaching needs.

The purpose of this book is to assist in further developing the knowledge, skills, and attitudes necessary for becoming more effective in teaching clients. In this text we have attempted to cull the information most helpful to the nursing student who recognizes teaching as an important aspect of health care, but for whom teaching is not or will not necessarily be a full-time occupation.

When considering the value of any text, the reader may benefit from an understanding of the authors' viewpoint. General systems theory and the nursing process are the basic theories we integrate throughout the text. The text is organized to follow the nursing process, i.e., assessing, diagnosing, planning, implementing, and evaluating *the client's learning needs*. We include analyses of clients' health potentials as well as deficits. This dual assessment approach is in keeping with our holistic approach to nursing diagnosis.

Education, whether formal or informal, occurs throughout life. It is the means by which individuals accomplish goals, expand intellectual processes, develop new skills, and form attitudes and values. It is a vehicle for growth and a unique experience for each individual. We believe that an important part of effective teaching is taking into account the needs of the learner. Learners possess a variety of educational backgrounds and life experiences. Each client comes to the clinical teaching moment with a body of concepts, facts, principles, and skills: a knowledge base upon which the nurse/teacher will build. Assessing the characteristics and needs of clients, and using this information to select appropriate content and teaching strategies greatly enhances teaching effectiveness.

Another value we hold is that nurses/teachers should model what they teach, especially in the areas of holistic health and human interaction. We have tried to present a view of teaching that is balanced, comprehensive, and clear and is sensitive to the needs of the reader as an adult learner. To accomplish this we have included cognitive, affective, and psychomotor aspects of clinical teaching. We address the cognitive aspects of teaching through presentations of theory. Four theoretic approaches to learning are reviewed: behavioral, gestalt, humanistic, and information processing. One of the text's unique features is the emphasis we gave to thinking within the framework of learning theories. Critical thinking is essential not only for nursing students but also for clients. Principles of learning have been derived from data contributed by adult learners.

We have summarized characteristics of learners at various developmental stages. We then discuss other biologic, psychologic, sociologic, and cultural aspects of learning. Learning objectives are based on the research done by education experts, and on the nursing process.

In the text we treat selection of content as an outgrowth of analyzing clients' learning needs using the domains of learning as established in the field of education. We present the technology related to instruction within the context of the planning and implementation phases of teaching. We use methods of evaluation that have practical application in clinical nursing.

Affective aspects of teaching are less concrete but no less important. According to Leininger, the essence of nursing is caring. Teaching is one aspect of caring. In order to care, the nurse/teacher must develop sensitivity and optimistic hope along with some measure of self-acceptance and acceptance of clients at the moment of contact. These characteristics are crucial elements in the sensing and exploitation of the "teachable moment." To develop the attitudes necessary for effectiveness, one must grow attitudinally, as a professional who can facilitate clients' decisions to change. To facilitate the process of attitudinal change, we have included some experiential exercises. We selected exercises that were identified by nursing students, nurses, and other health care providers as useful to their learning in the affective domain. Students reported that the exercises helped them gain deeper insights into clients' motivations, beliefs, and abilities. No doubt other teachers who will use this book have already discovered their own exercises that they find particularly helpful.

We also have included psychomotor aspects of learning through examination of learning principles and discussions of pertinent topics, such as the characteristics of a good demonstration. Knowledge about teaching and firsthand knowledge of the activity itself are not the same; therefore, practice exercises are included. One becomes better at doing something by doing it: with a model, coaching, feedback, and practice. Many aspects of learning theory are useful in helping an individual acquire or further polish a psychomotor skill. Throughout the book we introduce exercises that begin with a simpler tasks and progress to more complicated ones.

Speaking in public is a phenomenon that most individuals find anxiety provoking, even those who make a career out of it. Today's nurses report a wide variety of teaching experience. Many identify teaching as one of the most satisfying aspects of their careers. Others function as full-time health educators. Some report, "I feel comfortable teaching one-on-one with a client, but getting up in front of a group is scary!" Some nurses even find giving a change-of-shift report unnerving if it is done in a group setting. The idea of speaking to a group can be more intimidating than taking care of emergency situations and giving high-speed, highly technical crisis care. By the time the reader completes this book and does the exercises at the end of each chapter, he or she can expect to move a substantial distance along the continuum of expertise and comfort (in other words from Terrified Talker to Sophisticated Speaker). We hope that by learning and discussing relevant theories and practicing the steps of teaching the student will experience increased proficiency. This will lead to more skill and comfort with teaching in many settings and with a wider range of audiences. Nursing students find that as they practice speaking, their anxiety level lessens. Students have repeatedly offered us the feedback: "I hated it when you made us get up and speak, but it works, it's easier now. Be sure to make the next group do it, more often; that's the only way to get better. I'm even getting to where I almost enjoy it!"

Note to the Instructor

In the appendixes we have included a series of guidelines and forms that should help instructors prepare for a successful teaching experience. The instructor will find a variety of guidelines and forms (Appendixes, C, E, F, and G) that may be useful in teaching nursing students how to teach clients. To use this book to full advantage, the instructor may wish to discuss Appendixes A and B and assign them at the beginning of the course. Appendix A, the Reader Learning Profile, can be copied and distributed the first day of class. This profile will help the instructor assess the diversity in that particular group. Appendix B engages participants fully in the teaching/learning process by focusing attention on the content to be mastered. Appendix D contains examples of nursing diagnoses related to client teaching in the acute care setting.

We wish you as much fun and excitement in using this book as we have enjoyed while developing it.

Acknowledgements

The text is an amalgamation of contributions of our colleagues who have taught nurses how to teach clients since this subject was introduced about 2 decades ago. Dr. Mary A. Miller created the course and taught it for years, while continuing to nurture its evolution. Betty Marcom, Professor Emeritus, was a guest lecturer on the child as a learner until her retirement. Jan Buswell has been a guest lecturer on the readability of materials for several years. Professor Dorothy Babcock greatly enriched the course while teaching it for the past decade. This book also has benefited from other faculty, nursing students and nurses who have added, questioned, challenged, suggested, and otherwise helped to fine tune the content.

While we welcome this opportunity to express gratitude for all of our colleagues' contributions, we take the responsibility for the book's content, our views of teaching and learning, the emphases herein and in particular any errors or weaknesses. Suggestions to improve its clarity, readability, and utility are earnestly requested.

We gratefully acknowledge the editors for their expertise in polishing our work.

CONTENTS

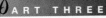

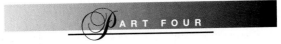

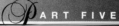

Evaluation of Learning 247

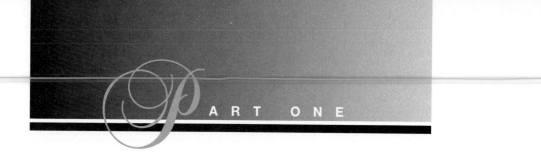

A Framework for Assessing and Teaching the Client

The Nurse and the Health Teaching System

Instead of looking at one thing
at a time, and noting its
behavior when exposed to one
other thing, science now looks at
a number of different and
interacting things and notes
their behavior *as a whole* under
diverse influences.

Lazlo, 1972, p. 6.

Objectives

Upon completion of this chapter you will be able to:

- Describe four purposes (goals) of health education.
- Apply the following system concepts to the teaching/learning process: input, process, output, feedback, suprasystem, subsystem, boundaries, and coexisting systems.
- Discuss the application of the nursing process to the teaching/learning process.
- Describe the effect of the National Consumer Health Information and Health Promotion Act of 1976 (Somers, 1976) and the recent publication *Healthy People 2000* on health education activities at the national, state, and local level.
- Identify and evaluate the significance of selected current events related to your role in client teaching.
- Discuss the statement, "The challenge of health education belongs to the nurse if she/he takes it."
- Identify two factors that limit teaching in today's environment.
- Propose three suggestions for increasing the frequency of client teaching.
- Distinguish among the following leadership roles: change agent, collaborator, resource person, and teacher.

Key Words

system	assess	feedback
input	analyze	suprasystem
high-level wellness	plan	subsystem
clinical teaching	implement	boundary
teaching/learning	evaluate	client
nursing process	output	

Introduction

This chapter introduces the theoretical framework of this book by examining two basic concepts from the perspective of health education: general systems theory and nursing process. The chapter clarifies related terms and describes the evolution of the health teaching/learning system. It concludes with an invitation to you to take a leadership position regarding client education.

The Teaching/Learning System

We will begin by defining some terms. There are many conceptual frameworks for examining the teaching/learning process. We chose general systems theory because it has widespread application, and because it can be a communication tool for individuals from diverse backgrounds. Ludwig von Bertalanffy (1968) is credited with developing general systems theory. He hoped that it would indeed become a general theory that could be used by researchers in many different fields of investigation for communicating with one another. We will describe selected aspects of his theory and explain how these aspects apply to teaching and learning of clients.

System

A system is a purposeful, complex whole composed of interdependent, interacting parts. Such a definition has several implications: (1) the system has a purpose, (2) it is complex, (3) the parts come together to form a whole, (4) the parts are dependent on each other, and (5) the parts interact. (See Figure 1-1.)

A system is complex. It consists of subsystems, which are systems within themselves. Each of these subsystems are purposeful and complex wholes.

They have boundaries that distinguish one from the other. With respect to one another, each of these subsystems is a coexisting system. They interact to form the system which is their suprasystem. Some other components of a system are input, process, output, and feedback. In the following paragraphs each of the components of a system will be addressed as it relates to the teaching/learning system.

Purposes or Goals

For you as a health educator, the main purpose of the teaching/learning system will be improved health behaviors of clients (Giardano & Dusek, 1988). These improved behaviors will lead to the highest level of wellness possible at every developmental stage and during each life crisis. In addition to facilitating movement toward optimum health, the purposes of clinical teaching include prevention of illness and disability, promotion of recovery, and optimum maintenance of function through rehabilitation.

High-Level Wellness

Health or high-level wellness is the optimum level of functioning that an individual is capable of achieving within the environment at any given point in time. This includes promotion of health, prevention of illness, and restoration of health. Continual

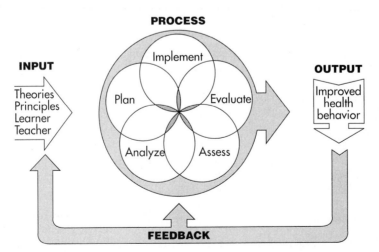

Figure 1-1 The teaching/learning system with the nursing process incorporated.

striving toward a higher level of functioning throughout the life cycle involves the biologic, psychologic, sociologic, and cultural influences of the individual interacting with his or her environment.

The Individual

The individual is a living, open, human system who performs multiple roles that affect and are affected by his/her environment. We think of the individual as a "patient" when she/he must depend on you for survival and other important aspects of nursing care, which you are learning. We consider the individual a patient when psychophysiologic impairments put him/her in your territory.

We use "client" in this text because our target is the consumer of health education. The client may be the family of the unconscious patient or the individual who is recovering from illness and needs information before she/he is discharged. In general, the client is more free to come and go from your presence and is free to refuse the services, counsel, and teaching that you will offer. Such encounters, for example, when you teach a CPR class to members of the PTA, may take place in the hospital, clinic, school, community, or home. In the context of teaching we emphasize the client's role as a responsible, thinking individual with the right to make choices about health.

Clinical Teaching

Clinical teaching is communication that facilitates learning by providing a structure within which clients are encouraged to assume responsibility for improving their health through changes in their attitudes and behaviors. The teaching role is generally accepted as an important aspect of responsibility for every professional in the health care field. In addition, we fully agree with Pender (1987) that illness prevention and health promotion are integral aspects of client care.

Input

Input consists of matter, energy, and information. In the teaching/learning system, matter includes equipment, audiovisual materials, and other physical objects that influence the teaching/learning system. Energy will be derived from you, the nurse/teacher, and from the client/learner. In the acute care setting, you will contribute much more energy than the client. In other kinds of health teaching—such as health promotion, illness prevention, and some stages of rehabilitation—the client may contribute much more energy than you.

In addition to matter and energy, information will be fed into the teaching/learning system. Information includes theories of learning, development, physiology, principles of learning, and hygiene. Other important sources of information include ideas, beliefs, and conclusions about the learning that is to take place. The perceptions of clients are as significant as your perceptions.

Process

Process is the dynamic activity undertaken by the various subsystems, which interact with one another to yield the system's product or output. The nursing process is a familiar model that we will use to further study the process of the teaching/learning system.

Assessment

In this phase, you will assess the biologic, psychologic, sociologic, and cultural influences on each client to determine each individual's learning style and capacity. Furthermore, you will decide if the client's situation is conducive or obstructive to learning. You also must assess how you fit into this process. It is important to establish whether or not you have the requisite knowledge, skills, and attitudes to facilitate each client's learning in the situation at hand.

Analysis

In this phase, in collaboration with clients whenever feasible, you will diagnose clients' learning needs. This includes analyzing both your perceptions and your clients'. Assessing needs also includes determining the kind of learning clients need. For instance, in which domain are your clients deficient? Do they lack information? Do they lack necessary skills? Is their developmental level a barrier to learning? Do they display attitudes that impair their optimum functioning? (McFarland & McFarlane, 1989; Lerner & Byrne, 1991).

Another way to approach clients is from the perspective of potential. What information do they desire? What new skills do they wish to learn? What opportunities for growth are inherent in their developmental stages? What attitudes are they ready to exhibit? What attitudes do they already possess that could motivate further growth? What strengths of mind, body, and spirit do they manifest that can help them in the inevitable transitions of life?

Planning

In this phase, you will outline the learning objectives. The planning phase should involve clients as well as their loved ones when appropriate. For example, if your client has Alzheimer's disease, then significant others, such as a daughter and son-in-law, should be included in the formation of plans. It is important to get feedback during the planning phase to discover if you and the clients are in accord with what is to be learned and how. Another step in the planning phase is deciding what needs to be learned and what strategies and materials will be most likely to facilitate achievement of the objectives.

Implementation

In this phase, you and your clients will carry out the actions that are most likely to facilitate the desired learning. During this phase you will need to elicit periodic feedback and stay attuned to behavioral clues that indicate clients' feelings of success or failure.

Evaluation

In this phase, you and your clients will compare the results with the goals: Did clients learn what was expected? Is their behavior more conducive to good health? Is their level of wellness higher? Are the problems with which clients needed help diminished, or are they coping with their problems more effectively? Two-way communication with the client will help you summarize and interpret results.

Although evaluation is presented as the final stage in the nursing process, evaluation takes place *throughout* the teaching/learning process. During the assessment phase, for instance, while identifying how clients perceive their problems, you will evaluate how well the two of you communicate. Are you understanding what the clients wish to convey? To find out, you might repeat back your interpretation of what they said. Do clients indicate that they were understood correctly? Do clients indicate that your words and actions make sense to them? Such transactions continue throughout each of the steps in the nursing process.

Output

The output of the system is its product; it is the result of the system's organization and activities. The success of the system can be measured by comparing the output with the purpose of the system (evaluation). Was the purpose of the system served? Did clients achieve improved health behaviors? Are clients perceiving themselves as more responsible for their own well being?

Feedback

Information gathered during evaluation is the feedback used for more input into the system. These data allow the system to continue on its course or provide ideas for changing the system so that it is better able to achieve its purpose. Output is used to reassess, replan, and reteach. Evaluation, output, and feedback are interrelated, as highlighted in Figure 1-1.

Suprasystem

The suprasystem is the larger system within which clients and caregivers interact. In the hospital, the unit is the suprasystem of the teaching/learning system. In community health-teaching the suprasystem is the home, the neighborhood, the school, or the larger community.

Environment

Environment is all that surrounds the system, an aggregate of things, conditions, and influences, both internal and external. The external environment includes all of the equipment in the patient's room in the hospital. It is similar to the concept of suprasystem. The internal environment is similar to the subsystem concept. The client's internal environment includes the respiratory system, the circulatory system, and the client's sensorium.

Subsystem

A subsystem is a system that is purposeful, receives input, and delivers a product. The subsystem interacts with other systems, forming a larger system. The respiratory system and the circulatory system are subsystems of the human system (individual). The teaching/learning system is one aspect (subsystem) of the nursing care system.

Boundary

The boundary is the edge of the system under focus and represents the limit of the system, beyond which the system ceases to be identified as itself. Boundaries mark the end point of one system and the beginning of another. Human beings are living, open systems. This means that we have boundaries, but those boundaries are permeable. There is communication between what is inside the boundary and what is outside. In the teaching/learning system, the clients (subsystems) allow information (outside the subsystems) to enter their knowledge base. In return, you (subsystem) will allow feedback from clients into your consciousness, which you use to shape the next transaction. If the client suffers from surface trauma, such as gaping wounds, the boundaries are inappropriately open to loss of internal resources (blood) and to entrance of hazardous invaders (infection). In that case your response to the client (subsystem) will be to give emergency care now and teach later.

Coexisting Systems

Coexisting systems are those that interact within a larger system. In the hospital the nursing care system coexists with the dietary system and the medical system. In the community the school system coexists with the health care system. The economic system and the political system are less tangible but equally important coexisting systems. Health insurance systems, for instance, greatly affect what health teaching is economically feasible.

The Context of Health Teaching

Why is health education important to today's caregiver? How is the teaching/learning system related to the national health scene? These are some of the questions addressed in the following paragraphs.

History

The tireless efforts of many pioneering investigators and public servants during the first half of this century have proved fruitful. As a result of such efforts the United States has enjoyed a great reduction in the incidence of infectious diseases. New knowledge regarding hygiene and isolation along with increased public pressure to make clean water available to most citizens were effective in improving individual and community health. Methods of waste disposal that protected the public from constant contamination were among the many public activities that improved our health and our chances of a "normal" life span (Zerwekh, 1992).

Making immunization a prerequisite for attending school pressured parents to provide this protective measure for their children. As a result, the incidence of early death from childhood infectious diseases has diminished. Many middle-aged nurses can recall the introduction in the early 1960s of the polio vaccine, which dramatically reduced the "scourge of summer."

Global immunization programs and efforts to provide clean water to the rest of the world have had gratifying results. One of the most remarkable of these achievements was the eradication of smallpox.

The third quarter of this century was characterized by a great influx of resources into the health care system. Dreams of The Great Society advocated by President Lyndon Johnson in the 1960s resulted in generous funding of institutions that trained health personnel, facilities to care for the ill, and programs that would make health care a right of all Americans no matter what their education, income, race, or creed.

Development of feedback was the hallmark of the 1970s, and the Alameda study, which was published in that decade, is evidence of its use (Bellock and Breslow, 1972). The Alameda Study investigated the health habits of 7,000 people for more than 5½ years in Alameda, California. The research revealed that men in their mid-50s who followed six or seven specific habits were in about the same physical condition as men 20 years younger who followed only three or fewer of those habits. Poor health habits were more closely related than income to the incidence of illness and early death. Furthermore, an American male's life is prolonged by 11 years and a female's by 7 years if they follow time-honored practices known as "Grandma's Rules." The rules include the following: do not smoke; drink little or no alcohol; eat breakfast; do not snack between meals; sleep at least 7 hours a night; maintain normal weight; and exercise regularly.

In 1976 the National Consumer Health Information and Health Promotion Act (Somers, 1976) was passed during President Gerald Ford's administration. With the passage of this act, the U.S. government officially recognized the importance of lifestyle in the health of its citizens. Furthermore, the Act committed the government to accept responsibility for educating the public about individual health actions that could raise citizens' level of wellness and reduce the risk of premature death.

Target Groups

The committee responsible for writing the act recommended targeting specific groups for health ed-

ucation. The target groups are listed below along with examples of how those groups are being reached today.

Patients

When people become ill, they are more amenable to health education than at many other times. Because you will be with clients when they are ill, you will be in an ideal position to reach them at their teachable moments.

School Children

Children are ideal audiences for health education, and such education can have a positive influence on children's behavior. Problems can be prevented by addressing simple activities, such as toothbrushing, or risky behaviors, such as experimentation with drugs and indiscriminate sex. The school nurse serves as the professional on the scene with the expertise needed for promoting learning or health teaching. In an effort to trim budgets, some communities have reduced the number of school nurses even though the number of children without private health care has increased (Disch, 1989).

Employees on the Work Site

Corporate America, which pays for much of this country's health care bill, is increasing its interest in measures for lowering care costs for sick and disabled employees. An occupational health nurse, who knows the employees and the health risks associated with their occupations, is in a unique position to design relevant health education strategies (Miller, 1989).

Communities

Numerous communities throughout the United States are now participating in public health education activities. Various supermarkets and food producers are providing information to their customers regarding the nutritional value of their products.

Citizens

The surgeon generals' reports, *Healthy People* (1979), a subsequent report entitled *Healthy People*,

2000 (1990), and recent national mailings regarding the hazards and prevention of acquired immunodeficiency syndrome are examples of how these officers are fulfilling the government's commitment of informing the citizenry.

Media Consumers

During the past decade there has been a proliferation of health programs via the media. These programs have been funded by government, private foundations, and commercial sponsors. News reports on items out of prestigious nursing, psychology, science, and medicine journals are now commonplace in daily newspapers and on television news programs.

Actions to Reach and to Teach

The Task Force on Consumer Health Education (Somers, 1976), recommended that specific actions be implemented to reach the six target groups mentioned above. Those actions and some results of their recommendations are listed below.

Information

Despite heavy lobbying to the contrary, the government has managed to inform the public that cigarette smoking is the largest single preventable cause of illness and premature death in the United States (Lesmes & Donofrio, 1992). Hazardous warnings that are now present on tobacco products are evidence that the government is to some extent assuming its responsibility.

Motivation

More research is needed to examine what motivates people to change. Bauman and Keller (1991) found that individuals who participated in a screening procedure, expressed more willingness to engage in risk-reducing behaviors when they perceived themselves at risk for diabetes II. Some preliminary findings have shown that threats, however severe and obvious, are of questionable value in the face of addiction or any kind of habitual behavior. Threats of breast cancer did not motivate women to do regular breast self-examination. Campaigns of self-disclosure, however, and "how to" lessons were catalysts for change (Detection and diagnosis of breast cancer, 1984).

Several times well-known and admired women have declared publicly: "I had cancer, I had it removed. I am well now. You, too, can check on your health." These brave role models inspired women all over the nation to examine their breasts and to report suspicious lumps to their caregivers. Breast self-examination classes and leaflets have also appeared to be more effective at motivating people than the use of threats.

Skill Development

Many classes now exist that teach people how to change their behaviors. These classes can be found in health maintenance organizations (HMO), in hospitals and in community education sites, such as the branches of the Young Men's Christian Association (YMCA). Education to enhance wellness and reduce personal health risks is now a big business.

Teaching Skills to Health Personnel

The committee that wrote the National Consumer Health Information and Health Promotion Act recommended that health personnel receive training in teaching. Nursing programs anticipated this mandate. Teaching has been seen as a nurse's responsibility since the beginning of the profession in this country (Nightingale, 1859).

Environmental Changes

The subject of environmental awareness is the most ambiguous. Although evidence mounts regarding the dangers of environmental pollution, such as cigarette smoking, subsidies to the tobacco industry continue. Furthermore, federal funding of watchdog agencies such as Occupational Safety and Health Administration (OSHA) and Environmental Protection Agency (EPA) continues to be reduced. This contrasts with the rhetoric that abounded at the 1992 Earth Summit in Rio de Janeiro, where world leaders gathered to examine the global effects of environmental pollution (Little, 1992).

A plethora of research and evaluation reports are available from numerous government and private sources, many of which were summarized by Bauer (1980). *Healthy People 2000* (1990) contains information from a broad spectrum of sources. Thousands of professionals from many disciplines, health advocates, and consumers were convened by the U.S. Public Health Service during a three-year period in eight regions throughout the nation. In addition to the results of that public testimony, the report contains compilations of many in-depth studies. Agencies such as the Kellogg Foundation, the U.S. Department of Health and Human Services, and the World Health Organization are sources of periodic summary reports (Little, 1992).

Toffler (1980) claimed that our society had entered a third wave of evolution. The first wave was that of agriculture, the second, the wave of consumption, and now the wave of the *prosumer*. Toffler defined a prosumer as one who both produces and consumes goods. An example is the nurse/writer, who buys a sophisticated computer, and then does much of the groundwork necessary for publishing on her own computer. Another example is the petroleum engineer who is laid off and uses the time to refinish the basement. Toffler characterized this third wave of civilization by acceleration of change, increasing mobility, increasing information exchange, increasingly intelligent environments, and the rising prevalence of consequential thinking.

Naisbitt (1990) and his staff traced trends in our civilization by carefully tracking the appearance and the disappearance of topics from the pages of selected newspapers and other periodicals across the nation. Trends that are having a salutary effect on our nation's health include salad bars in fast-food restaurants and sustained increases in aerobic activities. Naisbitt predicted that service professions, such as nursing, would remain relatively stable, while production tasks would be done by machines and relatively inexpensive labor in third world countries. Computers were expected to take over many of our routine filing tasks. What this means to you the nurse is that you will not have to handle lab reports to get them into clients' charts. Technology has already made it possible for you to see how your clients are doing without touching them or even going into their presence. Will these advances allow you to stay in better touch with all of your clients or will it tempt you to touch them less? (Backer, Frost, & Mason, 1985).

Naisbitt further predicted that, as a nation, we were reacting to a highly technologic society by showing the need for more human touch. The human growth movement, which included personal growth workshops and assertiveness training and the resurrection of massage as a respectable activity in this country, is a sign that human beings continue to need to express themselves and to touch. How many nursing programs still include massage in their curricula? In your program, will you learn how to routinely massage and otherwise touch your clients in caring ways with the intention to heal? The increasing interest in therapeutic touch is one indication that many nurses are again becoming aware of the power of healing touch (Krieger, 1990; Dossey, Keegan, Gouzetta, & Kolkmeier, 1988).

Our mortality rate, despite skyrocketing health care costs and technical sophistication, was unimpressive when compared with countries that have much smaller health care budgets. It has not improved much recently. According to one study, Japan had the lowest infant mortality rate, Sweden had the second lowest, Canada had the third lowest, Great Britain and Australia tied for fourth lowest, and the United States ranked fifth (Little, 1992).

Some of the other feedback included more encouraging signs. After the 1964 public delivery of the U.S. surgeon general's report regarding the hazards of smoking, 30 million Americans became ex-smokers (Bauer, 1980). This dramatic change showed that public education is effective for at least one third of the target audience. The Stanford Heart Disease Program was unique in that planned community education was accompanied by large scale research. The results of this study revealed that large scale, multifaceted educational efforts could result in sustained long-range improvement in health behaviors, which significantly reduce the risk that a population will develop heart disease and related illnesses (Bauer, 1980).

Current Trends

The acceleration of technology is giving rise to smaller and more portable systems of record-keeping. Whether you encounter the client in the hospital bed, the clinic, or the client's home, technology now exists that will allow you to access the entire data base on the client and add to the information with a small hand-held unit (Meyer, 1992). Although a more technologic environment should free you from routine tasks, other phenomena will encroach on your time.

Change in the sites of health care is evolving rapidly. Although two thirds of today's nurses still practice in hospitals, increasing numbers work in homes, surgical care centers, extended care facilities, shopping malls, health vans, and neighborhood ambulatory care centers. Increasing numbers of nurse widwives, anesthetists, and practitioners are entering the labor market. It has been shown that their performance is as effective as physicians' and their cost is lower (Disch, 1989).

In the next decade more than 25% of the recipients of health care will be older than 65. This will be accompanied by an increase in the number of Americans with chronic illness, which will in turn increase the demand for extended care units. At present it is estimated that 40 million Americans are uninsured even though two thirds of that group are employed (Hawken, 1990; Gold, 1989).

In 1992 the United States had 300,000 to 500,000 diagnosed cases of individuals who abuse drugs. Some of these drug abusers are violent and confused when they enter the health care system (Kurlowicz, 1990). The drug culture has been connected with the large number of babies exposed to cocaine and the resulting economic burden and loss of human potential (Sullivan, 1990). The use of expensive equipment and procedures is increasing our ability to delay death and prolong illness.

The measles epidemic of 1990 showed that the strides made in the first half of this century have broken down due to changing attitudes toward vaccination (Office of the Surgeon General, 1990). Other more hopeful trends are reflected in the rising popularity of do-it-yourself, home-testing kits for pregnancy, occult blood, and diabetes. Many clients now do their own preparations at home for these routine medical procedures.

The global economy and the loss of jobs in various industries are affecting the wage-earning status of nurses. Many nurses whose financial roles were secondary are now becoming the primary source of income for their families. Single individuals, single parents, or married couples are struggling with the changing economy. Nurses, most of whom are women, may be working because they must provide for themselves and their families.

Despite its drawbacks, nursing is attracting newcomers. Some are young students who have chosen nursing as their first career while others are older and are switching to nursing careers in the midst of raising families. Today's nurses and nursing students come from culturally diverse backgrounds. This diversity can greatly enrich the educational experience for the students as well as the teachers. At the end of the chapter on cultural diversity you will find some exercises that will guide you in learning from your peers and clients.

At this time the nursing shortage appears to be easing in some hospitals while in others it is reaching crucial levels (Hassanein, 1991). Women, who comprise most of the nursing force, now have many more career options from which to choose. Nursing is not known as an occupation that pays well in light of the amount of responsibility expected from its incumbents (Hassanein, 1991). That too is changing. In 1991 the California Nurses Association negotiated a 13% raise, which elevates the salaries of new nurses to more than $40,000, with a promise of a 9% raise the following year (S.F. pay jumps 13%, 1991).

How will these multiple changes in the United States influence the nursing profession as a whole? Moraldo (1992) predicted that domestic health issues will replace communism as a primary national concern, spiritual and emotional health will gain emphasis, nurse entrepreneurs will become more visible and assertive, home care and managed care will become the center of health care, national health insurance will become a reality, more nurse leaders will emerge, research into treating and preventing HIV infections will be funded, and increased accountability of health care providers will be demanded.

What are the implications of all this for you as a nurse? We believe that your job will change to teaching assisting personnel as well as clients. It is well known that hospital stays are shorter, and clients are being discharged sooner. As a consequence, more care is being delivered in the home by nurses, assisting personnel, and family members. Clients will continue to do more self-care. Increasing numbers of elderly clients will need varying degrees of support and education. With the increasing body of knowledge that is generated by research and advances in biomedical technology, your ongoing education will be critical. Continuing education in academia and in the workplace will be necessary for you to stay current. We must be willing to reshape ourselves and our institutions to deal with the new realities that will continue to emerge at an accelerating pace (Naisbitt & Aburdene, 1990).

Teaching as a Nursing Function

The challenge of health education belongs to you, if you take it. The education function has been within the scope of nursing practice since the beginning. The National League of Nursing Education (NLNE) (1918) defined nursing as the prevention of illness and the promotion of health especially in public health, child welfare, schools, home visiting, industries, hospitals, and social services. Pioneers, such as Lillian Wald and Mary Brewster, provided both social services and nursing care; in addition, they were politically active in pressuring the government and industry to improve living conditions and basic hygiene. Much of their activity took place in settlement houses (Kippenbrock, 1991). Two decades later the National League for Nursing (NLN) (1937) said that a nurse was essentially a teacher and an agent of health in whatever field the practice occurred. Nurse Practice Acts in many states include teaching within the scope of nursing practice. For 10 years the Colorado Nurse Practice Act has included the statement: "Practice of professional nursing shall include

the performance of such services as . . . (b) Health teaching and health counseling; (Colorado State Board of Nursing, 1991, p. 2)."

Because you will be with the client at the most teachable moment, you will be doing the most health education. Your background in anatomy, physiology, nutrition, psychology, sociology, anthropology, and other social and physical sciences makes you a very appropriate health teacher. Your education will teach you how the body can and should function and will teach you about the interplay among mind, body, and spirit. In addition, you have access to the behavioral research that can help people learn risk-reducing skills. This same body of research can be applied to help people change and maintain those changes in their health behaviors (Bauer, 1980). Your firsthand knowledge about the consequences of various life-styles will make you an authentic source of information. Your predecessors have earned the public's trust, and your own health habits can make you more believable as a health teacher and role model. Your clients will be coming to you better informed. This means they will be demanding more knowledgeable caregivers, and they will expect you to provide them with current and scientifically sound information. Many have done considerable reading about their particular health problem and consequently ask informed, sophisticated questions. Your credibility will be established by your answers. Consumers will continue to learn more about mobilizing their own immunoresponse systems, and they will expect you to help them do this (Houldin, Lev, Prystowsky, Redei, & Lowery, 1991).

The skyrocketing cost of medical care has caught the public's attention. The threats of HIV infection and substance abuse as public health menaces are real and growing. Consumer groups are pressing for more options in choosing health care providers and for more equitable distribution of illness costs. These groups are also making health care institutions more accountable for costs (Fein, 1992). Others recommend making those whose lifestyles contribute to their illnesses pay more for the treatment of the illnesses they incur. The theory is that higher insurance premiums may motivate people to learn more about how they can change their high-risk behaviors. Business and industry are encouraging dissemination of health information because such educational materials help lower illness costs. We are also seeing increased funding for health research. Moraldo (1992) says that enactment of a national health plan is inevitable. Books are appearing that describe the behaviors and attitudes of those who stay healthy in adverse circumstances and those who unexpectedly recover from serious illnesses (Siegel, 1986). In addition, the popularity of books that focus on various health-promotion topics is growing exponentially.

Because client education is mandatory (American Hospital Association, 1972), someone must be accountable for client teaching. If you do not exercise educational leadership in health and illness institutions, you may find yourself receiving guidance from individuals who do not know the clients and who know far less than you do about the content you must teach.

Third-party payers are recognizing the importance of teaching in the role repertoire of the professional nurse. Home visits by a professional nurse are now reimbursable only if those services include teaching and/or counseling (Huey, 1988). It behooves you to market yourself as the wellness educator with the best combination of solid scientific background and firsthand, day-to-day clinical experience.

Factors That Limit Teaching

Factors that limit the effectiveness of nurses' teaching include the nurses themselves, their clients, and the situation. Each of these factors will be explored in depth throughout the rest of the text. The amount of support nurses get in their teaching roles is one important variable. More and more hospital systems are being absorbed by for-profit chains in which cost containment is a reality. In the midst of the current nursing shortage, many nurses feel called upon to care for too many clients for too many hours. Increased workloads and diminished resources preclude anything more than basic and critical care. Institutions that used to enjoy heavy

endowment and rich funding now find it necessary to reorganize, streamline, and cut luxuries. Health-teaching can be seen as a luxury in the above circumstances (Prescott, Phillips, Ryan, & Thompson, 1991). Nurses, weighed down by today's demands, may be tempted to take the position of the mountain villagers in the following excerpt:

> . . . and thus [it came to be] with the story of the mountain villagers . . . their kind inhabitants labored day and night trying to resuscitate the large numbers of drowning people being continually swept down to them through the rapids of their turbulent river. A passing traveller asked why they did not repair the broken bridge upstream. The answer, he was told, should be self-evident. The daily care of the river's victims was already consuming much more time and effort than the village could afford. (Bauer, 1980, p. 177).

The Nurse as Change Agent

As nurses, you will function as agents of change. In the role of change agent you will assume responsibility for bringing about an alteration in the health delivery system and/or the level of wellness of individuals, families, groups, and/or communities (Chalick & Smith, 1992). When you persuade a client to move and breathe deeply after surgery, you are functioning as a change agent. When you join a public interest group to bring about policy changes to "mend the bridge upstream," you are functioning as a change agent. A study done two decades ago showed that nursing was the only health resource that made an apparent difference in outcomes on reducing community death rates (Miller & Stokes, 1978). Hughes and others showed that both public health nurses and nurse/midwives significantly reduced the morbidity and mortality that occurs in high-risk populations of mothers and their babies (Hughes, Johnson, Simons, & Rosenbaum, 1986).

You will learn to collaborate with others: professional colleagues, consumers of health care, and policymakers. In the role of collaborator, you will interact with individuals in open communication to accomplish agreed-upon purposes. It will be your responsibility to help plan and carry out health goals within the realities of the times (Califano, 1986). This collaboration will occur at the bedside, in the home, in the clinic, in the community, and at the national level. When you join a student organization or study with peers you are functioning as a collaborator. When you join a hospital committee to study quality assurance issues, you are functioning as a collaborator. When you sit down with members of a family to decide on how to manage in-the-home care of their loved one you are functioning as a collaborator. To collaborate, you need effective communication skills. Johnson (1990) and Smith (1989) describe several ways that nurses can participate as leaders in improving their own communities. It is important for you to perceive yourself as a partner in the process, to articulate well, and to bring to your clients, administrative personnel, colleagues, and legislators your thoughtful observations and recommendations for remedial action.

As a resource person your expertise will be used to aid and support clients by sharing knowledge, providing nursing skills, and/or assisting clients to access and utilize appropriate services and health care delivery systems. You will develop a rich background of scientific knowledge and sensitivity. When you combine this with daily personal caring and direct observation of the consequences of behavior on the quality of human life, you will indeed have much to offer. As the health professional who also functions in the home and in the community, you will be aware of the many self-help groups and community agencies that are available for myriad health concerns. When you connect clients with those resources, you are functioning as a resource person. When you offer to call the Cancermount volunteer for a client, you are functioning as a resource person. As the shift from hospital-dominated health delivery to a more community-based system occurs, your role as resource person will become even more important.

Summary

In this chapter we introduced the framework of general systems theory and nursing process upon which we will build throughout the text. We defined key words related to general systems theory and the nursing process and discussed the historical context of today's consumer of health care and your role as teacher in health practices and illness prevention. We followed this discussion with a description of some current trends and challenges. Political and economic forces may be perceived as obstacles; they also may be viewed as spurs to exerting leadership in the health education field. It is clear that besides teaching at the bedside, you must be engaged in education of families in their homes, in clinics, in schools, at job sites, in the media, and in your own neighborhood (American Nurses Association, 1991). Nursing's agenda for the year 2000 emphasizes the importance of professional nurses viewing themselves as health educators in many arenas.

DISCUSSION QUESTIONS

Purposes:

- Review information contained in this chapter
- Promote critical thinking

Directions:

- Form small groups.
- Choose which of the following issues your group will discuss (from questions one through four).
- Prepare a report that summarizes your discussion.

1. Identify the crucial behaviors identified in the Alameda study that prolonged life and health. Evaluate yourself as a health role model along each of those parameters.
2. "The challenge of health education belongs to the nurse if she/he takes it." Discuss this statement in terms of the following:
   a. What is the significance of the National Consumer Health Education and Health Promotion Act of 1976?
   b. Name target populations identified by the committee that drafted the act and discuss how nurses do or could take the initiative to reach them.
   c. Name the health activities identified by the committee mentioned in the previous question. Describe how nurses do or could perform each of those activities. You may use observations from your own clinical or student practice or personal observations.
   d. What is your opinion of the effect of that act now? Support your opinion with reports on relevant research.
3. Name five of the trends described in the chapter that you consider most important to the health care industry.
4. Explain how each of the items you selected in the previous question affect you as a:
   a. Wage earner and payer of taxes and insurance premiums
   b. Nursing professional
   c. Leader in the field of health promotion and education
   d. Consumer of health and illness services

PATIENT'S BILL OF RIGHTS

Purposes:

- Become more aware of the amount of teaching mandated in the Patient's Bill of Rights
- Compare and contrast the congruency between the bill of rights and its implementation in practice

Directions:

1. Obtain a copy of the Patient's Bill of Rights from a local hospital or clinic.
2. Analyze the contents of the bill of rights. Appraise its meaning, readability, and accessibility, in terms of the client population served at that facility.
3. Compare and contrast the theory of patient rights as they are outlined in the document with the way they are manifested in reality at that facility. You may also draw upon your observations as a student, client, or relative.
4. Bring copies of the patient rights documents to class and discuss them.

WAYS TO PROMOTE TEACHING

Purposes:

- Promote creative thinking
- Raise consciousness regarding clinical teaching

Directions:

1. Form small groups.
2. Discuss the following situation.
3. Take notes and prepare a report to be shared with the rest of your peers.

In the midst of many obstacles identified in this chapter some nurses are managing to teach their clients in mutually satisfactory ways. What are you doing to promote teaching? What client teaching have you observed by clinical instructors, supervisors, charge nurses, team leaders, and primary nurses? If you are not yet in the clinical area, seek out nurses in your school, hospital, or neighborhood and ask them what they are doing to promote teaching. Draw on your experiences as a patient, client, relative, or observer. In retrospect what do you think would have been helpful regarding the nurse's role in client teaching?

IDENTIFYING NURSING LEADERSHIP ROLES

Purposes:

- Review information presented in Chapter 1
- Promote critical thinking
- Apply theory to clinical situations

Directions:

- Following is a vignette of nursing students interacting with each other and an instructor. A number of leadership roles in various capacities are presented: change agent, collaborator, resource person, and teacher.
- Distinguish among the roles exhibited in the vignette. Use the descriptions of the leadership roles as explained at the end of this chapter to defend your analyses.

George Jones, nursing student, was very interested in the field of psychoneuroimmunology. He discovered that four of his peers were also interested in the subject. Together, they asked the instructor if they could get some credit for studying the subject further. The teacher said "Yes, why don't you do a group presentation for your classmates? I will help you get started."

1. During the meeting the four students and the instructor shared with each other their understanding of psychoneuroimmunology.
2. The instructor mentioned a recent article that reviewed the literature on the topic and gave the students information on how to locate the article.
3. The students used the references at the end of the article and the library retrieval system to locate more information. They agreed to divide the reading and preparation of the findings.
4. The students met at an agreed-upon time and pooled their knowledge. They divided

up the work required for preparing their paper and reached an agreement with the instructor on when to present their information to the rest of the class.

5. The students presented their findings to the class; they were delighted with the response of their peers, who found the presentation very informative, interesting, and thought-provoking.

6. The students were very pleased with their own initiative and with the instructor's receptiveness to input regarding course content.

References

American Hospital Association. (1972). *A patient's bill of rights.* Chicago: Author.

American Nurses Association. (1991). *Nursing's agenda for health care reform,* (PR-12-91). Author.

Backer, B., Frost, A. & Mason, D. (1985). High tech–high touch it's high time for nursing. *Nursing & Health Care,* 6(5), 263-266.

Bauer, K.G. (1980). *Improving the chances for health: Lifestyle changes and health evaluation.* San Francisco: National Center for Health Education.

Bauman, L.J. & Keller, M.L. (1991). Responses to threat information. *IMAGE: Journal of Nursing Scholarship,* 23(1), 13-18.

Bellock, N.B. & Breslow, L. (1972). Relationship of Physical Health Status to health practices. *Preventive Medicine,* 1, 409-421.

Califano, J.A. Jr. (1986). *America's health care revolution.* New York: Random House.

Chalick, T. & Smith, L. (1992). Nursing at the grass roots. *Nursing & Health Care,* 13(5), 242-246.

Colorado State Board of Nursing. (1991). *Colorado nurse practice act.* Denver CO: Author.

Detection and diagnosis of breast cancer. (1984). In *The Breast Cancer Digest* (2nd ed.). (NIH Publication No. 84-1691). Bethesda: National Cancer Institute.

Disch, J.M. (June, 1989). *Are we fostering excellence in practice?* Paper presented at the Nursing Education 89: The Conference for Nursing Faculty. Philadelphia: Medical College of Pennsylvania, Continuing Nursing Education.

Dossey, B.M., Keegan, L., Gouzetta, D. & Kolkmeier, L.G. (1988). *Holistic nursing: A handbook for practice.* Rockville MD: Aspen Publishers.

Fein, R. (1992). Health care reform: Is it time for our medicine? *Modern Maturity,* 35(4), 22-35.

Giardano, D.A. & Dusek, D.E. (1988). *Changing health behaviors.* Scottsdale AZ: Gorsuch Scarisbrick, Publishers.

Gold, A.R. (July 30, 1989). The struggle to make do without health insurance. *New York Times.*

Hassanein, S.A. (1991). On the shortage of registered nurses: An economic analysis of the RN market. *Nursing & Health Care,* 12(3), 152-156.

Hawken, P.L. (1990). NLN's national health strategy: A plan for reform. *National League for Nursing Public Policy Bulletin,* Fall 1990, 3-4.

Houldin, A.D., Lev, E., Prystowsky, M.B., Redei, E. & Lowery, B.J. (1991). Psychoneuroimmunology: A review of literature. *Holistic Nursing Practice,* 5(4), 10-21.

Huey, F. (1988). How nurses would change U.S. health care. *American Journal of Nursing,* 88(11), 1482-1493.

Hughes, D., Johnson, K., Simons, J., & Rosenbaum, S. (1986). *Maternal and child health data book.* Washington DC: Children's Defense Fund.

Johnson, P.A. (1990). National health insurance program: A nursing perspective. *Nursing & Health Care,* 11(8), 416.

Kippenbrock, T.A. (1991). Wish I'd been there: A sense of nursing history. *Nursing & Health Care,* 12(4), 208-212.

Krieger, D. (1990). Therapeutic touch: Two decades of research, teaching & clinical practice. *Imprint,* 37(3), 83, 86-88.

Kurlowicz, L.H. (1990). Violence in the emergency room. *American Journal of Nursing,* 90(9), 34-39.

Lazlo, E. (1972). *The systems view of the world.* New York: Braziller.

Lerner, H. & Byrne, M.W. (1991). Helping nursing students communicate with high risk families. *Nursing & Health Care*, 12(2), 98-101.

Lesmes, G.R. & Donofrio, K.H. (1992). Passive smoking: The medical and economic issues. *The American Journal of Medicine* 93(1), 385.

Little, C. (1992). Health for all by the year 2000: Where is it now? *Nursing & Health Care*, 13(4), 198-204.

McFarland, G.K. & McFarlane, E.A. (1989). *Nursing diagnoses & intervention, planning for patient care*. St. Louis MO: Mosby.

Meyer, C. (1992). Bedside computer charting: Inching toward tomorrow. *American Journal of Nursing*, 92(4), 38-44.

Miller, M.A. (1989). Social, economic, and political forces affecting the future of occupational health nursing. *Journal of the American Association of Occupational Health Nurses*, 37(9), 361-366.

Miller, M.K. & Stokes, C.S. (1978). Health status, health resources and consolidated structural parameters: Implications for public health care policy. *Journal of Health & Social Behavior*, 19(3), 263-278.

Moraldo, P.J. (1992). Trends to watch for in '92: Health highest on American agenda. *Executive Wire*. New York: National League for Nursing.

Naisbitt, J. & Aburdene, P. (1990). *Megatrends 2000*. New York: William Morrow and Company, Inc.

National League of Nursing Education: Standard curriculum for schools of nursing. (1918). Baltimore MD: The Waverly Press.

National League of Nursing Education: A curriculum guide for schools of nursing. (1937). New York: The League.

Nightingale, F. (1859). *Notes on nursing*. New York: Appleton-Century-Crofts.

Office of the Surgeon General. (1979). *Healthy people: The surgeon general's report on health promotion and disease prevention; background papers* (DHEW Publication No. 79-55071A). Washington DC: U.S. Government Printing Office.

Office of the Surgeon General. (1990). *Healthy people 2000* (DHHS Publication PHS No. 91-50213). Washington DC: U.S Government Printing Office.

Pender, N.J. (1987). *Health promotion in nursing practice*. Norwalk, CN: Appleton-Century Crofts.

Prescott, P.A., Phillipps, C.Y., Ryan, J.W. & Thompson, K.O. (Spring, 1991). Changing how nurses spend their time. *IMAGE: Journal of Nursing Scholarship*, 23(1), 23-27.

S.F. pay jumps 13%, starting now at $43,000. (1991). *American Journal of Nursing*, 91(8), 11.

Siegel, B. (1986). *Love, Medicine and Miracles*. New York: Harper & Row.

Smith, G.R. (1989). Community of caring. *Geriatric Nursing*, 10(5), 248.

Somers, A.R. (Ed.). (1976). *Promoting health, consumer education and national policy: Part III summary and recommendations*. Germantown MD: Aspen Systems Corporation.

Sullivan, K.R. (1990). Maternal implications of cocaine use during pregnancy. *Journal of Perinatal Neonatal Nursing*, 3(4), 12-25.

Toffler, A. (1980). *The third wave*. New York: William Morrow.

von Bertalanffy, L.C. (1968). *General system theory: Foundations, development and applications*. New York: George Braziller.

Zerwekh, J.V. (1992). Public health nursing legacy. *Nursing & Health Care*, 13(2), 84-91.

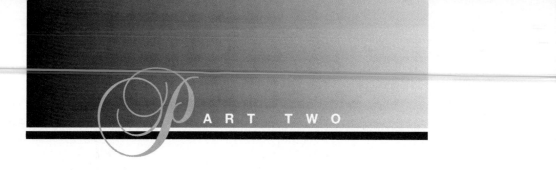

PART TWO

The Learning Process

The Learning System

To think critically is to show
that we are aware and reflective
of our place in the world, in
relation to things, events, and
other people. To think critically
is to examine assumptions,
beliefs, propositions, and the
meaning and uses of words,
statements, and arguments. By
clarifying both the means and
ends of living, critical thinking
helps to focus and sharpen
awareness.

Bandman & Bandman, 1988, p. 1.

Objectives

Upon completion of this chapter you will be able to:

- Analyze definitions of learning and formulate your own definition.
- Apply systems theory to the concept of learning.
- Differentiate among the cognitive, affective, and psychomotor domains of learning.
- Analyze definitions of thinking according to the following theories and formulate your own definition: stimulus-response, gestalt, humanistic, and information processing.
- Give clinical examples of the following types of thinking: scientific inquiry, problem solving, creative thinking, fantasy, reverie, and critical thinking.
- Identify at least two teaching strategies that help clients develop their critical-thinking abilities.
- Assist clients in the development of their own critical thinking.

Key Words

learning	psychomotor	creative thinking
learning system	domain	fantasy
cognitive domain	scientific inquiry	reverie
affective domain	problem solving	critical thinking

Introduction

In the previous chapter we considered aspects of the supra-system—namely, selected trends in today's society and other forces that impinge on health and illness teachers in the last decade of the twentieth century. In this chapter the focus shifts to the learning system and selected subsystems. We start by revisiting general systems theory as a way to view learning and examining three commonly accepted domains of learning. We then examine thinking: its definition, its relationship to four learning theories, the various types of thinking with particular emphasis on critical thinking, and the ways to promote thinking in clients.

The Learning System

Learning can be viewed as a living, open system. The learning system, illustrated in Figure 2-1, is a process that is dependent on an interchange between the learning individual and the environment. Learning is a purposeful activity and often results in a change in the individual's thinking, behavior, or both.

Thinking about the message in Figure 2-1 can help you avoid a common mistake. Some caregivers act as if telling the client a piece of information fulfills the client teaching obligation. Going over an informed consent form, doing preoperative teaching or giving instructions before leaving the hospital, often fit into this category. With your understanding of general systems theory, we hope you will take a more comprehensive view of the client's needs.

As shown in Figure 2-1, the *input* you draw from clients includes their expectations and interest in the learning at hand. You also need to be aware of yourself and the kinds of energy you bring to the learning process. Your knowledge of theories and relevant learning principles is another important contribution (input) to the system.

In the process aspect of the system you encourage your client (learner) to engage in the activities necessary to incorporate a new attitude, a new skill, or new knowledge. The client may do this by modifying and reorganizing formations already in place or by acquiring new ones. The client may need specific, new information or assistance in learning how to use known information to his or her best advantage.

The output is the result of the learning process. It is easiest to measure when it takes the form of a change in behavior. The client may be able to report the acquisition of new knowledge, demonstrate a new skill, or give evidence of a change in attitude. Lack of change may be a clue that you failed to clarify the fit between the client's goals and your professional goals, or maybe the client does not believe in the efficacy of your advice. Another possibility may be that the client is not hearing you because he or she is distracted. You may fail to learn the client's preferred mode for receiving and processing information. Output provides more feedback, which is used to alter the next phase of input. For example, you may modify the activities designed to facilitate the client's learning. Chapters 10 and 11 discuss learning activities in detail.

Domains of Learning

The person learns as a total system. When you learn, you are doing something; you are having thoughts

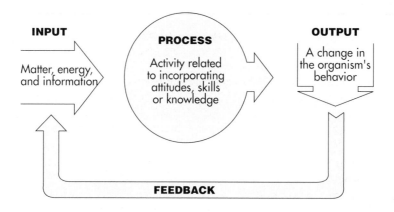

Evaluation of the output in terms of
the purpose of the learning process

Figure 2-1   The learning system.

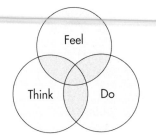

Figure 2-2   The domains of learning: cognitive (think); affective (feel); and psychomotor (do).

about learning, and you are also experiencing feelings about what you are doing and thinking. The doing, thinking, and feeling aspects of learning are clearly related, but they are not the same. When you decide to help clients learn something, one of your tasks is to decide in which domain clients need to focus most of their energy. The three domains that have received the most attention in educational literature in the United States are the cognitive, the affective, and the psychomotor domains (Bloom and others, 1956). Figure 2-2 illustrates the interactive, interdependent relationship among the domains. An explanation of each domain follows.

The Cognitive Domain

Cognitive learning is concerned with intellectual activities, also referred to as thinking. To think is to have a thought, to formulate in the mind. It means to judge, consider, believe, and recall. It also means to use the mind for arriving at conclusions, making decisions, and drawing inferences (Neufeldt, 1991). The mind and mental processes have been the subject of investigation throughout recorded history. Each new scientific discovery has provided more complicated answers as to what constitutes the mind and thinking. We will provide a fuller discussion of thinking later in this chapter.

René Descartes, who was born in France in 1596, brought a very interesting dimension to this investigation when he decided that the mind and body were two distinct entities. His famous dictum, "I think, therefore I am," proclaimed that the mind thus exists by a clearly observable fact. This di-

chotomy of the mind and body among Western theorists led to more than 300 years of investigation of the mind as an entity separate from the body. The pendulum is now swinging in the opposite direction; scientists in fields as diverse as psychology, neurology, and immunology argue that separating the mind and body is an erroneous pursuit (Benson, 1980; Siegel, 1986).

The Affective Domain

Affective learning refers to feelings or emotions. Affective behavior is conduct that reflects attitudes, values, beliefs, needs, and emotional responses (Davis, 1981). It has long been the experience of educators that affective learning is hard to teach, and even more difficult to measure. Because affective learning is not as concrete as behavioral change or cognitive achievement, it has received very little recognition in learning objectives. Despite these problems, few educators in caregiving professions, such as nursing, would deny its importance. Coletta has stated that "the nature of nursing demands that educators and practitioners pay a great deal more attention to the affective components of teaching and learning" (King, 1984, p. ix). She points out that educators, practitioners, and clients each approach the learning situation with certain beliefs, attitudes, and expectations.

The emotional climate affects all domains of learning, but attitudinal change is probably most vulnerable to the milieu. In stressful or threatening situations, clients are likely to close up and hold fast to their feelings and attitudes. In nurturing and supportive situations, clients are more willing to be open and entertain alternate views. For example, one client needed counseling regarding her rage and depression. The client needed to be heard and to feel that she was being understood. Each early encounter with her was marked by her tirades and my efforts to give her nonjudgmental and appropriate feedback. This experience of being heard and understood without pressure or judgment was healing to her. Later, after she began to trust me, she indicated readiness to entertain other ways of handling her pain besides emotional paralysis. As I offered alternatives, the client chose the option she was ready to consider. Slowly she changed her attitude. However, lengthy negotiations were necessary before the client was willing to commit to small behavioral changes.

Attitudes can be caught by associating with others and by participating in satisfying experiences. A vivid example is an association with the dental chair. An impoverished graduate student took advantage of the local university training lab for her dental care. She fainted while a dental student was thoroughly probing in her mouth. Fainting, however, did not repair her teeth. She persisted, sweating and suffering, wearing a green rubber dam over her mouth for interminable lengths of time. Eventually she tired of her own misery and noticed the enthusiasm with which the dental student was shaping the cavity he was repairing. Before inviting his supervisor over to inspect his work, he called to his classmates to come look at the work of art he had created in her mouth. Eventually, the positive attitude he conveyed eased the graduate student's fears and aroused her curiosity. Before their relationship was through, the client had managed to change her attitude toward dental work.

— Another method of facilitating affective learning includes persuasion from a trusted authority. For an example, observe how advertisers persuade consumers to purchase new drugs. Group participation in discussions sometimes helps, as does role playing. Another way to promote attitudinal learning is to induce conflict and then block old ways of solving the problem. This stimulates the learner to try a new approach. For example, in a counseling class each nursing student was assigned to talk about a real problem with a classmate. The classmate was instructed not to give advice. This is usually difficult because those who study nursing are expected to help by giving. A third classmate was assigned to observe the interaction. The listeners were told to sit on their hands to try and control their advice-giving behaviors. The observers watched to see if the listeners did indeed refrain from their usual mode of response. It is obvious that such maneuvers depend on the cooperation of the learners. This task is not completed without a lot of resis-

tance, which sometimes lasts for most of the semester. By the end of the class, however, the students realized the importance of listening. One nursing student, who worked on a very busy intensive care unit, summarized it by saying: "Last night a client told me he was afraid to die, and I ran away again; next time I'm going to stay."

The Psychomotor Domain

Psychomotor learning may be defined as the learning of a physical skill or procedure. This type of learning is the most concrete, the easiest to teach and observe, and the easiest to measure. Usually the learner forms a mental image of how the skill is performed and then translates that image into external behavior. An example of psychomotor learning is performing an insulin injection. This type of learning is usually done best in a step-by-step fashion, from the simple to the complex. The teacher shows the client how to perform, and then coaches the client through a return demonstration. The teacher corrects errors and reinforces correct responses. Practice is encouraged until the client and teacher are satisfied with the degree of skill.

Thinking

Thinking may be considered one of the most important subsystems of human learning. Thinking, learning, and remembering (recall) are integrally related. In this section we will expand on our definitions and discussion of thinking. A list of thinking skills will be followed by identification of various types of thinking, and we will conclude this section with a brief identification of strategies that you can use to promote thinking in clients.

Definitions of Thinking

Thinking is a personal, automatic, activity of the mind. It is essential to living but is a difficult term to define. You are not aware of how thinking occurs, yet you can observe the consequences of it. Although experts have long been concerned with the nature of thinking, few insightful definitions of it have been proposed. It is complex, multifaceted, and dynamic and involves the creation of images (Halpern, 1984). For example, when you wonder if the intravenous feeding is about to run out, you picture what the fluid level in the bottle looked like the last time you were in the room, and you think about the amount of time that has passed. In this sense, thinking is imagery accompanied by silent, internal speech.

Thinking and General Systems Theory

You can conceptualize thinking within general systems theory, that is, in terms of input, process, and output. For example, consider the input that stimulated you to think about a particular client. What caught your attention? Why did this catch your attention and not something else? As you ponder the situation to derive meaning, you are engaging in process. What is the significance of the information? Is it serious? Should it be reported? In this phase you form judgments and make decisions. Those decisions are what lead you to take action. These actions constitute the output of the thinking process. To illustrate, consider the nursing student who notices a large amount of sanguinous drainage on a client's dressing (input). The student investigates further to determine the full extent of the bleeding, notices the client's color, thinks about whether or not to take the vital signs, and listens to the client's description of how he feels (process). Based on what the nurse is thinking, she takes the vital signs, changes the dressing, and reports the situation to her supervisor (output).

The Relationship of Thinking to Learning Theories

A behavioral definition of thinking would be to consider it a covert behavior, which occurs inside the individual and which can be measured with various devices. The electroencephalograph (EEG) measures changes when a person engages in various forms of thinking. Minute muscular changes occur in the tongue of a vocalist who thinks of a song or in the arm and digit muscles of an instrumentalist who thinks of a musical piece. To the behaviorist,

thinking is symbolic trial and error. Individuals try out, in miniature and inconspicuous form, the behavior they anticipate performing (Dellarosa, 1988).

From a Gestalt frame of reference thinking is knowing, or understanding and achieving insight. It is the intelligent activity of human beings while they attempt to understand that which confronts them. Thinking persons confront their perceptual field as a whole and then attempt to differentiate those objects and events in that field (Lewin, 1955; Dellarosa, 1988). Individual conscious awareness is the focus of interest (Hall & Lindzey, 1957). You do not think in a vacuum. Rather, you think within an environment also known as a field. All that you have experienced affects what you perceive and think. You cannot consider the person's thinking as a separate activity. It must be this person's thoughts within context. For instance, a client who is hungry or who is in pain is thinking differently than when he or she is comfortable.

Clients you encounter in their own homes think and perceive differently than clients you meet in the hospital. Clients who know you as a neighbor because they have been coming to your clinic for years will think differently while in your presence than they would if you were a stranger.

To a humanist, thinking is the meaning that the individual makes out of personal experiences. The humanist sees thinking as a very dynamic process that keeps changing according to the individual's conscious experience at any point in time (Hall & Lindzey, 1957). You react to situations according to your perception of the situations, rather than the external reality itself. How closely your experience matches external reality is dependent in part on your level of self-actualization. The more self-actualized you are, the more open you can be to reality. You have less need to bend or twist reality to fit your preconceived notions.

Thinking may also be viewed as an information processing system. Information is received in the form of input, and it is processed, depending on the quantity of other data being simultaneously processed. Information is processed in short-term memory to be evaluated for meaning, worth, and association with other memories. If it is considered important enough, it will then be stored in long-term memory as electrochemical traces. If not, it will be forgotten (Slavin, 1988). Recall is the reconstruction of a memory: through stimulation of these trace deposits, the thinker brings forward to consciousness a reconstructed past perception.

Thinking Skills

Many current philosophers believe that the development of rational thinkers should be the goal of education today. It is their belief that our ability to survive as a democracy is directly related to how well people can think. Marzano and associates (1988) described various dimensions of thinking and how to teach thinking skills. These educators have identified thinking as a process consisting of a complex sequence of thinking skills as outlined in the box below.

Sequence of Thinking Skills*

1. **Concept formation:** organizing information about an entity and using a word to identify that thought
2. **Principle formation:** discovering a relationship between two or more concepts
3. **Comprehension:** understanding by associating new information with previous knowledge or by finding meaning in it
4. **Problem solution:** applying reasoning to resolve a difficult or perplexing situation
5. **Decision formation:** selecting from possible alternatives
6. **Research:** conducting scientific inquiry
7. **Composition:** developing a product that may be written, musical, mechanical, or artistic
8. **Oral discourse:** talking with others

*Modified from Marzano, R.J., Brandt, R.S., Hughes, C.H., Jones, B.F., Presseisen, B.Z., Rankin, S.C. & Suhor, C. (1988). Dimensions of thinking: A framework for curriculum and instruction. Alexandria, Va.: Association for Supervision and Curriculum Development.

Types of Thinking

In a general sense, thinking can be categorized into directed and nondirected. Directed thinking is goal oriented and purposeful, whereas nondirected thinking underlies our daily routine, such as getting dressed and ready for the workday (Halpern, 1984). Thinking has also been categorized as scientific inquiry, problem solving, creative thinking, and critical thinking. Many of these categories overlap. Thinking is just too complex to be broken down into one neat little definition.

Scientific inquiry is usually taught in courses devoted to the comprehension, evaluation, and execution of research. Emphasis is usually placed on learning and thinking skills, such as reflection, induction, and deduction; drawing careful inferences, discovering relationships between ideas, and ordering them toward conclusions. Researchers attempt to derive new insights from existing knowledge. Figure 2-3 illustrates induction and deduction as components of both scientific inquiry and critical thinking.

Critical thinking is "reflective and reasonable thinking that is focused on deciding what to believe or do (Ennis, 1985, p. 45)." This definition covers everything in your life because it includes behavior that emanates from what you believe or decide to do. Watson and Glaser (1964) saw critical thinking as a composite of attitudes, knowledge, and skills. Attitudes denote a frame of mind, or an attitude of inquiry, that recognizes the existence of problems. Knowledge involves weighing the accuracy and logic of the evidence—an understanding of the nature of valid inferences, abstractions, and generalizations. Skill in applying these attitudes and knowledge must be acquired. This definition is compatible with the domains of learning you will study in the next chapter. Attitudes, knowledge, and skill are comparable to affective, cognitive, and psychomotor domains. Paul (1990) defined critical thinking as "the art of thinking about your thinking while you're thinking so as to make your thinking more clear, precise, accurate, relevant, consistent, and fair" (p. 32). Bandman and Bandman (1988) define critical thinking as the following:

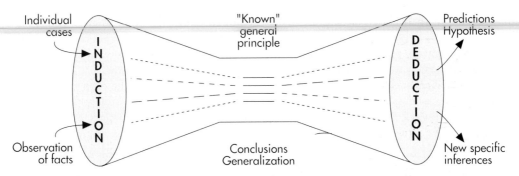

Figure 2-3   Scientific Inquiry. Induction is arriving at a generalization from observed facts and individual cases. Deduction begins with a conclusion, generalization, or a *known* general principle, and then derives new hypotheses or draws new specific inferences.

rational examination of ideas, inferences, assumptions, principles, arguments, conclusions, issues, statements, beliefs, and actions. This examination covers scientific reasoning, includes the nursing process, decision making, and reasoning in controversial issues. The four types of reasoning that comprise critical thinking are deductive, inductive, informal or everyday, and practical (p. 5).

Critical thinking involves the ability to identify central issues, to recognize underlying assumptions, and to recognize evidence of bias and emotion. The critical thinker evaluates the adequacy of the data that are presented to support assertions. The critical thinker attempts to be objective, while recognizing that the act of observing is itself a variable that influences both the observer and the observed. This type of thinking is crucial to the nurse researcher. The worthy scholar listens and reads with an open mind, considers other points of view and engages in self-evaluation (Trow, 1976). This particular way of thinking becomes more significant as you learn to care for clients from diverse cultures.

Critical thinking is contextual; that is, it involves the teacher, learner, content, strategies, environment, and learning domains (Miller & Malcolm, 1990). Take into account all of the variables that may be affecting your client. Consider family, friends, the learning setting, the client's

physical and psychological condition, yourself as a teacher, your teaching strategies, and the content to be learned. Each has some degree of effect that only you and the client can evaluate because it will vary for each client.

Problem solving may be defined as the application of critical thinking and scientific inquiry to a specific situation in order to understand, correct, or alleviate a problem. Problem solving consists of steps, such as identifying the problem, analyzing various aspects of the problem, hypothesizing about its cause(s) and a possible solution, trying out one of the hypotheses, and evaluating the results. To you, such a definition probably sounds similar to the steps of the nursing process. Saylor's (1990) beliefs about the reflection involved in problem solving is quite compatible with the evaluation phase of the nursing process. She believes that problem solving is an essential skill for intelligent practice and offers various ways to promote it.

One of the many reasons why it is important to promote careful thinking is that all knowledge changes and is likely to continue changing at an accelerating pace. If you perceive learning as continuous, you will be better prepared to cope with tomorrow than those who consider themselves as learned.

Creative thinking is the ability to go beyond current knowledge and think in a new way. The creative thinker is a careful observer and sees things the average person misses. Poets and painters entrance us because of their ability to describe anew familiar events.

The creative thinker tolerates ambiguity and uncertainty, adjusts easily to new and changing situations, and freely abandons old assumptions when confronted with new evidence. This type of thinker is willing to be "different." In our culture the artist is the one who has the most permission to look and act unconventionally.

Marzano and associates (1988) point out that it is not possible to distinguish between the critical and the creative thinker, because these traits are necessary in all good thinking. "Creative thinkers generate ways to test assertions; critical thinkers examine newly generated thoughts to assess their validity and utility. The difference is not of kind but of degree and emphasis." (p. 17).

Other ways of thinking include fantasy and reverie. Fantasy is the realm of wild, visionary, vivid imagination, or fancy (Neufeldt, 1991). It has also been defined as a mental image, a capricious or whimsical idea or notion, a dramatic fiction characterized by highly fanciful or supernatural elements. Reverie, a synonym for daydream, is similar to fantasy and means dreamy thinking, imagining, or fanciful musing (Neufeldt, 1991). In general, reverie has a more meandering, less vivid quality to it than fantasy. An example of reverie occurs when a lecture is boring. Your mind tends to wander to something more engaging like what you did last night, what you will do tonight or during an approaching vacation. Fantasy, however, is more directed. An example is when you help a client in labor relax during contractions by focusing her mind on warm, soothing waves of water rushing over her body. Another example of fantasy is when you mentally work through a difficult situation, such as fantasizing a discussion you plan to have with your supervisor. Suppose you want more time to devote to teaching your clients, and you anticipate that your supervisor will show some resistance to this idea. Fantasizing what your supervisor's arguments will be helps you prepare to counter them.

Become aware of how you think. How you think about things and how you go about your professional responsibilities are important insights. Although "thinking" per se may be difficult to define, you will become more skillful in your thinking and increase the efficiency of your thought if you monitor your thought patterns.

How effective are the outputs of your thinking? Are your decisions effective ones? Do you have sufficient data on which to make a good decision? Are the inferences you make accurate? What are your underlying assumptions relative to an issue and how did these focus your thinking? What influence do your beliefs and values have on how you framed the problem and selected the decision? Are the generalizations you made justified? By becoming aware of the input, process, and output of your thoughts, you can increase the efficiency of your thinking. Once you enact this critical thinking process yourself you will be better able to help your clients improve their thinking processes.

Promoting Thinking in Clients

As a health educator, you can assist clients in their thinking process. Note a client's frame of mind, readiness to entertain additional information and develop new insights, and thinking framework. Remember that you cannot completely change a person's thinking framework. You can, however, promote small and incremental growth, expand a client's perception of his or her circumstances and options, and facilitate problem solving.

How can you help your clients become more proficient thinkers? Showing that you respect and value your clients is fundamental for promoting critical thinking skills in your clients. Try to see life from the perspective of the client. This approach creates a safe environment for the client to experiment with new thoughts and behaviors. Such efforts can also make you a good role model for critical thinking (Brookfield, 1991). Clients watch your actions, which reflect your thinking process. You can teach clients a more effective way to think as you go about your professional activities.

When clients have shared insightful information or practiced critical thinking, reinforce this behavior. Praise them for their thinking process as well as the decisions they make. Reinforce even when they question your procedure or request. Responses, such as "I am glad you asked," and "Let me think, that is a complex question," and "That is a good point," are ways to reinforce thinking. "You are smart!" is a reinforcing response for children.

As you are conversing with a client, it may be helpful to mirror his or her attitudes, rationalizations, and habitual ways of thinking and behaving. As you reflect your observations back to the client, monitor the client's response. Are your comments being received? Are they annoying to the client? Be gracious and specific in your observations. If you encounter resistance, stop your intervention and assess what is happening.

As you teach, ask the client questions. It will let you know what is being understood and will give you an opportunity to stimulate thinking. For example, ask, "If that's so, then how do you feel about . . . ?" or "Will you explain . . . ?" Another fruitful line of questioning that helps clients anticipate consequences is "What will you do if . . . ?"

You can also assign tasks that involve thinking. For example, "Now that I've answered the questions in my nursing scope of practice, here's some paper and a pen so that you can write down the questions and concerns you have for your doctor, physical therapist, or health provider." The greater the participation of the client in the learning activity, the greater the likelihood of stimulating the client's thinking.

You will help clients develop critical-thinking skills by being explicit in the learning expectations you have for them. As you write behavior objectives, focus on what should be learned and how it can be best learned. As you share these objectives with clients, listen to their feedback. Do they understand the objectives as you intended? Do the objectives need to be modified to reflect the client's thinking?

When you teach stress management, pain control, weight reduction, blood-pressure control, and management of other stress-related diseases you can make good use of the imaginative forms of thinking, fantasy and reverie. Nurses who specialize in counseling and psychotherapy make intensive use of these strategies.

An example of fantasy used to teach pain control is a directive that a nurse gives to a woman in labor. The nurse says, "Picture your lungs filling with oxygen; picture the oxygen going to your womb and giving it the fuel it needs to push your baby out into the world." To another client who wanted to escape and who found the sounds of surf soothing, the nurse modified the image: "Picture the waves of the ocean rolling over you, flow with the waves. Listen to the surf. Smell the salty air. Feel the warm mist on your skin."

Role playing is based on recall and fantasy. It is an excellent diagnostic tool for discovering the client's way of thinking and approaching interpersonal problems. Role playing is also very helpful to the client who is learning to be more assertive. When used by the nurse psychotherapist, role playing may take on more intensity, such as that encountered in gestalt exercises, sociodrama, and psychodrama.

Summary

Conceptualizing learning as a system with various subsystems provides the framework within which you perform teaching functions. Learning itself is separated into three domains: cognitive, affective, and psychomotor. Cognitive involves the intellectual activities; affective deals with attitudes and values; psychomotor involves the learning of motor skills. Thinking underlies these domains. Thinking itself can be considered a vital subsystem of learning. We discussed thinking as it is defined within the context of four learning theories in addition to the different types of thinking. Because of the emphasis on critical thinking today, we explored this topic in greater depth. By developing your own thinking skills, you can also promote the thinking skills of clients.

LEARNING SYSTEMS

Purposes:

- Apply the concept of learning systems
- Relate the domains of learning to a clinical situation
- Generate strategies for stimulating critical thinking in yourself and in your clients

Directions:

- Join either group A or B.
- Carry out the directions as they apply to this situation.

The doctor told Mrs. Brown that her daughter, Linda, who is 13 years old, weighs too much. Her obesity has contributed to her newly diagnosed diabetes. The entire family is obese, but no immediate relative is known to have diabetes.

Group Assignment A

1. Design a model of clinical teaching that integrates systems theory, nursing process, and the goals of health education.
2. Define aspects of Linda's suprasystem that you consider important to include in the model.
3. Put the model on the chalkboard and explain it.

Group Assignment B

Act out a scene that incorporates some of the following:

1. Identify the three domains of learning (cognitive, affective, and psychomotor) that might be necessary to include in clinical teaching of Linda, her family, and her peers.
2. Identify two strategies you might use with Linda to help her begin to think critically about her illness and her role in treatment.
3. Give examples of how you might act as a change agent with this family in each of the following roles:
   a. Collaborator
   b. Teacher
   c. Resource person

USING CRITICAL THINKING SKILLS

Purpose:

- Expand your critical thinking skills

Directions:

- Divide into groups of four or five.
- Discuss the following situation and answer the questions.
- After you have completed the questions, rejoin the larger group and compare your group's answers with the answers of the other groups. How were your answers alike? Different? Discuss why the differences occurred.

A 23-year-old Hispanic woman had given birth to her second child and subsequently experienced kidney failure. On her fifth day of undergoing peritoneal dialysis, the client asked what the doctor had left in her body that the nurses and doctors were trying to wash out. She neither understood the treatment nor why it was necessary. Had she not asked the question, her misperceptions would never have been known.

Pretend you are the nurse in this situation. Answer the following questions:

1. Restate the problem from the client's perspective.
2. What is the problem from your perspective?
3. How is your frame of reference different from the client's?
4. What is the significance of this situation?
5. What is your goal in this situation, that is, what are you trying to achieve?
6. What assumptions has the client made?
7. What are your assumptions?
8. What evidence does the client have? What evidence do you have?
9. How has the client interpreted the evidence? How have you?
10. What inference(s) are you making?
11. What value judgments are you making?
12. What are the consequences or implications of this situation? For the client? For you?

References

Bandman, E.L. & Bandman, B. (1988). *Critical thinking in nursing*. Norwalk: Appleton & Lange.

Benson, H. (1980). *The mind-body effect*. New York: Simon & Schuster.

Bloom, B.S., Englehart, M.B., Furst, E.J., Hill, W.H. & Krathwohl, D.R. (eds.). (1956). *The classification of educational goals. Handbook I: Cognitive domain*. New York: David McKay.

Brookfield, S.D. (1991). *Developing critical thinkers*. San Francisco: Jossey-Bass.

Davis, C.M. (1981). Affective education for the health professions. *Physical Therapy*, 6(11), 1587-1593.

Dellarosa, D. (1988). A history of thinking. In R.J. Sternberg and E.E. Smith (Eds.), *The psychology of human thought* (pp. 1-18). New York: Cambridge University Press.

Ennis, R.H. (1985). A logical basis for measuring critical thinking skills. *Educational Leadership*, 43, 44-48.

Hall, C. & Lindzey, G. (1957). *Theories of personality*. New York: John Wiley & Sons.

Halpern, D.F. (1984). *Thought and knowledge*. Hillsdale NJ: Lawrence Erlbaum Associates.

King, E.C. (1984). *Affective education in nursing: A guide to teaching and assessment*. Rockville MD: Aspen Systems.

Lewin, K. (1955). *A dynamic theory of personality*. New York: McGraw Hill.

Marzano, R.J., Brandt, R.S., Hughes, C.H., Jones, B.F., Presseisen, B.Z., Rankin, S.C. & Suhor, C. (1988). *Dimensions of thinking: A framework for curriculum and instruction*. Alexandria VA: Association for Supervision and Curriculum Development.

Miller, M.A. & Malcolm, N.S. (1990). Critical thinking in the nursing curriculum. *Nursing & Health Care*, 11(2), 67-73.

Neufeldt, V. (Ed.). (1991). *Webster's new world dictionary*, 3rd ed. Cleveland: Webster's New World.

Paul, R. (1990). *Critical thinking: What every person needs to survive in a rapidly changing world*. Rohnert Park CA: Center for Critical Thinking and Moral Critique.

Saylor, C. (1990). Reflection and professional education: Art, science, and competency. *Nurse Educator*, 15(2), 8-11.

Siegel, B. (1986). *Love, medicine and miracles*. New York: Harper & Row.

Slavin, R. (1988). *Educational psychology: Theory into practice* (2nd ed.). Englewood Cliffs NJ: Prentice-Hall.

Watson, G. & Glaser, E. (1964). *Critical thinking appraisal manual*. New York: Harcourt, Brace & World.

Theories and Principles of Learning

The central task of education is
to implant a will and facility for
learning; it should produce not
learned but learning people. The
truly human society is a learning
society, where grandparents,
parents, and children are
students together.
In a time of drastic change it is
the learners who inherit the
future. The learned usually find
themselves equipped to live in a
world that no longer exists.

Eric Hoffer, 1973, p. 32.

3

Objectives

Upon completion of this chapter you will be able to:

- Apply the following learning theories to selected teaching/learning situations: behaviorism, gestalt, humanism, and information processing.
- Apply designated principles of learning in selected clinical situations.

Key Words

behaviorism	perception	information
stimulus-response	paradigm	processing
gestalt	humanism	theory
cognitive-field		principle

Introduction

In this chapter we start with a brief historical perspective on learning and then examine in depth four learning theories. These theories are behaviorism (stimulus-response), gestaltism (cognitive-field), humanism, and information processing. We will also consider principles of learning as derived from surveys of over 800 adult learners. This knowledge will be applied to the clinical situation in which the nurse is the primary teacher and clients are the primary learners.

Value of Theory

Nurses usually are pragmatists and eclectic thinkers. Like Dewey (1922), many nurses believe that what is good is what works. Nurses may freely select ideas from diverse sources and teach according to their experiences. For example, when you observe something, you try to make sense of it by fitting it into your mental and experiential framework. This is most effective when you are knowledgeable about what is observed and have had some experience with it. When you observe things that are outside your framework, that is, things for which you have neither explanation nor experience, you become curious and begin to seek answers. This search for answers to observed phenomena is the foundation of theory development. A theory helps you make sense of what you observe and is a way to view relationships and principles of observed phenomena that have been verified to some degree (Neufeldt, 1991). In the context of health education, theory development is a way to understand how clients learn. Theory-based teaching is a good way to organize your thinking, and to plan ways to conceptualize what you want to convey to other people. Theories are useful in other situations as well. Refer to the box below for examples.

Reasons for Theories

You Need a Theory When You:

1. Confront a new situation and what you already know does not apply to that situation.
2. Want to increase your understanding of something relatively familiar.
3. Face a familiar situation but what you already know is not working.
4. Wish to teach what you know to a colleague or a client.
5. Question the validity of a cherished belief.
6. Explore new hypotheses.
7. Observe events for which you can find no explanation in your present way of thinking.

Historical Perspective

Aristotle (384-322 B.C.), the famous pupil of Plato, declared, "We learn by doing." For instance, men became builders by building and lyre players by playing the lyre. So, too, you become just by doing just deeds, temperate by acting temperately, and brave by behaving bravely.

Aristotle also considered reason to be the most essential human characteristic. In addition, he acknowledged that our minds are necessarily affected by external things, such as poverty, calamity, and sorrow. Food and a moderate amount of physical comfort make it easier to exercise reason. In many ways, Aristotle anticipated three of the learning theories—behaviorism, gestaltism, and humanism—we will explore. The fourth theory, information processing, is related to society's involvement with the computer.

Theories of Learning

Behavioral Theories of Learning (Stimulus-Response)

Behavioral theories were among the first to be widely stated and used in the American educational system; in fact, they are so pervasive that when the term "learning theory" is used, it usually refers to the body of knowledge accumulated by researchers in the field of behavioral psychology.

Pavlov (1849-1936), a Russian physiologist, is famous for his classic work with a hungry dog. He discovered that when meat powder is placed in a dog's mouth, the dog automatically salivates (unconditioned stimulus). When a bell is sounded simultaneously with the offering of meat powder, the bell (conditioned stimulus), becomes paired with the dog's salivation. Eventually the bell by itself will stimulate the dog to salivate. It is important to note that if the response is repeatedly presented without the accompanying unconditioned response, it will eventually extinguish. That is, if the bell is presented often enough without the accompanying meat powder, eventually, the dog will stop salivating (Slavin, 1991; Davis & Hurwitz, 1977). Pavlov's experiment has been repeated in many ways and is the basis for much of behavioral theory.

Although his theories preceded behaviorism, Thorndike (1874-1949) contributed many basic tenets to the field. Thorndike hypothesized that learning was an association between sense impressions and impulses to action. This hypothesis has been credited with being the original stimulus-response psychology of learning (S-R). This theory of learning is also known as connectionism (Hilgard & Bower, 1966).

Thorndike noted that the most characteristic method of learning for both animals and humans is trial and error. The organism confronts a problem and selects from a number of possible responses the response that seems most likely to lead to the goal. Much random behavior occurs until the goal is met. On each successive trial, the random behavior decreases and the goal-directed behavior increases. This forms the basis for the principle of positive reinforcement that Thorndike called the Law of Effect. The principle was later refined by Skinner and associates (Dellarosa, 1988).

Edwin Guthrie (1886-1959) was an early behaviorist. One of his contributions is known as the *Law of Contiguous Conditioning*. He said, "A combination of stimuli which has accompanied a movement will on its recurrence tend to be followed by that movement" (Guthrie, 1935, p. 26). Simply stated, it means that events that occur together in time tend to become paired. He proclaimed, as do behaviorists today, that a science of psychology must be based on a study of what is observable: behaviors, bodily changes, data that can be detected by an observer and/or a measuring device. All data are admissible except introspection, which can only be reported by the client.

Skinner is probably the most familiar of the behaviorists in the United States. He is famous for his Skinner box, an experimenter-controlled cage in which the behavior of animals (rats and pigeons) was studied. Skinner acknowledged two kinds of learning. The first is respondent behavior—which is in response to a known stimulus, such as the knee jerk in response to the hammer of an examiner. The second type of learning is an operant response. When a response is reinforced, whether random or

planned, the behavior tends to be repeated (Slavin, 1991; Gage & Berliner, 1992). That statement is a simple way of explaining operant learning. Most human behavior is the result of operant learning. This chapter outlines a number of propositions of behavioral theory as it is understood today.

Propositions of Behavioral Theory

1. An event that is regularly followed by a specific response may be considered a stimulus to the response. When smokers inhale, they anticipate a lift. They have learned to expect the cardiovascular response because nicotine is a stimulant.
2. Behavior that is followed by a reinforcer tends to increase in strength. When a client attempts to transfer from bed to chair, the nurse in attendance smiles, praises, and encourages. This praise reinforces the client's behavior and increases the likelihood of further attempts to transfer.
3. Behavior that is followed by punishment tends to be suppressed. For example, a young man is very compliant with his father's commands because the young man is afraid of his father. The son complies because he has learned that rebellion or questioning will stir his father's anger.
4. Behavior that is followed by the removal of a negative stimulus tends to increase in strength. Deep breathing relieves tension during an asthma attack and thus decreases the severity of the attack. When a client experiences the difference proper breathing can make, the client is motivated to attempt this type of breathing during any subsequent attack.
5. Behavior that tends to recur is in some way being reinforced or is itself reinforcing. An infant crawls and gets into things because it is fun and satisfies the infant's curiosity.
6. Frequently recurring behavior may serve as a reinforcer to strengthen another behavior. In the past, chronic schizophrenics who were heavy smokers could be persuaded to act more appropriately for a time period in

exchange for doles of cigarettes. For example, if the client sat in his chair in a group therapy session for 10 minutes, he would be given a poker chip. The chips could be exchanged after the session for cigarettes.

7. Irregular and inconsistent reinforcement of a behavior strengthens the persistence of that behavior. Parents who try to resist a whining child's complaints or demands but who eventually give in are inadvertently strengthening the whining behavior with the most powerful method known: intermittent reinforcement.

8. Immediate and consistent reinforcement of a behavior strengthens that behavior most rapidly. A breast-feeding baby soon learns that sucking satisfies hunger.

9. Rewards that are specific to and desired by the client are more powerful than general or routine rewards. One teenage client may respond well to the nurse offering compliments. Another may respond better to the nurse matching wits with the teen.

10. Rewards and punishments that are clearly connected to the behavior are more powerful than vague or inconsistent responses. The client who moves in certain ways after surgery quickly learns which motions produce pain. This principle also helps explain why eating disorders are so difficult to change. The pleasure or relief that the overeater experiences outweighs the hazards because the pleasure is more immediate and the hazards are more remote. The effects of overeating do not show on the body and scale for days, and the health hazards may not become evident for many years. The connection is also vague and inconsistent because other variables, such as genetics and exercise, are thought to add to or reduce the health risks.

11. Behavior that receives no response and meets no biologic need tends to extinguish. Children bring home new words that they hear in the outside world. Some of the words may include language the family does not

sanction. Children who experience no response when they try out the new vocabulary tend to lose interest in those words. (Gage & Berliner, 1992; Slavin, 1991).

Behavior modification is the application of learning theory, as exemplified in the above propositions, to modify a behavior by changing the stimulus that elicits it or by changing the consequences that follow it. Classical conditioning emphasizes that whatever came before a behavior influences that behavior. An antecedent (beforehand) event influences the responding behavior.

Operant conditioning stresses that the behavior is also influenced by the response that follows. A behavior that is followed by a negative response will be diminished, while a behavior followed by a positive consequence will be increased. When both of these theories are applied together, behavior is seen as a result of an antecedent event, and that behavior is further influenced by the consequences that follow it. This is illustrated in Figure 3-1.

To decrease an undesirable behavior you can eliminate or change the antecedent event that tends to evoke the behavior, you can punish the behavior after it occurs, or both. To increase a desirable behavior, you can change the antecedent event to one that is more likely to evoke the desired behavior, reinforce the desired behavior when it occurs, or both. An example of controlling antecedent be-

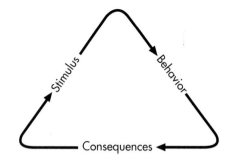

Figure 3-1   To change a behavior you can change the stimulus that elicits it and/or the consequences that follow it.

havior is the advice given to the person learning weight control: "Shop on a full stomach and use a shopping list." The antecedent event of being hungry makes a person with weight problems vulnerable to unwise shopping, such as buying too much food, buying high-calorie food, and buying of handy snacks that are low in nutrients. When that same person shops for food after eating a nutritious meal, that person finds it easier to shop wisely. Shoppers are also more likely to select items more prudently if they use a shopping list that was prepared ahead of time. The antecedent events of a full stomach and a prepared list influence shoppers' behavior in the desired direction: wise shopping for wholesome food.

An example of using the above concepts to decrease negative consequences is illustrated by a woman in labor. She is anxious, scared, thrashing about, moaning, and groaning, both during and between contractions. To alter her behavior, the nurse stays with the client, and talks soothingly to her, while placing warmed hands on the woman's abdomen. The nurse uses suggestion and direction to get the client to focus on something that the client finds encouraging or soothing. This is an example of changing antecedent events. While performing effleurage the nurse feels a contraction starting. With a soft but firm voice and direct eye contact, the nurse says to the client: "Breathe with me slowly and easily. Take in fresh air and gently blow out the stale air. Watch me and breathe with me."

The nurse, with firm and gentle reassurance, interferes with the client's previous behavior—tightening up. The result of following the nurse's directive is increased comfort or decreased pain. In addition, the client experiences increased control in a situation that can be perceived as overwhelming. An increased feeling of control is reinforcing for most human beings.

If the nurse stays with the client and coaches her through some more contractions, the client is likely to feel more control, more comfort, and less fear (changed consequences). It is likely she will continue this behavior on her own as long as the nurse returns periodically to reinforce the behavior and to encourage the woman during her labor. Another, even more effective option is to teach the above procedures to the person accompanying the laboring woman.

When you deal with clients, you must find out what each one considers reinforcing. Clients are unique, and all do not find satisfaction in the same thing. To find out what is reinforcing to your clients you can ask: "What do you do to give yourself a treat when you're pleased with yourself?" "How do you celebrate when you achieve a goal?" To a child you can say: "Tell me your three favorite things, people, or toys." Another way is to observe the circumstances under which you see clients smile, relax, and appear pleased.

To the behaviorist, behavior is a response to a stimulus. Something in the organism, such as an unmet need, or something in the environment causes tension. An action ensues that lowers the tension. Learning is a change in behavior. It is brought about by eliciting a new response to the need that also lowers the tension. Repeated practice of this new response leads to the formation of a new habit.

Teaching is the arrangement of stimuli that are most likely to elicit the desired behavior and the subsequent application of the contingencies of reinforcement (Bigge, 1982). The teacher directs the learning and retains most of the responsibility for the learning. The teacher specifies the target behavior and stimulates the client to comply by producing this desired response. When the desired behavior occurs, the teacher reinforces it. Immediate reinforcement increases the likelihood that the behavior will recur. Over time, the teacher moves from reinforcing the behavior every time it occurs to an intermittent reinforcement schedule. This gives the new behavior more stability.

Teachers have discovered that punishment is not a long-term solution to undesirable behavior. Punishment may indeed suppress it, but if the behavior is meeting some need, that behavior is likely to return as soon as the threat is removed. Another possible consequence of punishment is erratic and unpredictable response. The most effective way to eliminate an undesirable behavior is to find out what need the behavior is meeting, and to reinforce a more desirable method of meeting that need. The example used in Proposition 7 was a whining child. It could be applied just as easily to a whining client. Many possible reasons, such as habit, fear, and loneliness, exist for the whining. You will find that frequent, pleasant, and predictable attention along with encouragement and assistance often reduces the whining. More information on behavior modification can be found in many counseling texts (Okun, 1987).

Gestalt Psychology (Cognitive-Field)

The gestalt view of learning embraces frames of reference, which are also known as cognitive-field theories. Wertheimer, Koehler, Koffka, and Lewin are some of the pioneers in this field. They developed their theories in Germany before they immigrated to the United States (Koffka, 1935). They insisted that behavior was much more than a conditioned response and that perception and memory can be studied by introspection in addition to external observation. *Gestalt* is a German word that means "the whole or totality." In the field of psychology the concept means that the whole is more than merely the sum of all of its parts. Gestalt psychologists hold that psychologic phenomena are irreducible wholes, which cannot be derived just from analysis. If the configuration of a particular perception is dissected, the meaning is lost (Neufeldt, 1991).

Perception refers to the act of becoming aware of something, by the use of any of the senses, such as hearing or seeing. To perceive means to take notice of, to observe, to detect, to become aware of in one's mind, to achieve understanding of, to apprehend. Perception refers to the portion of the world that is grasped mentally through sight, hearing, touch, taste, and smell (Neufeldt, 1991). The gestaltist sees perception as an active, constructive process rather than a passive reflex as proposed by the behaviorists (Dellarosa, 1988).

Our perception of any object is very much affected by the context in which we become aware of it. Clients who are in a strange hospital and who are in pain will perceive your messages differently than clients who greet you in their homes. Our per-

ceptions of any event are also affected by all of our life experiences and interests.

A philosophy professor, after recovering from five-way bypass surgery, had this to say:

> I had a very positive experience while in intensive care—feeling awfully good—and had a breakthrough in my consciousness to the richness of the transcendent area often called the cosmic! Here I was, a neophyte adventurer, kicking my feet up and out and into the cosmos, bouncing, paddling, playing. A wonderful joyous awakening to another level!
>
> With great enthusiasm I shared that ecstacy with my 'transpersonal thought' friends who came to visit me in the hospital, and they were most interested. As a minister I have many religious friends with a more traditional set of mind. To them I described it as experiencing grace as I never had before. The phrase "amazing grace" had taken on a much greater depth of meaning.
>
> A few weeks later, in my home, I was sharing my episodes of rapture with one of my colleagues, a psychiatric nurse interested in holistic health and familiar with altered states of consciousness. After I had told her all about my experience, she sat back in her chair and said: "Yeah, that morphine's great stuff, isn't it?"

Gestalt and cognitive-field theories of learning take into account both the learner and the learning context—all of the individual's experiences and perceptions. The familiar vase/profiles seen in Figure 3-2 exemplifies the importance of figure/ground relationships. The context in which the figure is viewed affects the perception of the observer. If the dark area is perceived as ground (background or context), the figure is perceived as two profiles facing one another. If the white area is perceived as ground, then the dark area is perceived as a vase. You may be able to see both possibilities when you view the figure. The two configurations seem to shift back and forth while being viewed. This particular example is often used because it is so flexible; most people can see both possibilities.

In many circumstances individuals' perceptions are dissimilar, and other possible perceptions

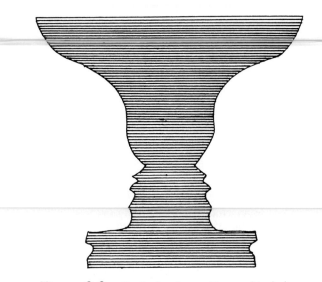

Figure 3-2 Study this figure. If ground is dark area, you perceive two profiles. If ground is light area, you perceive a vase. Your perception may shift over time.

are not easily seen. Even individuals who experience the same event at the same time may have different perceptions of that event. Because you tend to assume that others perceive events the same way you do, you may not even be aware that others see something differently than you do.

It is distinctly possible that you and your client may not perceive the same stimulus the same way. An equally important factor to consider is that you may not even be aware of your disparities in perception. It is very important for you to look for clues to these differences and to address them. Reconsider the example of the 23-year-old Hispanic woman from Chapter 2 who had given birth to her second child and subsequently experienced kidney failure. On her fifth day of undergoing peritoneal dialysis, the client asked what the doctor had left in her body that we were trying to wash out. She neither understood the treatment nor why it was necessary. Had she not asked the question, her misperceptions would never have been known.

Kurt Lewin, a physicist who joined the gestalt movement, expressed his concept of a person's perceptual field using physics and mathematics. He viewed the person and the environment as parts or subsystems of the same psychologic field. He proposed that behavior is a function of the field or life space that exists at the moment in which the behavior occurs. Analysis begins with the situation as a whole.

Lewin made it clear that the environment to which he referred was the environment as the individual interprets it, and that this environment does not necessarily correspond with reality. Lewin's topology, a form of nonmetric mathematics, is very similar to the general model used in system theory. Lewin used topology and a drawing to portray an individual in his or her environment—both internal and external (Hall & Lindzey, 1957). Although Lewin's formula is considered obsolete, the idea that the individual can be understood only within the context of that individual's total perceptual field is widely believed by learning theorists today.

Koehler was another pioneer in the field of gestalt psychology. He, like the behaviorists, studied animals. However, the animals Koehler chose were not rodents; rather, he studied great apes. Two of his most famous experiments were done using bananas as lures. The apes in the studies figured out how to use a box as a leaping platform, and to put two sticks together as extension poles to reach the fruit (Koehler, 1958). From his observations he claimed that these animals were capable of insight, and they could make the intellectual leap from problem to solution without trial and error behavior.

Piaget (1972), a French psychologist, focused his detailed studies on the thinking processes of children. He conducted one-on-one transactions during which he presented various stimuli to infants and children. He then observed and recorded the children's responses to the experiments. The responses led him to believe that thinking and learning are active processes and not merely passive, or trial and error, responses to stimuli as the behaviorists believed. As the children grew old enough to speak, Piaget spoke with these children as he conducted his experiments. He concluded that intellectual development is a gradual process and that it evolves over time.

Learning is a transactional process in which individuals gain further understanding, new insights, or more developed cognitive structures. Two ways of learning that Piaget identified were assimilation and accommodation. Assimilation is a way of learning in which new ideas are incorporated by association with known ideas, concepts, and memories. Individuals may assimilate new ideas into their current beliefs. If the knowledge is quite different from what they already know, they may respond with the intellectual process known as accommodation, which is more difficult than assimilation. When accommodating the new idea, individuals may need to give up former beliefs or substantially change their frame of reference or both. Accommodation may also occur after a person has assimilated so many new concepts that the concepts can no longer be contained in the person's old structure. A paradigm shift then occurs as the aftermath of an accumulation process. Figure 3-3 illustrates assimilation and accommodation.

A paradigm is the way a given community views the world (Choi, 1985). A paradigm shift that occurred a few centuries ago involved the shape of earth. Our predecessors moved from the notion that the world is flat to the notion that the world is round. A more recent paradigm shift with which many of us are struggling is the move from viewing the best patient care as the most efficient and uniform care. Slowly some of us in the health care industry are beginning to realize that our patients are really clients who must be consulted during the formation of their care plan. The number of clients who think differently than we do is increasing. These clients challenge our notions of care. They teach *us* (Siegel, 1986).

You will frequently deal with clients when they are undergoing life transitions such as experiencing birth or death, becoming parents, becoming single, and experiencing assaults to personal integrity, which include physical assault, accidental loss of sight or limb, loss of a way of life, and surgical removal of an organ or significant part. Such transitions can force clients into the need for reconstructing and reorganizing their perceptions of themselves and reality (Selder, 1989). When clients struggle with the issues of "Who am I?" and "What is life about?" they also are going through the process of accommodation.

The following is an example of the use of gestalt psychology in teaching children. The nurse who is involved with preoperative teaching of young children, arranges for them and their parents or main caretakers to come to the day-surgery area for a visit. While the children are in the unit, they see a video that portrays surgery from a child's perspective. "You wear green pajamas with a hat and socks to match. You get a shot (ouch) that makes you sleepy, and you ride on a table with wheels. The ceiling and people look funny when you ride flat. When you wake up you'll be sore, but you'll get more shots that will make the soreness go away."

Following the video the children are led to a room with numerous pieces of equipment, drapes, and surgical clothing with which the children are invited to play. Dolls rigged up with various kinds of typical equipment (without real needles) are also within reach so that children may handle them and play "operation." The nurse observes the children and their conversations, using their responses as clues to what further teaching might be needed.

The main goal of the gestalt perspective is to promote understanding and insight. The teacher diagnoses the client's perceptual field and designs a situation most likely to stimulate interest and understanding. The teacher attempts to organize the

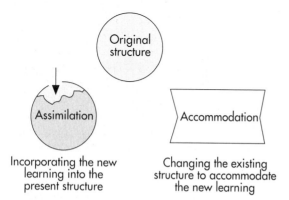

Figure 3-3 Assimilation vs. accommodation.

learning design to fit the client's developmental stage, previous experiences, and learning ability.

Humanistic Psychology

Humanism was the name given to a cultural and intellectual movement during the Renaissance and is characterized by an interest in the person and his or her capabilities. Humanism followed the rediscovery of the literature, art, and civilization of ancient Greece and Rome. Humanism also means a philosophy or attitude that is concerned with the achievements and interests of human beings, rather than the abstract beings of theology, or the respondent creatures of behaviorism.

The Association for Humanistic Psychology was founded by Carl Rogers, Kurt Goldstein, Andral Angal, Abraham Maslow, Henry A. Murray, and many others as an outgrowth of gestalt psychology and, in some ways, as a reaction to the more analytic and scientific theories of the behaviorists. While acknowledging the importance of the individual's developmental history, these theorists focused on contemporary experience and conscious awareness in the present. The uniqueness of the individual is central to many of their hypotheses (Freedman, Kaplan, & Sadock, 1975; Rogers, 1969). These humanists believed that human beings have much more potential than was previously realized. They believed that the study of the human being should go beyond the study of human nature, behavior, and problems by including self-actualization, creativity, joy, love, and levels of transpersonal experience.

The humanists' vision of the human experience is closer to the frameworks of Eastern theorists and their understanding of the higher levels of consciousness. This "third force" in psychology is concerned with topics such as love, creativity, self, growth, being, becoming, joy, transcendence, play, humor, affection, naturalness, autonomy, responsibility, extrasensory perception, and peak experience. In many ways humanism is a very holistic way of regarding human behavior.

Maslow, who many consider to be the father of humanistic psychology, is the author of the famous hierarchy of needs (Maslow, 1954; Shaffer,

1978) with which so many nurses are familiar (see Figure 3-4). Maslow's beliefs include the concept of the human as striving toward self-actualization, a condition that is more possible when the individual's basic biologic and sociologic needs have been met.

Humanistic psychology is identified with the human potential movement of the 1960s and 1970s and was the dominant force in American education in the early 1970s. The movement is a successor to John Dewey's progressive movement of the 1920s and 1930s. Humanistic psychology is less concerned with an area of research and specific investigation and more concerned with an attitude or an orientation toward psychology as a whole (Slavin, 1991; Shaffer, 1978). Three characteristic beliefs of humanistic educators are important for you to know. First of all, humanists believe that learners should have substantial involvement in directing their own education, in selecting content, and in the method of studying the content. The goal behind this belief is to make learners self-directed and self-motivated.

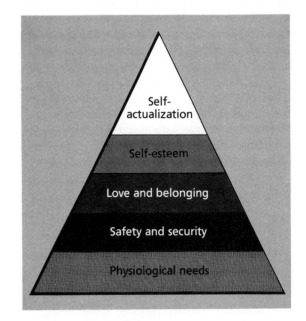

Figure 3-4 Maslow's Hierarchy of Needs. Used with permission from Rice R: Home Health Nursing Practice: Concepts and Application, St. Louis, 1992, Mosby.

Second, humanistic educators value affective learning as much as cognitive learning. They believe the goal of education is not only to produce knowledgeable individuals but also responsible, caring adults. The third belief is that education should teach people to learn and value learning for its own sake (Slavin, 1991). The basic tenets of humanistic psychology are found in the box below.

From a humanistic perspective, individuals react to situations according to the sense they make out of them. Individuals are free to choose the attitudes and actions they adopt in response to life and its limitations and opportunities. Individuals are responsible for the choices they make in life.

To the humanist, then, learning is the development of one's full potential in the direction of self-actualization. The client is actively involved in the process by choosing what, how, and from whom to learn. The client initiates the learning. In the end it is the client who also evaluates whether or not the learning was useful. The essence of learning for the humanist is the meaning that the client derives from the experience. Information will affect a client's behavior only in the degree to which the individual has discovered its personal meaning for him or her (Slavin, 1991).

The teacher's role is to respond by attempting to meet the client's requests. The client, rather than the teacher, is the initiator of the learning experience. Regarding the client as a person, rather than

subject matter, is the focus of the teaching and learning. The teacher is apt to engage in self-disclosure, by communicating past experiences, which are relevant to the task at hand, to facilitate the present learning. For instance, while teaching counseling methods, the teacher is likely to share personal stories of counseling triumphs and disappointments.

Information Processing

Another theoretic framework that has begun to appear in the educational literature is the view that learning is a very sophisticated form of information processing. The first component of the information processing system is the sensory register. This component decides whether or not to notice or register on an external sensory bit of datum, such as an odor, a flavor, a touch, a sound, or a visual stimulus. This same component decides whether or not to register bits of data that are internal, for example, an itch, a chill, a peristaltic wave, a headache, or a memory (Slavin, 1991).

Humans can often describe stimuli that they did not notice if they are asked to do so immediately after the stimulus. However, they are unable to do this after a couple of seconds have passed. In addition, people will retain less if they are bombarded with too many diverse stimuli at one time (Slavin, 1991).

The storage capacity of short-term memory appears to be limited in most individuals. Only five to seven thoughts can be held in short-term memory at one time. As if they were bowling pins, ideas in the mind can be crowded out by the introduction of more items (see Figure 3-5). These thoughts can be related to what the person is feeling, doing, or thinking at the moment, or they can be related to thoughts that are stored in long-term memory and are associated with some current stimulus.

The above mentioned theory is illustrated in the following example. A nurse admits a small child who is tightly clutching a teddy bear. While observing the child's color, breathing ability, alertness and the parent/child interaction, the nurse might also re-

---

Basic Tenets of Humanistic Psychology

1. Conscious experience is an important and primary source of data for the psychologist.
2. The essential nature and integrity of the human being as a whole must be addressed.
3. The essential freedom and integrity of the human being is valued but individual limitations must be taken into account.
4. Human nature cannot be fully defined. Human nature is more than what people do; it includes what people are.

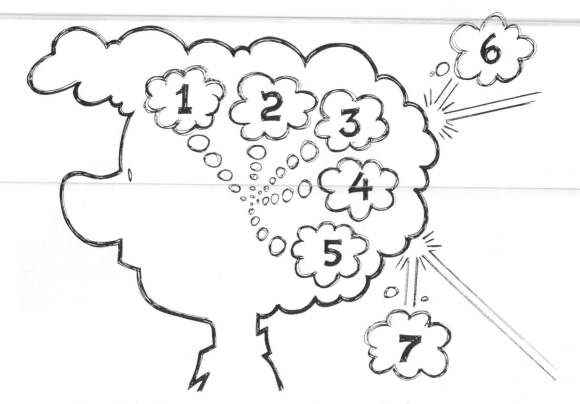

Figure 3-5   Short-term memory is limited to five to seven thoughts in consciousness at any one time.

member his or her own teddy bear from years ago, or that of a small daughter or son at home. Such recollections might make the nurse more sensitive to the child at hand. If too many memories impinge on the nurse's consciousness, however, the memories may detract from the nurse's ability to note and track all of the currently available data about the young client and the client's family.

While holding an idea in short-term memory, the client decides on the idea's meaning, importance, and novelty and begins the process of dismissing or encoding the idea. The thought itself is not stored. Rather, a shorthand sketch of the idea and its related associations is conveyed throughout the brain in the form of a series of electrochemical messages. How it is stored is not well understood, but the notion that it is retained in some manner is widely accepted.

For example, a computer screen can display hundreds of words and calculations, which are formed by a rather simple process: either there is or there is not an electrical charge in a given space on the computer disk at any given point in time. This description of the electrical charges in the computer bears some resemblance to the electrochemistry of the brain. Neuroelectrical traces, which result in retention of the information about facts, impressions, or sensations, are thought to occur throughout the brain.

The information processing model is used to describe the encoding of information and its subsequent dismissal (forgotten) or processing into long-term storage (retained). In computers the storage is achieved in the form of minute changes on a hard or a soft disk. In the human brain, outlines of the encoded information are thought to be stored as sketchy electrochemical deposits, which, when stimulated, are capable of producing charges that can be reconstructed into memories. This results in the ability to recall information, such as past feelings or sensations. The more often these impressions are recalled the more electrochemical deposits are thought to occur. The more these particular pathways are accessed, the more stable and accessible the path becomes. This theory fits with the life experience of most people: repetition promotes learning.

At this point the computer analogy falls short because human beings think and learn with much more complexity. How humans store information also appears to be much more complex than previously realized. Unlike the spot on a disk, a brain cell is capable of responding differently to each electrochemical stimulus it encounters (Bolles, 1988).

The information processing model is particularly useful for teaching a process, such as a nursing procedure, which must be done in an orderly sequence. The processor obtains available data and, based on known variables, chooses a path to follow. This conceptualization is also useful for teaching an individual who works with and enjoys computers. The teacher can point out the learner's errors, gaps, or misperceptions by using computer jargon.

Your job from an information processing point of view is to program the client with the new information. Divide up the learning into steps that are compatible with the client's hardware (basic neurologic and physiologic health and intelligence) and the computer's software (previous experiences with this type of learning). Assist the client in accessing current beliefs (information) that will enhance or inhibit the learning task at hand. Translate the message into a program that the client will be able to process.

Many fine examples of programmed instruction now exist in the literature (Mager, 1984). An example of using the information processing model in a verbal transaction follows. "Today we are going to add to your program on insulin injections. You have done a good job of learning to give yourself the shot. Now I would like to help you process some information on calculating the dose. Have you ever taken algebra? What is already in your file (pointing to head) about that kind of math?"

Table 3-1 summarizes the four views that have been presented for describing learning. Each model has advantages and disadvantages depending on the type of intended learning and on the learner/teacher interaction. When you are selecting a model, ask yourself the following questions: What is the purpose of the learning? Who initiates the learning? What is the role of the teacher and of the client? Who evaluates whether or not the learning has been effective?

The responsibilities of the teacher vary depending on the learning model used. In each of the

TABLE 3-1
Four Views Regarding Thinking, Learning, Teacher, and Learner

Views of:	Thinking	Learning	Teacher	Learner
Behaviorist	Covert trial and error	Changes behavior	Directs	Complies
Gestaltist	Knows, perceives	Understands	Designs	Participates
Humanist	Discovers meaning	Actualizes	Responds	Initiates, evaluates
Processor	Processes information	Registers, retains, recalls	Programs	Inputs, outputs

above four views the teacher's role is that of either the director (behaviorism), the designer (gestaltism), the responder (humanism), or the programmer (information processing). The main goal of the learner in each of the above is to change behavior (behaviorism), understand (gestaltism), self-actualize (humanism), or register, retain, and recall information (information processing).

Principles of Learning

A principle is a fundamental law or truth (Neufeldt, 1991). In this context principles that are based on direct observation of teachers and learners will be presented. Regardless of their theoretic inclinations, most teachers agree on the following principles. These principles, which are summarized in the box below, have been derived from research (Slavin, 1991) and from data obtained from more than 800 adult learners over a period of 10 years.

Focusing intensifies learning.   Individuals vary in the ways they help themselves complete tasks. Learners depend on eye contact with the teacher;

Principles of Learning

1. Focusing
2. Repetition
3. Learner control
4. Active participation
5. Individual styles
6. Organization
7. Association
8. Imitation
9. Motivation
10. Spacing
11. Recency
12. Primacy
13. Arousal
14. Accurate & prompt feedback
15. Application
16. Personal history

---

they focus on the teacher's verbalizations and body language. Others make images of what is being presented. Kinesthetic learners are people who learn through the sensation of bodily position. Some write images on paper or write notes to stay actively involved.

While studying, some learners need a certain kind of music to help them concentrate. Others need a minimum of auditory or visual distractions. Others have a number of rituals through which they go to help themselves focus. Some of these rituals are meditation, sharpening pencils, preparing a snack, or going to the bathroom. Most learners can enhance their ability to retain and recall by developing a pattern that provides for physical comfort, a comfortable level of arousal, and a clear mind.

Repetition enhances learning.   The learner repeats the lesson until he or she is able to produce it from memory. Periodic practice will stabilize the learning. This is true for the memorization of facts as well as the mastery of a psychomotor skill.

Learner control increases learning.   Learners do better when they feel in control of the learning process. They are more likely to choose methods of approach that will work for them. Our experience has shown that nurses are very successful adult learners who can verbalize what they need to enhance their chances of mastering new information and skills. They take more responsibility for their own learning process and do better when they encounter teachers who acknowledge this in both actions and words. This same principle applies to learners of any age. Older learners in general need more time to absorb new information. They do better when they are in control of both the pace and the increments of learning.

Active participation is necessary for learning. Learning is an active process. Most people find that the more they are able to involve themselves in the learning, the more they are able to learn.

Learning styles vary.   Some find it easier to comprehend verbal discourse. Others comprehend visual clues more easily. Still others seek hands-on experience to fathom the meaning of the learning. The Preferred Learning Channel(s) self-analysis exercise at the end of this chapter will help identify your preferred mode of learning. Many find that a combination of verbal, visual, auditory, and kinesthetic experiences is most effective. You need to pay attention to your own learning style because it is the style you are most likely to use when you teach. You also must pay attention to your clients' learning styles so that you can modify your approach to enhance their learning potential. The skill in teaching and learning is to find an effective match.

Organization promotes learning.   When learners highlight readings, synopsize paragraphs, explain their assignments to others, and ask questions about material they do not understand, they are actively organizing the material. This personal intellectual activity makes the learning meaningful to the individual and thus easier to retain. Methods of organization vary. To be most effective, the organization of the material fits both the content and the learner. Affective learning frequently is best organized around the principle of low-risk to high-risk behaviors from the learner's point of view. Psychomotor skills are enhanced by teaching from the simple to the complex. A cognitive task, such as learning history, is facilitated by using chronology.

Association is necessary to learning.   In order to retain any new information or skill, the learner must be able to associate the new learning with phenomena already within his or her repertoire of experience. Association provides relevance to the learner.

Imitation is a method of learning.   Imitating is particularly useful for mastering psychomotor skills, but attitudes and beliefs can also be incorporated if the learner observes a model the learner values.

Motivation strengthens learning.   It is easier for you to grasp facts, learn new skills, and change attitudes when you anticipate benefits from the effort involved. Becoming aware of a need that provides a learner with benefits is a way of strengthening motivation.

Goal setting is an essential aspect of motivation in terms of both determination to learn and evaluation of self. For example, a plumber shared the following story. "I had trouble passing the Master Plumber test. Being a Master Plumber will make it easier for me to find a good job. I told myself if I want to pass that test, I am just going to have to memorize the rules and codes." He motivated himself with visions of better vocational and financial health; he studied and passed the test. Motivation varies among individuals. Common motivators are a decrease in pain, fear of the consequences of not learning, expectations of pleasure and increased self-esteem, curiosity, the ability to feel more effective, and the hope of living a longer and healthier life.

Success and the expectation of success are powerful motivating forces. Learners retain more and can make better use of the material they have mastered if they are learning in a positive atmosphere.

Spacing new material facilitates learning. Smaller amounts of new material that build on each other are easier to grasp than larger amounts presented at one time. Many learners prefer to keep up with the reading and assignments on a regular basis. This approach allows them to grasp more of the material as they progress through the learning experience and to ask the teacher questions within a time frame that is more closely related to the learning. Some learners prefer the "indigestion" method of study. They study intensively at a few sessions (cramming) and depend on the principle of recency to get them through the test.

Recency influences retention.   The more recently the learner has been exposed to information or practice of a skill, the greater chance the individual has to recall it correctly. Retention is grasping or holding onto information or skill.

Primacy affects retention.   Learners tend to learn the first few items best. More attention is paid and more energy devoted to the first items in a learning package. The human mind appears capable of retaining a limited number (five to seven) of new bits of information. Once these new bits of information have been associated with other more solidly retained memories, learners can move on to grasp and retain another set.

Arousal influences attention. Arousal is affected by novelty. The human mind is attracted to change and glitches in patterns. Other sources of stimuli besides novelty include sensory intensity, emotional arousal, and other sources of tension. A certain amount of tension enhances the learner's ability to focus on the current task. This tension can be caused by things such as fear, anger, anxiety, curiosity, and amusement. When tense, a person's neurochemistry changes. Chemicals are released that improve circulation, provide sugar to the brain and muscles, and enhance visual acuity. Individuals vary in how much tension is ideal for them. This is illustrated in Figure 3-6. For example, too much tension interferes with learning. Individuals may become immobilized or restless and engage in behavior that further obstructs the learning process. Fear of punishment usually impedes learning and interferes with the ability to apply that learning to new situations.

Accurate and prompt feedback enhances learning. Learners want to know how well they are meeting the objectives of the learning. Consider how frequently periodicals, such as newspapers and magazines, include self-scoring tests and questionnaires. People are curious about how well they have learned a variety of attitudes, skills, and facts. Clients particularly need this feedback because they may not be able to tell how well they are doing. Prompt feedback provides a feeling of satisfaction if the client is successful. Even when correction is necessary, feedback can reduce tension because the learner then knows what is learned and what has not been mastered yet.

Application of new learning in a variety of contexts broadens the generalization of that learning. Application broadens the generalization of learning. An example is practicing crutch walking and applying the skill in practice settings, such as walking up and down steps. Exposure to a particular concept, attitude, or skill under varying circumstances will assist the learner to retain the

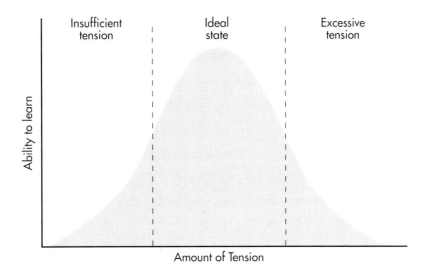

Figure 3-6 Arousal and learning. A moderate amount of tension enhances learning. Too little tension fails to engage learner's attention. Too much tension interferes with learning.

new material and will help the learner develop the ability to use the material in a wider variety of situations.

The learner's biologic, psychologic, sociologic, and cultural realities shape the learner's perception of the learning experience. Our health affects our energy level and ability to concentrate. Our self-esteem and previous experiences with learning affect our willingness to risk, our tolerance for temporary failure, and our expectation of success. If clients are at a developmental level in which they can focus only on memorization and processing information in somewhat shallow ways, you must respect that. If all they want to know is what to do, you must respect their intuitive wisdom about how much they can handle.

Societal norms and learners' previous experiences with institutions affect their ability to learn in a variety of settings. Your attitude toward learning, the amount of personal responsibility for health attainment, and the climate in which you learn best are all strongly influenced by our culture. More information about culture can be found in Chapter 8.

Summary

This chapter focused on theories and principles of learning. Four theoretical frameworks were presented through which we examined the process of learning. Each view has advantages and disadvantages, and each is of value in certain learning situations. You must use judgment in matching the needs of clients with the appropriate theoretic framework. This contrasts with principles of learning, which are of value in all teaching/learning situations. The chapter provides examples of the above information as it relates to the clinical situation.

LEARNING CHANNELS

Purposes:

- Facilitate your awareness of your own learning channel
- Explore ways of expanding your learning repertoire
- Become familiar with a tool to be used with clients

Directions:

- Take the learning channel inventory below.
- Discuss the results with your peers.
- Discuss ways you might use this instrument/activity with clients/peers.

Survey of Preferred Learning Channel(s)*

DIRECTIONS: Read the following statements. If the statement is mostly true for you, then circle the letter that follows the statement.

1. Once I've done something, then I've got it .... K
2. I must look directly at the speaker to understand him or her V
3. My handwriting is quite good .... K
4. I enjoy silent films, pantomimes or charades V
5. I can spell words out loud better than when I have to write them down .... A
6. If someone asks me to spell a word, I have to write it down to answer V
7. I would rather listen to tapes than view slides .... A
8. I remember a lecture better than what I read .... A
9. I understand material better if I read it out loud .... A
10. I am often the last person to notice that something has been added to a room .... A
11. I learn better if I see and hear the material at the same time .... V&A
12. I often need to ask people to repeat what has just been said V
13. Sometimes in a lecture I tune out when I am really trying to pay attention V
14. I use my hands a great deal when I speak .... K
15. I have had speech therapy V
16. I can tell if I'm doing a new physical skill right by the way it feels .... K
17. I would rather demonstrate how to do something than explain it .... K
18. I have trouble remembering unless I write things down .... V&K
19. A page full of print is confusing to me .... A
20. The easiest way(s) for me to learn something is to:
    a. read it V
    b. hear it .... A
    c. try it .... K
    d. write it in my own words .... K
    f. explain it to someone .... A
    g. draw a picture or diagram of it .... K

TOTAL EACH OF THE LETTERS YOU CIRCLED: V's _____ A's _____ K's _____
V's indicate visual channel. A's indicate auditory channel. K's indicate kinesthetic channel. Add up the number of A's, K's, and V's. The highest total indicates your preferred learning channel.

*Adaptation of the Swassing-Barbe Modality Index from *Teaching through modality strengths: Concepts and practices,* Columbus, OH, 1979, Zaner-Bloser.

INTEGRATING LEARNING THEORIES AND PRINCIPLES

Purpose:

- Integrate learning theories and principles in preparation for client teaching

Directions:

- Divide into groups and choose which assignment(s) your group will prepare.

Group Assignment A

What learning theories and principles would you apply in each of the following nursing situations? Act out one of the following scenes.

1. You are going to teach self-catheterization to a client after abdominal surgery before she goes home.
2. As a nurse working gynecology clinic, you are to teach breast self-examination to groups of women in the waiting room.
3. As a public health nurse, you are to teach a group of young parents at a day-care center about behavior modification, using the propositions of behavioral theory. The main point is to translate the most important concepts into plain English and give practical examples.

Group Assignment B

You are a group of nurse entrepreneurs who have been granted an interview with a station program producer. Select two members to collaborate in playing the role of station program producer.

1. Your task is to talk the station program producer into buying your television program package. Prepare the following information.
   a. Identify the target audience. Are audience members viewers of general television? Are they in schools? If so, which grade level? Are they in industry? If so, which one(s)? Why did you choose this audience?
   b. What population trends make your program feasible?
   c. Suggest how often your program should be shown. Daily? Monthly? What day? What hour? Provide your rationale.
   d. List the topics you would cover with your target audience.
   e. Identify the sponsors you would approach.
2. Place yourself in the role of the producer. Identify questions and doubts you have. Consider things such as profit; market acceptability; risk; controversy; sensitivities of various cultural, ethnic, and age groups; and timeliness. Present these concerns to the nurse entrepreneurs.

Group Assignment C

Conduct the following activities on your regular television health program.

1. Your first guest is a self-styled fitness expert or nutritionist who is very popular but whose scientific base you question. Conduct the interview in a way that will promote critical thinking in your audience.
2. Create a commercial break in which you:
   a. Market nurses as health educators, consultants, and care providers.
   b. Advertise a health product/system with which you would like to be associated.
3. Interview your other guest, a nurse colleague, about the changing trends in health care and what that means for the average citizen.

References

Bigge, M. (1982). *Learning theories for teachers* (4th ed). New York: Harper & Row.

Bolles, E.B. (1988). *Remembering and forgetting: An inquiry into the nature of memory.* New York: Walker and Company.

Choi, M.W. (1985). Preamble to a new paradigm for women's health care. *Image: The Journal of Nursing Scholarship, 17*(1), 14-16.

Davis, H. & Hurwitz, M.B. (Eds.). (1977). *Operant-Pavlovian interactions.* Hillsdale NJ: Erlbaum.

Dellarosa, D. (1988). A history of thinking. In R.J. Sternberg & E.E. Smith (Eds.), *The Psychology of Human Thought* (pp. 1-18). New York: Cambridge University Press.

Dewey, J. (1922). *Human nature and conduct.* New York: Holt, Rinehart & Winston.

Freedman, A., Kaplan, H. & Sadock, B. (Eds.). (1975). *Comprehensive textbook of psychiatry* (2nd ed). Baltimore: Williams & Wilkins.

Gage, N.L. & Berliner, D.C. (1992). *Educational psychology* (5th ed.). Boston: Houghton Mifflin.

Guthrie, E.R. (1935). *The psychology of learning.* New York: Harper & Row.

Hall, C. & Lindzey, G. (1957). *Theories of personality.* New York: John Wiley & Sons.

Hilgard, E. & Bower, G. (1966). *Theories of learning* (3rd ed.). New York: Meredith.

Hoffer, E. (1973). *Reflections on the human condition.* New York: Harper & Row.

Koffka, K. (1935). *Principles of gestalt psychology.*

New York: Harcourt, Brace & World.

Koehler, W. (1958). Gestalt psychology today. *American Psychologist, 14,* 727-734.

Mager, R.F. (1984). *Preparing instructional objectives.* Belmont CA: Lake.

Maslow, A.H. (1954). *Motivation and personality.* New York: Harper & Row.

Neufeldt, V. (Ed.) (1991). *Webster's new world dictionary* (3rd ed.). Cleveland: Webster's New World.

Okun, B.F. (1987). *Effective helping: Interviewing and counseling techniques* (3rd ed.). Pacific Grove CA: Brooks/Cole.

Piaget, J. (1972). Intellectual evolution from adolescence to adulthood. *Human Development, 15,* 1-12.

Rogers, C. (1969). *Freedom to learn.* Columbus: Charles E. Merrill.

Siegel, B. (1986). *Love, medicine and miracles.* New York: Harper & Row.

Selder, F. (1989). Life transition theory: The resolution of uncertainty. *Nursing & Health Care, 10*(8), 437-451.

Shaffer, J. (1978). *Humanistic psychology.* Englewood Cliffs NJ: Prentice-Hall.

Slavin, R.E. (1991). *Educational psychology: Theory into practice* (3rd ed.). Boston: Allyn & Bacon.

Swassing, R. H. & Barbe W. (1979). *Teaching through modality strengths: Concepts and practices.* Columbus, OH: Zaner-Bloser.

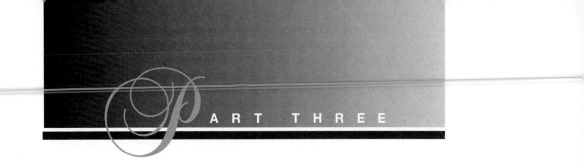

PART THREE

Assessing a Client's Readiness, Abilities, and Needs

Fundamentals of Assessment

If you think communication is
all talk, you have not been
listening.

Anonymous.

Objectives

Upon completion of this chapter you will be able to do the following.

- Explain how your perceptions and those of the client will affect the teaching/learning situation.
- Identify three facets of readiness to learn.
- Describe how the client's level of wellness affects teaching/learning: acute illness/trauma, convalescence, long-term illness, and health.
- Describe the interrelationship between teaching/learning and a client's psychosocial adaptation to health.
- Discuss the bearing of a client's level of education upon the teaching/learning process.
- Identify four types of communication difficulties on the part of the client, yourself, or both that affect teaching/learning.
- Describe strategies to cope with each type of communication difficulty.
- Identify the influence of seven factors in the physical environment on teaching/learning.
- Compare and contrast the effect of the following environmental settings on teaching/learning: hospital, clinic or clinician's office, client's home, school, and industry.

Key Words

perception	adaptation	socioeconomic
experiential readiness	stages of recovery	factors
motivation	levels of wellness	communication
developmental	denial	patterns
readiness		teaching/learning
		environment

Introduction

The first part of this book, from a general systems frame of reference, focused on the *structure* of the teaching/learning system in terms of its goal (improved health behavior), its informational input (theories and principles of learning), and its suprasystem (the historical and political realities of the situation in which client teaching takes place).

In the next several chapters we will focus on the *process* of the teaching/learning system. Process refers to the interaction of matter, information, and energy and results in output (improved health behavior). The nursing process is the model used to study this aspect of the teaching/learning system.

In this chapter we examine some fundamental concepts that are inherent in the assessment process. The first concept is the role of perception in assessment. Next is readiness to learn. The effect of psychophysiologic processes on readiness is analyzed, as are socioeconomic factors. A discussion of communication difficulties as they influence assessment follows. We close the chapter with assessment of the teaching/learning environment,

—Continued next page

55

which includes the client, you, your relationship with the client, and the physical environment in which client teaching takes place.

Dynamics of Assessment

Role of Perception

The first phase of the nursing process is assessment. Your assessment of the client will be greatly influenced by your perception of that system, whether it is a person, a family, or a larger unit. Perception is the ability to receive stimuli through the senses of sight, hearing, taste, touch, and smell and to give meaning to those sensations. Your perceptions will be shaped by the amount of meaningful clinical and/or teaching experience you have accumulated, as well as your individual interests. An experienced nurse would notice changes in a client's condition that are imperceptible to a neophyte.

Your perceptions not only shape the way you view your clients but also influence clients' self-perceptions. Clients tend to perceive themselves in response to how you react to them. What you know about clients' readiness to learn and your perceptions of their biologic, psychosocial, and cultural characteristics will greatly influence how you perceive them. You react differently to clients you perceive to be dumb or smart, unmotivated or motivated, hopeless or hopeful, uncooperative or cooperative, a pain or a pleasure to treat, and ignorant or knowledgeable.

Your perceptions, the parts of the universe to which you attend, are shaped by your own physiologic, psychologic, sociologic, and cultural history. For instance, Christine was an 18-year-old client who came into the street clinic. She lived on the streets and was known to the clinic staff as someone who frequently smoked marijuana and took stimulants and depressants. During her visit she had dysuria and frequency of urination and was diagnosed as having a urinary tract infection. The doctor prescribed antibiotics. I instructed her about the medication and how it should be taken, told her to take all of the medication and not stop taking the medication even if her symptoms subsided. She had a difficult time accepting that and wanted to know difficult time accepting that and wanted to know what would happen if she failed to take it as prescribed. To Christine, the antibiotic represented the medical system, and she did not want to be harmed by a physician error. She perceived smoking marijuana and taking uppers and downers as a regular part of her way of life, a way that was safe.

Your perceptions are also affected by your attitudes. When you are feeling confident and self-actualized, you are able to take in more of the environment. When you become defensive, you perceive selectively. You pay attention to things that are important to you and neglect those things in your environment that you do not value. It is easier for you to hear messages that already fit in with your belief systems and messages that come from people whom you like or respect. In the box below and on the next page, a number of variables that affect our perceptions are listed, particularly those that affect the way we listen.

Readiness to Learn

Readiness, or the ability to engage in a given learning activity, depends on three major aspects: an aroused interest or motive, relevant preparatory training, and physiologic maturation (Kaluger & Kaluger, 1984). In the following paragraphs, we have listed a number of questions that should help you assess clients' readiness.

Motivation refers to an aroused interest. Are clients willing or sufficiently motivated to learn?

Listening and Perception

We Hear:

1. What we expect to hear.
2. What we want to hear.
3. Through the perspective of our reference group.
4. One way when the speaker acts friendly.
5. Other ways when the speaker acts mad, sad, or scared.

Readiness for Listening	
The Amount We Hear Is:	
More	**Less**
When we feel OK	When we do not feel OK (mad, sad, scared)
From a person on our level	From a person above or below our level
When an idea or speaker is important to us	When an idea or speaker is not important to us
When an idea fits our beliefs	When we do not believe what is said
When the message makes sense to us	When the message does not make sense to us
When we want to hear	When we do not want to hear
When we pay attention	When we are distracted with other concerns

Motivation concerns clients' confidence in themselves as learners, their perception of their chances of success, and their willingness to make the effort to learn. Do clients see themselves as responsible for learning what you consider to be valuable? Do clients consider themselves instrumental in their own healing? Do they feel capable of learning that which you expect them to learn? How much support will clients receive from their friends, family, co-workers, or culture for learning the new behaviors? How meaningful is the support that will be available from you and the physician?

Are clients willing to learn behaviors that will have long-term, favorable consequences (smoking cessation, caffeine reduction) and cause immediate discomfort? Are they willing to admit to the hazards of their present life-style (using recreational drugs, enjoying too much fattening food)? Clients are more likely to be ready if they understand the goals of learning and how these goals will be personally beneficial, but it is clear that comprehension is not enough. Consider the frequency with which well-informed nurses continue behaviors they know are self-destructive.

Experiential readiness refers to the client's relevant preparatory training or previous associations. Has the client sufficient background from previous experiences to make sense out of the new learning? You will assess the client's skills, attitudes, and cognitive abilities. Can the client grasp the meaning of the lesson and perform the required behaviors? An example of the importance of experiential readiness or relevant preparatory training follows. While a graduate nursing student, I worked at a naval hospital in a large port city and conducted a resocialization group with young sailors who were hospitalized with psychiatric disturbances. I wanted to help them plan a trip into the center of the city. It was my hometown, so I was quite familiar with such an activity. While assessing these young men, I discovered that one had never used a pay phone. He grew up in a small town where all calls went through Aunt Matilda who did all of the dialing through the switchboard.

The fact that he confided he did not know how to use a dial phone was a major step in establishing a therapeutic relationship with me. I did not view him as stupid but did wonder about the relationship of his psychiatric disturbance to his struggle with culture shock. We spent some sessions dealing with a pay phone in a phone booth until he gained the necessary skill and confidence to use the instrument. It also became clear that he needed additional preparatory training before he would be ready to take the subway train into town.

Psychophysiologic Processes

In addition to sufficient past experience, clients must be psychophysiologically ready to learn.

Levels of Wellness

When clients are acutely ill, their concern is with physical survival. The stage of acute illness is frequently accompanied by pain, confusion, physical disability, and fear. Acutely ill people regularly receive medications that cloud the sensorium. Most clients in hospitals are receiving numerous drugs, which may produce interactive problems. Clients at this level of illness are receptive to very little formal teaching. They benefit from information that will ease their fears and help them maintain orientation to their condition, surroundings, and time of day. Coaching that will make them more comfortable and allow them to breathe more easily is, of course, welcome. In the case of very ill people, the family may be the client that will receive teaching.

McHatton (1985) identified several stages of emotional adjustment to trauma and related them to Maslow's hierarchy of needs (1954). The first stage, impact, is characterized by extreme anxiety, loss of control, despair, and discouragement. Concerns about physiologic and safety needs are paramount at that time. The next stage, regression, is characterized by denial, flight to a more comfortable time, and a need for love and belonging. The third stage, acknowledgement, is characterized by self-negating statements and doubting of confidence and competence. Teaching can begin during the acknowledgement stage. The final stage, reconstruction, can be identified by expressions of clients' needs for self-actualization and for realizing their potential. During this stage clients are more open to trying out new approaches. McHatton's model (1985) presents an interesting view of psychosocial adaptation to trauma. Such adaptation can save you time, energy, and frustration. It is an excellent model for assessing readiness to learn in the client who has suffered trauma—either accidental or surgically induced.

Some clients become ill and recover in a more gradual progression as described in Suchman's model of adaptation to illness: symptom experience (client becomes aware that something is wrong), assumption of the sick role (client states or acts as if he or she is sick), medical care contact (client legitimizes illness by contacting a culturally recognized medical authority), assumption of the dependent patient role, and recovery or rehabilitation (client is ready to resume normal citizenship role) (Suchman, 1965). In Suchman's model, the rehabilitation phase is the one in which the major por-

tion of teaching occurs. During the rehabilitation phase, the client is interested in learning how to speed recovery as well as acquiring information, attitudes, and skills that will help the client avoid a repeat of the illness.

Convalescence seldom occurs in the hospital setting today. In the hospital you will see this phase of recovery much less than you would have a decade ago. Clients are frequently dismissed just after the acutely ill stage. During community health nursing you will encounter clients who were still seriously ill when they were sent home. These clients and their families need much support, supervision, and teaching. Families need instruction in learning to do procedures that were previously done by highly skilled physicians and nurses. Convalescing clients and their families are likely to be interested and motivated learners. They are usually motivated to learn whatever is necessary to resume normal life as soon as possible. In general it is believed that people recover more quickly in their own territory surrounded by familiar support systems.

Successful teaching of clients with chronic illnesses depends on the clients' reactions to the reality of their illnesses. Clients with long-term illnesses may have much more experience with these illnesses than you. Today's clients, many of whom show deep interest in their diseases, can intimidate you with their level of knowledge about their own illness and expertise in their own care. In such a situation you may find it more profitable to take the role of learner, while supporting clients' attempts at mastery.

Many chronic illnesses wax and wane. When the effects of disease are exacerbating, clients may indeed be weary of the discouraging changes. In addition to emotional responses to their deterioration, clients may experience failing energy resources. Your role in such situations will be one of listener and then collaborator. Together you and the client will experiment with adaptations designed to make the best of the client's remaining abilities and energies. Clients are likely to be more motivated when their symptoms are subsiding.

In addition to teaching clients who are recovering from illness, you will encounter clients who are interested in preventing illness and in promoting their own health to its fullest potential. Many people now realize that the way they conduct their lives is directly related to their health, longevity, and well-being. You encounter potential clients among visiting friends and relatives of clients in the hospital, in their homes, in free-standing surgical and medical clinics, and in workshops and classrooms. You also encounter them in your neighborhood.

In the first chapter of this book we described some of the changes underway in this nation. For example, at the college where we teach, the department of nursing has for years offered a nutrition course as a service to the general college community. In the last 2 years, enrollment in that course has tripled. We believe the change indicates a widespread interest in learning more about nutrition and a growing awareness of the connection between health and nutrition habits.

Figure 4-1 illustrates how a client's needs and learning ability change depending on the level of wellness. When a client is acutely ill and has little energy, his or her learning needs are very limited and concrete. During convalescence, clients are interested in what they can do to promote their own recovery and return to optimum health. Those with chronic illnesses are greatly affected by the reality of their illness. Those in good health are open to a wide range of health teaching.

Socioeconomic Forces

In addition to assessing biologic factors that impinge on the teaching/learning process, you should address sociologic factors. Individuals with financial and emotional resources can purchase services and rely on support systems to sustain themselves through their recovery and to augment whatever functions they have left. Individuals without such resources are much more bereft and at risk for reaching less than their potential level of functioning.

The meaning that altered functions has to

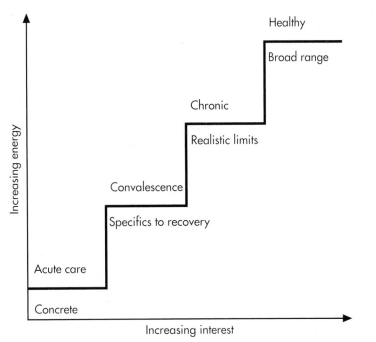

Figure 4-1 Levels of wellness. A Client's energy and readiness to learn increases as his or her level of wellness increases. Courtesy Maureen Sullivan, RN, BS. Used with permission.

clients and their families greatly influences their psychosocial adaptation. For instance, an engineer finally was admitted to the hospital after severe weight loss, which had occurred within a month. Both he and his wife, who was a nurse, were scared and anxious about the cause. His problem was eventually diagnosed as cholecystitis. He was still very alarmed by his rapid weight loss when his physician deemed immediate surgery necessary. His perception was quite different than that of the medical staff and his wife who were greatly relieved to learn that his problem was cholecystitis and not pancreatitis.

In addition to socioeconomic factors impinging on illness, clients' illnesses can impinge on their socioeconomic well-being. Individuals who are suffering the effects of AIDS find that their diagnosis is a barrier to employment, health insurance, social freedom, and other sources of socioeconomic support. At the same time, many are suffering devastating losses of their friends to AIDS (Carmack, 1992). At this point, the clients along with their caregivers are struggling together to find methods of adaptation to their multiple losses (Feinblum, 1989; Froman, Owen, & Daisy, 1992).

Educational Level

Another aspect of psychosocial assessment is the client's educational level. Such an assessment provides clues pertaining to the client's general knowledge level. The client's level of education is often related to general knowledge about health and illness. The higher the level of education, the greater the knowledge base. Furthermore, the higher the level of education, the more likely the individual is to engage in health-promoting behaviors, such as exercise, proper diet, and smoking cessation (Thompson, McFarland, Hirsch, Tucker, & Bowers, 1989).

The vocabulary that clients use is to some extent a measure of their educational level. Those with large vocabularies are more apt to comprehend what you are saying. Clients with less education are less likely to comprehend the more abstract and technical language you might inadvertently use. Con-

crete answers and examples are more likely to be meaningful to those with less education. We wish to caution you, however, that intelligence is often correlated with vocabulary no matter what the educational level (Slavin, 1991). Clients with given health problems can be extensively informed in their particular field of interest. Nurses are reporting this phenomenon more often in the new era of increased information availability. Keep in mind that people do not necessarily read at their educational level (Doak, Doak, & Root, 1985). The mean literacy level in this country is tenth grade. Normal literacy rate and years of education are only approximations of what the individual client can grasp. Clients and their families have repeatedly reported to us that their anxiety level and other concerns interfered with their ability to comprehend material that would be quite understandable under normal circumstances. Cultural phenomena can also have an effect on an individual's vocabulary and willingness to communicate. This topic is discussed further in Chapter 8.

Adaptation

Adaptation is a process that the individual initiates to counter stress, and reduce and/or neutralize its effects in order to maintain a steady state during biologic, psychologic, social, and cultural changes. All of these factors are interrelated within the individual. The client is a living system, continuously adapting to all of the internal and external factors affecting him or her. All living systems adapt continuously in order to go on living. The change in humans is more noticeable when they change their behavior. Even if we cannot perceive change, it is occurring.

At one end of the coping spectrum are individuals who adapt to illness by facing it and concentrating on recovery, the functions they have at their disposal, or both. At the other end of the spectrum are individuals in denial. There are times when denial serves the psyche well. When a person must mourn the loss of a limb, a function, or any other loss, denial is a necessary defense. People protect themselves from being overwhelmed with the changes in their lives by denying the magnitude of these changes. Ersek (1992) asserts that as people move along in their crisis and grief they can exercise control over the amount of reality they are ready to confront. They are able to relinquish more unrealistic hopes as they find more realistic ones. This may occur when you provide them with support and assist them in finding new, more realistic hopes.

Denial serves another purpose. Many cardiac clients who denied the seriousness of their illnesses fared better than clients who were passive and compliant with the regimen laid out by their physicians. In fact, cardiac care has been revolutionized by those researchers who were willing to learn from these survivors (Thompson, McFarland, Hirsch, Tucker, & Bowers, 1989; Folks, Freeman, Sokol, & Thurstin, 1988; Winslow, 1985; Shabetai, 1983).

However, denial can also be a very destructive force. The client who is in the denial stage may distort or suppress whatever teaching you attempt to do (Hickey, 1986). Solutions vary. You may wait and gently present small amounts of reality, or you might focus on affective assessment and learning. Direct confrontation is a method used in rehabilitation settings. Taking the initiative to directly engage clients and confront their denial is sometimes necessary to move them beyond apathy, denial, or both. Such an approach is likely to arouse their anger. Anger is a very unpleasant emotion for both clients and you. However, anger is much more energizing than depression. When we are angry our circulation stirs and our blood pressure rises. We become more alert. Our muscles are nourished with more oxygen, sugar, fats, and hormones. It is much easier to learn in an aroused state. Anger is much more motivating than apathy and despair.

Clients' adaptation to their current stressors and their illnesses depends on their self-concept before they became ill. People who see themselves as individuals of intrinsic worth are likely to respond to illness differently than individuals with low self-esteem. For example, people who value themselves respond to tragedies and other life crises as challenges to overcome or lessons to learn. People with low self-esteem are more likely to remain overwhelmed and give up.

In her moving story, *First You Cry*, Betty Rollin (1976) reveals how her breast amputation affected her life. Sharing her experience with the public was courageous and generous as well as a statement about her self-esteem. One of the observations credited to her mother was that Rollin had no previous experience with adversity. It took her a while, and she learned to deal with this new challenge positively. A film star, whose low self-esteem was legendary, was reportedly unable to cope with a similar crisis and took her own life. Of the two women who faced devastating blows to their body images, the woman with the good self-concept found a way to cope, while the woman with poor self-esteem killed herself.

The severity of the illness and its effect on the client's life-style also affect the client's psychosocial adaptation. A sore throat is a more serious affliction to a professional singer than a construction worker. A fractured leg would be more serious to the construction worker than the singer. A writer who had arthritis in colonial days would be affected differently than a writer today who owns a word processor.

The tasks of reorganization and rehabilitation of clients are greatly affected by the adaptation of clients' families. A family often goes through dynamic phases of adaptation to a loved one's illness. In families, these phases may parallel the ill person's adaptation and/or take place in an out-of-phase disharmony. Your sensitive explanation of the dynamics may help the family find its way through the crisis.

Illnesses that wax and wane are very wearing on clients and their families. Reintegration becomes necessary after each exacerbation. In general, however, well-informed clients tend to become better adapted as they learn to cope with recurrences of diseases.

Communication Difficulties during Assessment

To assess clients accurately, you must be skilled at communication. Pohl (1981) points out that there are many communication difficulties that can interfere with teaching. These difficulties can come from the client as well as from you.

Hearing Impairment

Clients who have long-standing hearing deficits can teach you what modes of communication work best for them. One adaptation you can make is to ensure that the client's hearing aid is in and turned on and that the batteries are working. Creating other means of sound augmentation, such as cupping your hands around the client's ears or using the stethoscope in reverse, are other options. Be sure to position yourself so the client can see your face and read your lips. Communication tools, such as flash cards, and pencils and pads, are all helpful to the client who knows how to write and has the strength to do it. The most important point is that you find a way to elicit responses that help you assess the client's hearing abilities and comprehension.

Vision Impairment

People who have been blind for some time develop other senses, particularly hearing, to compensate. Their acute listening skills make being shouted at a painful experience, and it does not aid their comprehension. Clients who are blind are unable to make use of body language or lipreading. If you are used to conveying meaning with your hands and head shakes, you must be alert to the fact that such clues are unavailable to the blind client. We recommend that you learn to use more verbal description and tactile learning than might be necessary with a sighted client.

Blind people can often discern whether a door is open or closed by the echo in the room. A door halfway ajar, however, can be deceiving as well as dangerous. We recommend that you close the door or open it all the way. It is also courteous to announce your presence and state your business:

> *Example:* "My name is Fred Jones, and I'm your nurse for today. I'm going to . . . , then later I'll. . . . Tell me what things help you get oriented to the food tray, the bathroom, and the door."

Language Impairment

Another communication difficulty is related to the use of language. In Chapter 8, we address communication with the person who speaks little or no English. If your client has a form of dysphasia as an aftermath of stroke, consult with the psychologist and neurophysiologist to select the best ways to assess the client's learning abilities. One client may very well understand your words and not be able to answer. Another may not be able to understand your words but can interpret your pantomime, singing, drawings, flash cards, or objects. These variables are determined by the location of the brain lesion. Clients who cannot hear, understand English, speak, or see each have unique communication difficulties. They share a common bond: shouting is not helpful to any of them.

Nurses' Contributions to Communication Difficulties

The final communication problem we wish to raise at this point is the one you might inadvertently create. When you mumble, use technical jargon, or talk when you should listen, you interfere with communication. Learn to recognize signs of client confusion: confused facial expressions, lack of attention, and questions that indicate the client has not understood your message.

Some suggestions to reduce this barrier include the art of active listening and observing. While listening and watching body language, you will develop a sensitivity to other communication clues. What kind of metaphors does the client use? Auditory? Visual? Kinesthetic? Does the client wave her hands as she speaks? While listening to an artistic hand-waving client, the nurse noticed that the patient was having difficulty finding the words to express herself. After receiving a large pad of blank paper and some pens, the patient immediately began sketching a recurring dream. This led to a very fruitful exploration. Seeing her thoughts drawn in her own style allowed her to study them in more detail and depth than she could as they flitted through her mind.

The Teaching/Learning Environment

We view the teaching/learning environment as a system composed of the teacher, the learner, the relationship between them, and the physical environment in which this relationship takes place. As a nurse, you will be responsible for assessing the teaching/learning environment. Furthermore, you will be responsible for choosing and modifying the environment as much as possible to facilitate the client's learning.

The Teacher

In this part of the chapter we wish to emphasize the assessment of you as a crucial subsystem in the client's teaching/learning system. You are a composite of biologic, psychologic, social, and cultural influences that affect your client. The associate degree nurse is expected to teach individuals and sometimes their families, particularly in the acute care setting. The baccalaureate degree nurse is expected to have beginning skills in assessing health education needs, analyzing domain deficiencies and potentials, planning health education, delivering this education in various settings, and evaluating the results of the learning as well as the process itself. You must also be ready to teach in group settings.

The Teacher/Learner Relationship

The relationship between you and the client greatly affects the success of the learning. The psychologic climate is a vital part of the teaching/learning environment. You are expected to create an environment of warmth, caring, and mutual respect (Leininger, 1988). The information and examples throughout this book are intended to help you achieve that goal.

The Physical Learning Environment

Another responsibility of yours is to take control of the learning environment, to make it as conducive to learning as possible. Factors we address include space; temperature; visual, auditory, and olfactory stimuli; equipment; resources; furniture arrange-

ment; physical comfort; and time as shown in Figure 4-2. You need enough space so that you can get maximum use of your teaching materials. This is true whether you are speaking to an individual, a family, or a group in a living room or an auditorium. Examine the space for sound and sight barriers. Pillars will make it difficult for clients to see you. Partitions in the ceiling may act as sound barriers that will prevent the sound from getting past the partition.

Temperatures that are too hot or too cold can also interfere with learning. Clients distracted by the heat spend their time fanning themselves, or if cold, by clutching their arms instead of listening to you.

Visual stimuli can be distracting and interfere with vision. Do not place yourself in front of a sunny window. The glare behind you will turn you into a shadowy figure. Your audience will be squinting and wanting to look elsewhere. Try to pick a spot where you can control the appearance of the learning situation. If you cannot control all of the stimuli, look for ways to control the corner in which you intend to teach. In the hospital you may draw the curtain around the client's bed. One way to modify sound in a client's room is to hang a sign on the door:

Example: "Client teaching in progress: Please return in . . . minutes. Thank you."

If your client is a family, you may be able to cordon off a corner of the waiting room. In a dining area of an extended care facility you may be able to attach a long clothesline from one wall to the other and pin sheets to it. Auditory stimuli may or may not be under your control. Olfactory stimuli produced by others are usually not under your control. If the nearby odors are very distracting, you might be able to get a quiet fan going to deflect the odors. You could try cutting a lemon or putting a drop of cinnamon oil on a nearby heated surface, such as a light fixture.

Equipment and resources will of course influence your options. One of the attitudes we hope to promote is curiosity. We invite you to find out what equipment and expertise is available in your hospital, community, or both to enhance the teaching you wish to do. See Chapter 11 for more information on materials.

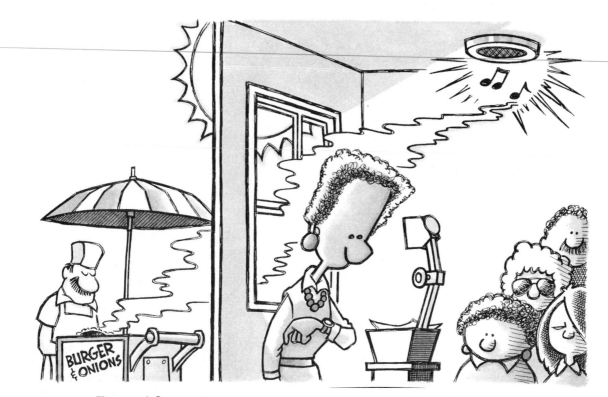

Figure 4-2 Physical environment affects both the nurse/teacher and client/learner.

Furniture, unless it is nailed to the floor, may be arranged in a way most conducive to the learning you wish to encourage. Be sure to take into account your objectives. Do you plan to have the clients interact with each other? Do you wish a relative to see everything you are doing for the client? Move the furniture so that it enhances your teaching. Some foresighted nurses at one hospital influenced the planning stage of a new intensive care unit by asking for glass walls that open completely on the side facing the nurses' station. Their request was granted. These walls allow them a great deal of flexibility in moving clients and equipment. The nurses also requested and received an attractive, spacious waiting area for clients' families. As a result, this unit is very conducive for teaching. Clients and their families often comment on the level of comfort and caring they perceive.

Physical comfort is an important variable in enhancing the teaching/learning environment. You may decide to teach a client after he or she has had a bath or once she or he is settled in a chair after getting out of bed. You will find that your client can learn better during a particular phase of the medication cycle: medicated enough to be undistracted by pain, but not too sleepy to pay attention. Lighting and temperature also affect comfort. You will want the lighting to be bright enough to allow lip readers to see your face but not so strong that it creates glare.

Time is one factor you must take into consideration. The main mistake we have seen busy nurses make is trying to jam too much information into the time available. They operate as if clients will absorb everything they say, no matter how fast they say it.

Teaching/Learning Settings

In the acute care setting, clients need to be oriented to surroundings, given honest, hopeful appraisals of their condition, and instructed on what they can do now to survive, cooperate, and be more comfortable.

There are times when urgent anticipatory guidance becomes necessary. Catastrophically burned clients may need immediate support and information. Such clients have very little time to decide on how they wish the staff to respond to their conditions before they become unable to communicate.

A woman who was alert during her cardiac arrest and subsequent emergency procedures needed repeated anticipatory guidance to alert her to the traumatic stress syndrome that would follow. At the time she could not understand the staff's insistence on her making contact with a psychiatric nurse consultant. Later, when she moved into grief, the relationship she had already established with the nurse allowed her to confront and move through her grief smoothly.

In the United States today, most convalescent care occurs in the home. Clients go home from the acute care setting with increasingly complex treatment and learning needs. Families are expected to learn skills and information that, only a decade ago, were reserved for highly educated medical personnel. Clients often find it easier to learn in familiar surroundings. You will be the guest, and the territory belongs to the client. During home health nursing it will be easier for you to be realistic in your teaching because you can see the reality of the client's environment. Family dynamics that may enhance or impede recovery will be more evident in the home, which means you will be more likely to be realistic in your direction of teaching the family as well as the client.

The school is an ideal learning environment because its main purpose is learning. With learning aids located nearby, the school is an ideal setting for teaching prevention and providing anticipatory guidance. Nurses are ideal for addressing today's concerns about ways to avoid human immunodeficiency virus (HIV) infections associated with lifestyle choices, and substance abuse. This education must begin in the grade schools. Occupational health nurses can provide many services to both management and employees. For example, these nurses can provide consultation about cost-effective insurance plans, infection and accident control, health promotion, and maintenance programs. You can also conduct physical assessments, teach prevention to employees, provide screening services, produce health newsletters, and do research on the major health hazards in that setting. The political system within the industry greatly affects your ability to be helpful. Self-help groups for alcoholism, smoking cessation, stress management, prevention of accidents, and safety precautions are all worthy topics of consideration.

If you plan to teach in an unfamiliar setting, such as a community center, you must assess the environment more conscientiously than would be necessary in a familiar work setting, for example, the hospital where you work or your child's classroom. In addition to the physical setting—chalkboard, electrical outlets, window covers, sound system, acoustics, and flexibility of seating—we recommend that you focus on the psychosocial environment. We have listed a number of questions for you to ask yourself as you enter the classroom as a guest speaker. What is the culture in that room? For instance, are the students accustomed to discipline and to giving polite attention? Are they able to sit and listen? Will the teacher help maintain order? Will you need to take over that function? What methods of communication and discipline does this group understand?

Summary

Your assessment of clients and their teaching/learning needs is greatly influenced by your perceptions of their ability to learn. They, in turn, are influenced by your perceptions of them as well as their own perceptions of you and themselves. A client's readiness to learn is dependent in part on his or her past experiences, motivation, level of wellness, and the coping mechanisms used to deal with health problems. Selected communication difficulties related to client impairments, mumbling, and the use of jargon can impede communication. The teaching/learning environment is also affected by your characteristics, the relationship you build with the client, the physical learning environment, and various teaching/learning and physical settings.

PERCEPTION IN ASSESSMENT

Purposes:

- Raise your consciousness about the importance of perception in assessing clients
- Recognize how easy it is to let your own biases affect what you see and hear in your interactions with clients

Directions:

1. Share one example in which the client's perception of his or her health status was significantly different from yours.
2. Describe a situation in which it was easy to relate to a client. What factors in you and the client made it easy to relate to the client and understand his or her perceptions?
3. Describe a situation in which it was difficult to relate to a client. What factors in you and the client made it hard to relate to the client and understand his or her perceptions?
4. How did this affect your assessment of the learning needs of this client?
5. Think of a situation in which you saw a client as much smarter or much less intelligent than your colleague did. What do you think was going on? Examine the differences in perceptions you suspect may have biased your peer's view or your view of the client.

EMOTIONAL AND EXPERIENTIAL READINESS

Purpose:

- Apply knowledge of experiential and emotional readiness to clients

Directions:

1. Differentiate between experiential readiness and emotional readiness.
2. Give an example of each.
3. How will you apply this knowledge as you prepare to teach a client about diabetes care?

ADAPTING TO CHANGE

Purpose:

- Become sensitive to the personal struggle involved with behavioral change

Directions:

- Divide into dyads.

- Share with your partner a life change you made or identify one health-related behavior you have succeeded in adopting.
- Answer the following questions about your change:

1. Why did you adopt the behavior?
2. Identify the factors related to your readiness to change.
3. What information did you need to make the change?
4. What experiential training did you need to have?
5. What was the hoped for outcome that motivated you to change?
6. What did you say to encourage yourself?
7. What was the trigger, that is, what finally got you started?
8. How can you use this to help clients get started with health behavior changes?

References

Carmack, B.J. (1992). Balancing engagement/ detachment in AIDS-related multiple losses. *IMAGE: Journal of Nursing Scholarship*, 24(1), 9-14.

Doak, C.C., Doak, L.G. & Root, J.D.H. (1985). *Teaching patients with low literacy skills.* Philadelphia PA: Lippincott.

Ersek, M. (1992). Examining the process and dilemmas of reality negotiation. *IMAGE: Journal of Nursing Scholarship*, 24(1), 19-25.

Feinblum, S. (1989). Pinning down the psychosocial dimensions of AIDS. *Nursing & Health Care*, 7, 255-257.

Folks, D.G., Freeman, A.M. Sokol, R.S. & Thurstin, A.H. (1988). Denial: Predictor of outcome following coronary bypass surgery. *International Journal of Psychiatry in Medicine*, 18, 57-66.

Froman, R.D., Owen, S.V., & Daisy, C. (1992). Development of a measure of attitudes toward persons with AIDS. *IMAGE: Journal of Nursing Scholarship*, 24:(2), 149.

Hickey, S.S. (1986). Enabling hope. *Cancer Nursing*, 9(30), 133-137.

Kaluger, G. & Kaluger, M. (1984). *Human development: The life span.* St. Louis, MO: Mosby.

Leininger, M. (Ed.). (1988). *Care: The essence of nursing and health*, Detroit: Wayne State University Press.

Maslow, A.H. (1954). Motivation and personality. New York: Harper & Row.

McHatton, M. (1985). A theory for timely teaching. *American Journal of Nursing*, 85(7), 798-800.

Pohl, M.L. (1981). *The teaching function of the nursing practitioner.* Dubuque IA: Wm. C. Brown.

Rollin, B. (1976). *First, you cry.* Philadelphia: Lippincott.

Shabetai, R. (1983). Cardiomyopathy: How far have we come in 25 years, how far yet to go? *Journal of the American College of Cardiology*, 1, 252.

Slavin, R.E. (1991). *Educational psychology: Theory into practice*, 3rd ed. Boston: Allyn & Bacon.

Suchman, E.A. (1965). Stages of illness and medical care. *Journal of Health & Human behavior*, 6, 114-128.

Thompson, J.M., McFarland, G.K., Hirsch, J.E., Tucker, S.M. & Bowers, A.C. (1989). *Mosby's manual of clinical nursing*, St. Louis MO: Mosby.

Winslow, E.H. (1985). Cardiovascular consequences of bed rest. *Heart & Lung*, 14, 236.

When the Client Is a Child

All I really need to know about
how to live and what to do and
how to be I learned in
kindergarten . . . Share
everything. Play fair . . . Put
things back where you found
them . . . Live a balanced life—
learn some and think some and
draw and paint and sing and
dance and play and work every
day some . . .

Fulghum, 1988.

5

Objectives

Upon completion of this chapter you will be able to:

- Select, in a given situation, teaching content appropriate to each developmental level of the child client.
- Describe teaching strategies appropriate to each developmental level of the child client.
- Discuss teaching/learning implications for the child.

Key Words

caretaker
caregiver
psychosocial
   development

cognitive
   development
biologic
   development

infant/environment
   learning system

Introduction

In addition to an aroused interest or motive and relevant preparatory training, physiologic maturation affects readiness to learn. This chapter, therefore, will deal with assessing developmental readiness. Developmental readiness in interaction with experiential readiness, emotional readiness, health, strength, and environment all affect the child's ability to learn. In this chapter we begin by offering several frames of reference for assessing the child and the child's caretaking system, the caregiving (medical) system, and the situation. We will consider general systems theory, behavioral, gestalt, and humanistic perspectives, and the information-processing viewpoint with respect to children. We will apply knowledge about growth and development, Erikson's theories on psychosocial development, and Piaget's theories on cognitive development to stages of childhood, and we will discuss possible relevant nursing interventions.

Ways to View Human Development

General Systems Theory

Environmental Influences   General systems theory offers two relevant assumptions. First, all that surrounds the child internally and externally makes significant contributions to the learning process. The child's internal environment—biologic potential, state of health, temperament, and intellectual capacity—greatly affect the situation. The external environment is composed of the physical world, temperature, and material goods (or lack thereof), and caretakers. Caretakers' biologic realities—such as IQ and state of health, as well as attitudes, perceptions, and skills—enhance or inhibit a child's ability to realize his or her potential. These caretakers may be the child's biologic parents, grandparents, aunts, uncles, or adopted relatives. Today the most important caretaker(s) may be babysitter(s) or nursery employee(s). Besides the relationship of these important people to the child, other socioeconomic and cultural factors shape the perception of the child. The caretakers' places in society and how they feel treated will, in turn, affect how they treat the child. The infant's system is depicted in Figure 5-1.

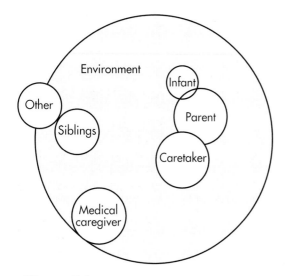

Figure 5-1   The infant/environment learning system

The physical surroundings that first affect the child are those in the uterus. The health and lifestyle of the mother can greatly alter the biologic potential of the child. For instance, mothers who are very young, poor, or who use cigarettes, alcohol, or other substances, are more likely to produce babies of low birth weight (MacGregor et al, 1987; Stein & Kline, 1983). Two-thirds of all babies who die in infancy have low birth weight (less than 2,500 grams) (National Commission to prevent Infant Mortality, 1988). Other more positive aspects of the environment also seem to have an effect on unborn babies who react to music with increases in heart beat (Kaluger & Kaluger, 1984).

As soon as they are born, babies experience numerous new stimuli. Even babies who are only 6 days old can distinguish between different odors. For example, one study showed that neonates spent significantly more time turned toward breast pads that had been in their mothers' bras than clean breast pads (Anderson, 1989).

The psychologic environment is created by the child's caretakers: parents, other relatives, the babysitting system, peers, teachers, neighbors, and society in general. The family's socioeconomic status and cultural experiences also influence the child's growth and health. For example, homeless infants in New York City had a mortality rate that was double that of their peers. Homeless children have inordinately high rates of common acute pediatric problems (Berne, Dato, Mason, & Rafferty, 1990).

Transactions   Learning or change is a transactional process between the child and those in the environment. The child is influenced by the caretakers and they in turn are influenced by the child. In general, mothers and other female attendants tend to coo and smile at babies, while fathers and other male attendants tend to juggle and physically move their babies (Schuster & Ashburn, 1986). Parents and others are also influenced by the babies; attractive, smiling, and cooing babies get more attention from those around them. Mothers who spent time in skin contact with their babies find that their breast milk flowed more abundantly and freely (Anderson, 1989). The mutuality of the baby and caretakers is symbolized in Figure 5-2.

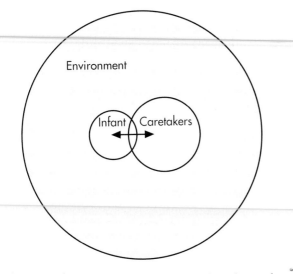

Figure 5-2 Transactions between the infant and the environment.

In addition to viewing the infant and caretaking system, you need to look at yourself, the nurse, as part of the caregiving system. You and all of your colleagues and equipment in the caregiving setting affect the parents or other caretakers and the child.

Behavioral Theories

When using behavioral theories you will notice that behaviors that bring pleasure (approval and need satisfaction) tend to be repeated and are incorporated into the child's repertoire of responses. An example is the development of the rooting reflex during the first few weeks. Rooting soon evolves into the skill of hunting for and finding the nipple. Behavior that brings pain and disapproval tends to be suppressed, and behavior that brings no response tends to be extinguished. Many children who fail to thrive are sad examples of this last proposition.

Imitation plays an important role in the learning of very young children as soon as their vision is clear enough to focus (Meltzoff & Moore, 1989). Observe the behavior of most adults when they feed a young child. Most people automatically open their mouths while approaching the infant with a spoon. This semiconscious adult behavior suggests the awareness at some level of the infant's penchant for

imitation. Poulson, Kymissis, and Reeve (1991) document this possibility that children can engage in imitative learning as early as 6 months. Others (Meltzoff and Moore, 1989) believe this ability develops much earlier but there is more controversy about that hypothesis.

Caretakers' behaviors are also shaped by babies. Caretakers intuitively hold babies closer to their faces than is comfortable for adult vision. This close distance is a result of the baby's greater activity when the distance between the caretaker and child is shorter. The shorter distance accommodates for the infant's immature visual ability.

Gestalt/Cognitive Field Theories

A child's cognitive field widens over time, and children's developmental milestones are related to their ability to learn at various stages. Emile Rousseau wrote that children learn by the natural unfolding of their innate capacity. Rousseau's claims have since been substantiated by numerous studies (Reinisch, Rosenblum, & Rubin, 1991). Piaget, the Swiss psychologist and world renown researcher of cognitive development in children, also adheres to the belief that the child's ability to think and reason is a stage-dependent process (Ginsburg & Opper, 1979).

Children are more like each other than they will be as adults; still, they are still very much individuals. Although the patterns of biologic development are recognizable in any culture, the timetable of each child is controlled by the child's inherited chromosomes. Internal, genetic programming is, in turn, influenced by various phenomena in the child's environment, such as biologic (nutrition), psychologic (emotional warmth), sociologic (attention), and cultural (patterns of nurturing) (Smith & Nix, 1991; Ingalls, 1991; Schuster & Ashburn, 1986). In addition to neurologic maturation, children's mobility increases their opportunity to explore, learn, and exert themselves on ever-widening fields of interest. For instance, a toddler of 18 months recently discovered many interesting properties of oil (the kind one finds in a garage). Her caretaker was then inspired to experiment beyond her usual repertoire for removing stains.

Humanistic Frame of Reference

The humanistic view is a very holistic approach to personality development. The developing individual is considered a total person. The personality is viewed as the integrating factor. Ideally, those in the environment support the young human being in striving for control over the environment to satisfy basic needs. The measure of success experienced by the young person influences that individual's self-esteem and level of self-confidence. This self-concept is also influenced by significant others in the environment. The child learns what is valued by parents and caregivers and what is not valued. The child then reacts accordingly. The ideal self is the image that the individual forms as a result of the interplay of those forces (Kaluger & Kaluger, 1984).

A recent phenomenon that exemplifies the holistic intermingling of physiologic, psychosocial, and cultural variables is the clinical research that nurses are doing in Sweden, Norway, Finland, Denmark, and Germany with *Kangaroo Care*. A nurse educator was sent by the United Nations Children's Emergency Fund (UNICEF) to study the practice of having mothers and fathers come to intensive care units to lay their premature babies against their bare skin. Several photographs illustrate the pleasure experienced by the parents and the total relaxation experienced by the babies. The babies' respiratory and circulatory competence improved and their weight gain was better than expected. This experiment originated in Bogotá, Colombia, where there was a lack of incubators (Anderson, 1989).

Information Processing

From an information processing point of view, the infant is born with a simple set of hardware that will become more sophisticated in time. The hardware and its evolution is spelled out in the genetic code. Over time the child also accumulates numerous software programs in virtually unlimited numbers. Programs for breathing, eating, and attracting attention evolve. Programs for talking are particularly interesting. Children all over earth with similar hardware (brains and tongues) learn to speak many different languages. Even the way people sneeze is culturally influenced.

Temperament and Sex

The research on temperament has provided relief for this generation of parents. It is no longer necessary to feel totally responsible for babies' dispositions. Their general attitude toward learning and any kind of change is greatly influenced by the arrangements in their genetic code. Repeated studies have shown that some children are easy to deal with, while others are more hesitant in any new situation. Some children, who act out of sorts and generally uncomfortable, are difficult to deal with in general (Saudino & Eaton, 1991; Garcia Coll, Halpern, & Vohr, 1992).

Sexual differences, aside from obvious anatomic characteristics, are under investigation for explanations of how and when males and females learn. It is extremely difficult to differentiate between biologic and environmental influences, because they influence each other. Females' brains develop thicker corpus callosum and expend 20% more energy than males. Males develop more cortex (Bingham, 1987). The cause, meaning, and outcome of these differences are at this time speculative. Some behavioral differences that are well established include the females' accelerated biologic timetable. Females, in general, have a greater verbal ability, which becomes most marked in adolescence. Males in general lag behind females in biologic development and attention span. They surpass females during adolescence in strength. Boys also tend to outdistance girls in visual-spatial ability and in mathematical pursuits. It is important to note, however, that maturational timetables may have as much influence as sex (Reinisch, Rosenblum, & Rubin, 1991).

Developmental Factors and Stress

There are critical periods in the maturational process during which it is easiest to learn certain tasks. Most learning is incremental and developmental.

Few children go from lying on their backs to managing the antigravitational feat of standing. They usually go through several smaller stages: learning to push with their hands, to turn over, to crawl or scoot, and to steady themselves on furniture before fully balancing themselves. Most other learning is similar in that it builds on previous experiences.

Illness and handicaps as well as parental abilities and attitudes can interfere with children developing according to their own maturational potential. Some deficits appear amenable to eventual remedy. For example, nutritionally deprived children can make great leaps in catching up. Deaf parents that have a hearing child cannot expect the child to learn language by listening to a radio or watching television. The child must interact with another person to acquire language skills (Sachs & Johnson, 1976). Language can be acquired more readily if it is taught before puberty. Some aspects of language may be more difficult to learn later (Johnson & Newport, 1989).

In addition to parents' anxiety as an aftermath or contributing factor to the condition of their offspring, parents are in their own developmental stages. They have their own capacity to grasp reality, their own values, and their own experiential readiness for parenting imperfect children.

Receiving information in itself can be stress relieving. A brief review of growth stages relevant to general parent education follows (Keepers & Babcock, 1986).

When the Client Is an Infant

The parents or other caretakers must be involved in the entire process, for it is they who will use your teaching. It is important to assess the parents' anxiety levels. The higher the stress for the parents, the more need there is to tend to the parent's stress as a first priority in the teaching process. What is the parents' reaction to the situation? Parents who display their emotions freely may be easier to evaluate than stoics (Fisher, 1992). No matter what their emotional style, it takes skill and patience to assess parents' stress levels, and their readiness to learn.

Be cautious regarding your own assumptions of which illnesses are most stressful to parents. Nurses who work with extremely ill babies have told us that it was easy for them to view certain problems as non-life-threatening and correctable; and, hence, fail to tune in to the magnitude of the parents' distress. Parents who were expecting perfect babies may be upset by any flaw; they may not be able to judge the seriousness of the problem. Furthermore, they may have very strong personal, historical, or cultural experiences impinging on their consciousness as they encounter the medical system. It is important that you discover these perceptions before planning your teaching.

Another important variable to assess is the caretaker-child relationship. With whom will the child be spending convalescence? What does the child mean to each parent? How is the fit between this child and each of the parents? Is this child's illness related to or exacerbated by the parental relationship? Are the parents in separate households? Is this child's problem an aftermath of parental distraction and diminished alertness? Were the parents under stress already before the medical crisis occurred? Accidents increase under circumstances that are likely to distract parents. Such stressors include moving and marital discord (Keepers & Babcock, 1986; Coppens, 1990).

Psychosocial Characteristics

According to Erikson (1963), the issue of trust vs. mistrust is the first major dilemma that children must solve. They develop an emerging sense of trust balanced by a growing realization that all is not perfect. They respond by smiling at familiar faces within 5 or 6 weeks of birth, and they become emotionally symbiotic with the main caretaker. Their individual temperaments emerge in the earliest weeks. Their main needs at that time consist of rest, exercise, love, and physical strokes. Their cuddliness is part of their temperament and varies greatly.

Cognitive Characteristics

According to Piaget, infants are in the sensorimotor stage, learning mainly through their bodies and receiving sensory input. The sucking reflex starts developing into a definite skill within 2 weeks. At 2 to 3 months of age, most babies look toward sounds. At about 8 or 9 months, object permanence is evident. Keepers and Babcock (1986) believe that the young baby first thinks in pictures.

Language Characteristics

When they reach about 6 or 7 weeks of age, babies purposely produce prelanguage sounds. They are more likely to do this when they are in a good mood, and act as if they enjoy the effort. They tend to increase this activity when they experience responses from their caretakers. They are thought to be developing inner language. Babbling begins in the third or fourth month. Their audio and visual receptive powers develop earlier than their expressive skills. For example, babies recognize spoken words before they can produce them.

Teaching Implications

The caretakers are the targets of teaching activities. These individuals should be the ones with whom the baby will spend the most time. It may be a parent, a grandparent, another relative, a neighbor, or some combination. Try to figure out who is most invested in the child's well-being and be sure that person is included in your teaching. You must calibrate for the caretaker's tolerance level for information, his or her developmental level, and culturally related beliefs (Fisher, 1992). Anticipatory guidance is appropriate regarding temperamental differences, usual developmental milestones, safety, and the importance of stimulation—both physical and verbal (Cain, 1988; Curran, 1985).

Check with the caretakers on the nature of the authority system through which this advice will be filtered. To be effective, your advice must be compatible with that of the main advisor within the family. If you give advice that is contrary to the authority figure in the home, the parents are going to be in conflict. They are most likely to follow the advice of the people who are always available and on whom they depend for support.

Whoever learns the sophisticated technical procedures that will continue at home needs to be involved in the infant's care as soon as possible. You can begin teaching even before the parents are ready to focus on learning any procedures, by the use of indirect methods. You can explain to the baby what is going on and why it is needed. You will thus model the place of auditory stimulation in the nurturing of an infant. The parents grasp as much as they can tolerate. Because the "lessons" are not yet directed to them, they can listen with less tension. You can facilitate this process and model appropriate nurturing of the child simultaneously.

When the Child Is a Toddler

Psychosocial Characteristics

According to Erikson (1963), the main psychologic dilemma that the toddler must resolve is autonomy vs. shame and doubt. It is during this stage that the balance of love and hateful feelings, cooperation and willfulness begins to emerge. "No!" is a very popular word with the young child, who hears it often. Ambivalence is common in words and behavior: "yes - no - yes!" These words reflect the disposition of toddlers who are frustrated by personal and external limits. It is an age of egocentrism. Toddlers can be very bossy and their bedtime rituals can be very rigid.

Mobile toddlers explore places and things. In Figure 5-3 the toddler is exploring the physics of motion. Children develop remarkable ability to conduct scientific investigations. The toddler studies the effects of gravity with the determination of a conscientious scientist: "Does the liquid always go down when I up-end the cup?" This same toddler eventually moves into social experiments: "What does Mommy/Daddy/nurse do when I up-end the cup?" (Keepers & Babcock, 1986).

Toddlers can obey commands like "Kiss grandma goodbye," and "Put your arm out." Play with peers at this early stage usually ends up in tears because they have yet to learn much about delayed gratification, tact, or rules of sharing and fair play.

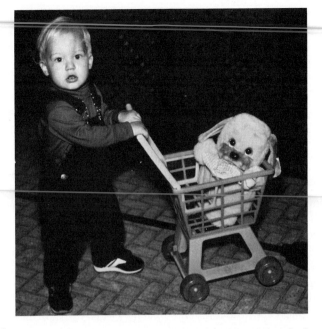

Figure 5-3   The toddler. *From Whaley, L. and Wong, D.* Nursing care of infants and children, ed 4, Mosby–Year Book, 1991.

Cognitive Characteristics

Toddlers are at a more advanced level of sensori-motor development than infants. They still think in pictures until language is well established. Representational levels of development (use of symbols and images) are evident when imaginary friends appear between the second and third year. The appearance of imaginary friends indicates a measure of intellectual development as well as personal creativity (Harter & Chao, 1992). Not all children are open about telling others of the existence of their imaginary companions.

Other indications that they have reached representational levels of development can be seen in their playing tea. They stir something and then bring it to the caretaker or caregiver. The adult is expected to drink from something, which may be a real cup, a play cup, a stone, or an invisible object (Keepers & Babcock, 1986).

By the time children are 3 years old they have a sense of time and know the meaning of "pretty soon" and "when it's time." Children who watch television and who experience much time structure in their lives will be more conscious of it than children who are raised with less structure in their lives.

Language Characteristics

Children speak in one- to three-word sentences, starting with single syllables. Those syllables that are reinforced tend to increase in frequency. Other words that occur early are imitations of what they hear. Sometimes logical but unexpected results occur. Whenever an infant boy showed interest in an object, his father said things, such as "This is a ball," "This is a blanket," and "This is milk." The child's first words were, "This is." As soon as the father heard the results of his approach, he was able to make use of the feedback. He changed to just nouns and verbs; his son soon acquired the names and actions of the objects. The father learned by trial and error what the research has shown: children who are just learning to talk do better with slow, simplified speech (Fernald & Kuhl, 1987). Verbs (catch), nouns (bottle), and adjectives (soft) are words that have meaning for the child and are among the early acquisitions.

Teaching Implications

Most teaching of toddlers is still done through the parents or main caretakers. Today's pediatric care facilities acknowledge the importance of the caretakers' roles in promoting children's healing. The child's needs for safe play space, love, and security are paramount. Before the parents leave, ask about routines that the child can do and finds comforting. Because toddlers are at the peak age for nightmares, ask what the child finds soothing after awakening from a nightmare.

Special words for bodily functions are usually important. Ask what commands the toddler will obey at home. Information on the child's exposure to television and favorite programs is important information. Children may be able to listen and learn better from a favorite television character in the form of a puppet. We wish to caution you, though, that imagination is very vivid, and the child may use your words to build a very frightening scenario. Pay attention to the words you use to describe procedures. "Cut" and "knife" are familiar words but they are also much more frightening than "fix, sew, and make it go away." "Bandaids" are probably more familiar than "dressings." Not only do Bandaids have magical healing properties, but they keep people from bleeding to death (by covering the hole). If possible, leave nondangerous equipment with the child so the child can manipulate it. This allows the child to work through in play the task of integrating this new, and often unnerving, experience.

Picture books and tapes can be used for children who are more sedate and mature. Puppets help some children focus on the message. Doing the procedure to the teddy bear first will help the child grasp what is coming. To help bring the child's imagination closer to reality, try using role play. When children go through anticipated procedures in play, they get a clearer picture of what to expect and they have the opportunity to do some mastery learning, to develop some coping mechanisms. Give positive simple commands and expect cooperation. The presence of a comfort toy can make a difference in the child's ability to cope with stress and pain and to learn.

Parents who need information on normal growth and development may welcome guidance. In addition to the needs mentioned above, children should experience a balance of restraint and freedom. They should be able to experiment without becoming victims. They should not be set up for failure. They learn letter when caretakers manipulate the environment to improve their chances for success.

A number of good books on child care are now available (Cain, 1988; Keepers & Babcock, 1986; Curran, 1985). These books are written for different readability levels. Parenting classes through family care centers, maternity centers, and community colleges are available in many communities. Advise young parents or other interested caretakers to browse through the books available looking for one that makes sense to them, does not undermine their self-confidence, and does offer suggestions that are practical for their circumstances. You may find simpler pamphlets on specific subjects at the local health department. Another source for non-English pamphlets and simply written pamphlets is the U.S. Government through the Superintendent of Documents. See the list of resources in Appendix G.

One common dilemma that parents face is teaching their children to deal with anger. It is important that children identify anger as a legitimate feeling. They also need to learn ways for expressing anger that are acceptable in their family. You can use the topic as a way to assess the family's comfort with negative emotions.

> *Example:* "Some of Joey's treatment is likely to make him angry and scared. We want to support his learning to deal with these emotions. What is he allowed to do when he's mad at home?"

If their answer indicates an intolerance of negative emotions, you can use the dialogue as an opportunity for anticipatory guidance.

> *Example:* "All children and, of course, adults need ways to express all of their feelings. We certainly want to help Joey learn ways he can use at home, at school, and at play. Some of the methods we use here are . . . Can you imagine any of those methods working for you at home?"

It is equally important that you acknowledge the feelings and needs of the parents. Parents may need reassurance that they also have rights and that they need not try too hard to be perfect parents or to avoid conflict (Keepers & Babcock, 1986). Today's parents are expected to handle much sicker children on their own (Donar, 1988). You will start teaching as soon as you encounter the parents. As soon as the parents are willing, an apprentice style of learning is begun. Initially you will want to concentrate on establishing rapport. This is vital to parents' feeling they have your support.

When the Client Is a Preschooler

Psychosocial Characteristics

The main psychosocial dilemma that Erikson believes that children ages 3 to 6 must solve is initiative vs. guilt. They attack tasks for the sake of being on the move. Their excess energy and desire to dominate may lead to frustration and anger. In general the preschooler moves around more freely, communicates better, and gives evidence of an expanding imagination.

This is an out-of-bounds stage. Children approach life with avid enthusiasm. They run full tilt greeting the world, up on the trampoline, down in the holes, into the puddles, and onto the tricycles as seen in Figure 5-4. A child's curiosity is consuming and his or her ability to act on impulse increases daily. Along with increased agility and expanded social world, preschool children's growing imagination leads to many fears: strangers, separation, disapproval, pain, punishment, and aggres-

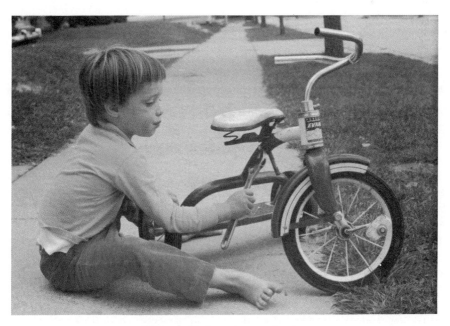

Figure 5-4 The preschooler.

sion. Keepers and Babcock (1986) believe that nightmares are related to situations that children have learned are unsafe but have not yet developed the self-control and other skills to handle. Two prevalent themes that Keepers and Babcock encountered in their clinical practice were sex and aggression. Fear of violence was the theme that Babcock encountered most. Fear of loss of body integrity is the preschooler's greatest fear, which affects the child's encounters with medical personnel (Smith, Goodman, & Ramsey, 1987).

Learning their social roles and deciding on tentative scripts are other major psychosocial tasks characteristic of the preschool child. We can observe children's perceptions in their play and in their conversations.

Example: "Boys do. . . . Girls do. . . . When I grow up I'm gonna be. . . ."

During this phase the rudiments of conscience become evident, and rudimentary self-control begins. An overly zealous adult may inflict too rigid and intimidating a conscience on the young child. On the other hand, children may decide all by themselves that their illness is punishment for their sins of commission or omission.

Much play between preschoolers is parallel. They talk at each other rather than engage in listening and exchanging observations. They give little evidence of seeing another's point of view.

Example: "The teacher told *me* to . . . , then she told *me* to take a nap," no mention of *us*.

Cognitive Characteristics

Cognitive development is evident in preschool children's expanded imagination. They are moving into preoperational thought as their ability to handle concepts is rapidly growing. Their richness of life experiences influence how quickly and how thoroughly they are able to put related concepts together. They still think differently about the world than do most adults. The box at the top of the next column contains some examples of children's magical thinking.

Examples of Children's Magical Thinking

1. The sun and moon follow you when you walk.
2. Anything that moves is alive.
3. The names of objects reside in the objects themselves.
4. Dreams come in the window at night (some cultures believe that the spirit leaves the body to go on an adventure; trouble can ensue if the soul cannot find its way back).
5. Stones, clouds, and other objects have feelings.
6. If a child imagines a monster, it exists.

Many preschool children can differentiate between safe and unsafe situations and they can specify preventive actions (Coppens, 1990). The cognitive attainment, however, according to the clinical experience of Keepers and Babcock (1986) may not be followed by congruent behavior. In other words, children may tell you the safety rules but may not actually follow them.

Language Characteristics

The language of 4- to 6-year olds rapidly expands. Their proficiency with meaningful sentences mushrooms. Most children by the age of 5 can use the language and syntax of their main caretaking systems. Children in bilingual families are fluent in both languages. By this age they can separate the languages, mix them together, or both as they hear done by the grown-ups in their households.

Teaching Implications

Much of the teaching concerning the preschool child is still through the parents, particularly during these times of rapid discharge. Your role may be teacher, consultant, or model, depending on the parents' capabilities and anxiety level. When you assess the learning ability of the preschool child you will base your teaching on your observations of the child's abilities to communicate, to relate to others, to perform appropriate tasks, and to follow instructions. This will help you determine how much instruction the child can absorb.

Children at this age need very simple concrete explanations.

> *Example:* "You will see. . . ." "You will smell icky perfume."
> "When you wake up you'll be wearing a big white boot, with long pipes propping it up like Jimmy's over there."

They can benefit from watching videotaped travelogues of real children going through an experience that is similar to their upcoming procedures.

While you teach, you are modeling for parents how to explain complicated and possibly frightening events and procedures. Timing is an important consideration. Children need enough warning to gather themselves together, but not enough so much time that they panic themselves with dire fantasies. Role playing the upcoming procedure with their teddy bears may be helpful. During procedures children do better if they feel connected to someone or something. It will help if you hold their hands, ask them to hold the bandage, or tell them a short story about a child going through what they are experiencing. An alternative is to tell a wild story that will capture the imagination and allow the child to escape from the present and a painful procedure (Donnelly, 1988). Children should be given only as much control as they can handle. For instance, they may be able to choose which limb will receive the injection, but they may need to be held during a prolonged and painful procedure.

During illness children can be expected to regress. Regression is a natural defense, which helps them to weather the crisis and to accept the dependency that usually accompanies illness. They may need specific instructions from you on safe ways to express feelings.

> *Example:* "Keep your leg very still and quiet, but it's OK for the rest of you to cry."
> "I know you are scared. Want to hold your teddy?"
> "Want me to hold your hand?"

They may need specific reassurance that they are not responsible for their misfortune. They may have been told they are at fault, or they may have decided that by themselves (Willitt, 1988).

If you can support the regression and think about the positive tasks that are appropriate to that age, you may help the child to recycle earlier tasks and arrive at a better resolution than he or she did originally. Trust is a good place to begin. When you are honest, positive, and warm and validate all of the child's feelings as legitimate, you can help the child have a good experience despite adverse conditions. If you are teaching a child who has a long-term, chronic illness you need to be particularly creative about designing substitute experiences that will enhance his or her developmental needs (Smith & Nix, 1991; Ingalls, 1991).

Groups of children, such as those found in preschool settings, are ready for basic health teaching. They do better with short programs, hands-on experiences, and active participation. Simple songs, puppet shows, and large muscle activities related to the theme are very effective. Stories accompanied by colorful pictures are also very useful. If you wish to learn more about teaching children, we suggest that you watch high-quality children's programs such as *Mister Rogers* and *Sesame Street* for ideas on how teach them in groups.

When the Client Is School-Age

Cognitive and motor development has progressed in children of 5 to 7 years of age to the point that many societies begin formal training of their children during this developmental phase. This formal training takes place in all societies whose life-styles are above the subsistence level (Kaluger & Kaluger, 1984). The information and muscular and cognitive skills that children learn during these years will be shaped by their society and the subculture in which they mature. The child in a suburban school that is equipped with computer technology (Figure 5-5) and television will develop a substantially different repertoire than the child in New Guinea who plays outdoors much of the time and sits at the feet of an elder to hear the legends of the tribe.

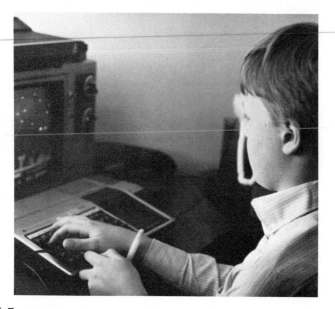

Figure 5-5 School age learner. *From Whaley, L. and Wong, D. Nursing care of infants and children, ed 4, Mosby–Year Book, 1991.*

Attitudes, values, and perceptions of the world are similarly shaped. Visions of space ships and plastic toys to match stimulate differently than the impressions gained from listening to and copying real adult role models all day and listening to oral history.

Psychosocial Characteristics

Erikson has identified the dilemma of this age as one of industry vs. inferiority. School-age children have developed the intellectual and motor coordination that allows them to do many things. They attain numerous skills and become aware of their own special talents. They gather data about the world outside their immediate neighborhoods. They compare their own family's rules with those of other families, and they refine the "conscience." They may have an embryonic faith that sustains and comforts them.

Growing older is very exciting. They are ready and willing to learn. Boys tend to know who is tallest, fastest, and toughest. Girls continue to be more aware of who is "best friends" with whom.

Both sexes develop attitudes toward cooperation and competition that are compatible with the older models to whom they are exposed. Peers and adults outside the home become more important influences. By the time they are 10 years old, most children can see another's point of view. However, some researchers believe that ability is present much earlier (Slavin, 1991).

Cognitive Characteristics

Piaget has labeled the type of thinking school-age children do as concrete operations. They have mastered concepts, such as conservation (an object such as clay weighs the same rolled into a sausage as it would rolled in a sphere), reversibility (milk is the same amount in this tall thin glass as it would be if poured back in the short wide one), and inferred reality (if the experimenter puts a black filter in front of the red car, the car remains red (Flavell, 1985; Flavell, Green, & Flavell, 1986). Other psychologic tasks of elementary school children include learning to separate fantasy from reality and developing more fully their cognitive operations of memory, reality testing, and problem solving.

Children are able to engage in inductive reasoning and solve problems in concrete ways regarding situations and materials with which they are familiar. For instance on a trip the family wanted to meet a latecomer at a specific location within a large park. They talked about drawing a map indicating where they would be. They hoped there would be a pay phone and guard at the entrance to the park. The adults started scrambling for a piece of paper and reminded the designated drawer to look at the terrain to map it accurately. David, who was 6 years old, suggested they ask at the entrance to the area if there were maps already printed. David had not been there before but somewhere in his experience he had noted that people sometimes give out little maps at entrances.

Giving up magical thinking in deference to reality thinking is a lifelong process. In the first few years of school, many children are reluctant to give up some cherished beliefs even when they have much data to the contrary. They mix fact and fantasy for fun, for practice at imagining and for spicing up conversations. Most children have begun developing permanent memory by the age of 4; some show evidence of it much earlier and some do not develop it until they near 8 years of age.

Language Characteristics

The vocabulary of school-age children continues to grow, depending on the words to which they are exposed and the reinforcement they receive for using them. In their speech, outgoing children give evidence that memory, reality testing, and problem-solving abilities are increasing.

This is a time of using language as a tool and as a toy. Children use language to ask why and to argue. They repeat stories or make them up, mixing fact and fantasy freely. Joking and teasing styles vary according to the family and culture. Repertoires increase as children mature. They employ language to fool each other, and they can enjoy playing with the language in making up rhymes, limericks, and telling jokes.

Teaching Implications

School-age children are ready for direct formal teaching from you. They welcome basic factual information about what is wrong, how the procedure will feel, how long it will take, how it is done, and what it will accomplish. Their vocabulary and ability to repeat information in their own words will give you clues as to how much they comprehend. Their expanding intellect, memory, and attention span allow them to focus on more complicated explanations for longer periods of time. Assessment of their reading ability is a prerequisite to choosing appropriate reading materials. They may find it easier to draw pictures of their perceptions than to tell you with words. Drawing pictures is an excellent way to convey emotionally laden material with all age groups. It is also a way to heal from the psychologic effects of trauma.

School-age children should know the safety rules for all of the activities in which they engage: walking, climbing, swimming, camping, biking, hiking, and softball. The should know general rules of preventing accidents, and they should know what to do in case of emergencies. Even very young children can benefit from programs and instructions such as "Hug a Tree," (staying put when lost) "Hug for Life" (a juvenile term for the Heimlich maneuver) and "Stop, Drop, and Roll" (if one catches on fire).

By the time they complete later childhood, children should be able to perform all aspects of their own personal hygiene. They should recognize the signs and symptoms of illness. They can also learn to handle impressive amounts of their own care, including complicated procedures. The more control they can exercise over their situation, the more competence and self-esteem they develop. Children need to know what they can do to promote their own well-being. They can choose nutritious menus when they are given the opportunity to learn healthy eating patterns. One way to teach children about health is to incorporate it into their current interests. Cabbage Patch Kids became a very important part of the American culture in the recent past. Innovative caregivers in a clinic created a

"Cabbage Patch Clinic" to attract youngsters. Girls from the ages of 7 to 12 came to the clinic, where creative staff and pediatric nurses elaborated on the well-known principle of using toys and puppets to relate to youngsters. The Cabbage Patch Clinic was started by two young girls coming into the community clinic located in a low-income housing unit. These girls asked for baby-bead bracelets to identify their dolls to protect them from being stolen. The receptionist, instead of brushing the girls off, seized the teachable moment to encourage the girls to talk about their "babies'" health and made appointments for the girls to have their babies checked. The nurses joined in and developed an impressive list of teaching opportunities in response to detailed expectations of the children. Each "mother" made an appointment for her baby. Each "baby" received a physical examination and a booster shot. The young mothers then brought up their own concerns, such as fever, diarrhea, and ear infections. As might be expected, word of the clinic's new service spread rapidly. The theme spread into the nearby day-care centers and proved to be a wonderful metaphor for health promotion (Crowe, 1986).

Children with specific chronic diseases should be well informed about their part in the disease process (Smith & Nix, 1991; Pidgeon, 1989). They can benefit from learning how to handle their problems through group classes. Not only does it help them feel less different but also peer pressure becomes increasingly important to them as they mature. On the other hand, they may need privacy if they are likely to lose control during disturbing procedures. They are able to learn stress-coping techniques, such as relaxation and self-hypnosis. Youngsters find these skills quite beneficial also when they must deal with adversity beyond their control. By teaching relaxation and self-hypnosis, you are enabling children to lower their risk of contacting stress-related chronic diseases as well as improving their health and resistance to disease. These lifetime tools are also useful in coping with chronic disease (Brophy & Mitchell, 1989).

Social resistance can also be learned at this age. Children can be taught to resist peer pressure through role playing. Programs that combine emphasis on improved self-esteem with refusal skills

have been very useful. Group teaching of school-age children should take into account specific ages, verbal ability, writing ability, and attention span. You will need to assess the children in the group to include appropriate opportunities for physical expression of the learning under consideration.

A group of nursing students taught a class in cardiac fitness to a group of school-age youngsters. At that time, a song that began with the sound of a heartbeat was popular. The nursing students captured the song on audiotape and used it as their theme. When the youngsters came into the gymnasium, it was dark. All they could see was a heart model, that was lit by an angled flash light and was placed on a black velvet-covered chair. All they could hear was a heartbeat. The children were mesmerized. The heart then "talked" and gave the children some information on how to keep their hearts fit. Later in the lesson, the nursing students turned on the lights and switched on the bouncy song that began with a heartbeat. The nurses then led exercises to this music, and they all had a wonderful time.

When the Client Is an Adolescent

Adolescents are in transition between childhood and adulthood. In our culture it is a prolonged period of time, accompanied by much turmoil for many adolescents and their families. This is particularly evident in the earlier period from ages 11 or 12 to 14, when there is great variation in the biologic and psychologic maturation. Middle adolescence is a period of biologic completion for the earlier developers. Late adolescence, from the age of 19 and older is affected by heredity and by cultural expectations regarding emancipation.

Psychosocial Characteristics

Erikson has identified the adolescent dilemma as one of identity vs. role confusion (1968). The more complicated one's society and options become, the more complex the decisions regarding, "Who am I? Why am I here? Where am I going?" Erikson believes that as childhood ceases and youth begins, young people become primarily concerned with how they appear to others and how they can connect their skills and abilities with career choices as they see them. In Figure 5-6 a teenage boy practices shaving.

Adolescents need to develop new and more mature relationships. They are expected to become emotionally independent from their parents, and they need to learn how to choose associates wisely. Sexual identity becomes solidified during this stage. Some prepare for marriage and family life. Economic and career planning is a necessity for both sexes. Hopefully they develop a workable value system and make tentative decisions about their social responsibilities.

These years are characterized by periods of mood swings and ambivalence in this culture. Adolescents' two main fears are loss of face and loss of control. They go through several periods of personality disorganization, reorganization, and consolidation. Recycling is one way of looking at that process and its purposes (Keepers & Babcock, 1986). From a systems theory point of view, disorder must occur to build a better, more adaptive order.

As adolescents move toward emancipation, the opinions of their parents become less influential. They look for models outside the home. Some of these models may be adults with whom the adoles- cents have formed trusting relationships. Particularly in the earlier phases, they are very vulnerable to the opinions of those whom they view as models, for example, their peers and particularly the leaders within their peer group.

Cognitive Characteristics

From Piaget's theoretic perspective, adolescence is the stage of transition from the concrete operations of later childhood to the application of formal operations in reasoning. Adolescents become able to use logic and abstract reasoning, to grasp the simultaneous influence of several variables, to invent a systematic procedure for keeping track of results of experiments.

They can apply formal principles of logic to situations they have never encountered, and they can argue more than one side of a debate. They can do deductive reasoning—from the general to the specific—as well as inductive reasoning, which was possible much earlier. These capabilities can be taught if they do not spontaneously appear.

Language Characteristics

Adolescent vocabulary is dependent on intellectual capacity, cultural influences (including adolescent

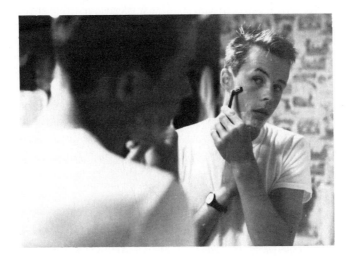

Figure 5-6 Adolescent. *From Whaley, L. and Wong, D. Nursing care of infants and children, ed 4, Mosby-Year Book, 1991.*

and neighborhood subcultures), and the socioeconomic group. Adolescents' vocabulary development is also influenced by their motivation and reading ability. Subgroup slang is one of the characteristics of adolescent development. In general it tends to be quite temporary and changes along with fads in clothing and in hair styles.

Teaching Implications

One of the first challenges to you, the nurse, will be developing a trusting relationship in which mutual respect can evolve. Tact and thoughtfulness on your part can help ease an adolescent's fear of losing face. One way to do this is to provide privacy for personal discussions.

Ask for the meaning of slang words; treat the adolescent as a consultant on what today's adolescent (or teen or young adult) thinks about. This type of indirectness is often a useful way to get at information that the teen is not yet ready to share directly. Many who work well with teenagers have talked about the importance of "reading between the lines," to be on the lookout for a topic that a teen may be trying to bring up.

Although teens are trying to protect themselves psychologically, they do not honor such a need in their caregivers. They expect you to be honest, open, and as straightforward as possible. You need to be prepared for sudden mood shifts, which may or may not be related to anything explainable. There is usually a cause, however, which may be related to a hormone shift, a phone call, or any number of possibilities that the teen may or may not be able or willing to explain. The important thing for you to do is not take it personally.

Peer teaching is very effective. Teens benefit from visiting others who are coping successfully with similar problems. Group instruction/discussion is a very powerful way to help teens belong to a group. Within appropriate groups, teens are more likely to confront their own health challenges and to consider significant behavior changes. Groups can be very effective in helping peers to deal creatively with their health problems in common teen situations (Frey & Denyes, 1989).

Assessment of their knowledge should help you decide where to begin teaching. Relevant lessons on anatomy and physiology may be woven into science reports they could use at school. Teens appreciate being told about upcoming procedures, their effects, and what they can expect in the way of results.

Control is an important issue. All decisions that can be shared with the teen should be. For hospitalized teens, wearing their own clothes and having significant gear from home can help them feel some measure of control. Stevens (1987) identified the feeling of choice to have surgery and adolescents' perceived abilities to handle pain as very significant factors in how well they bounced back from surgery. Youngsters who were confident of their ability to handle pain fared much better postoperatively than those who perceived pain as out of their control. These youngsters might benefit from learning that indeed they have more control than they realize. Step-by-step lessons in guided imagery and other relaxation techniques would be very practical for increasing an adolescent's feeling of control.

Being allowed visits from friends, if medically possible, should be checked out with the teens. This gives adolescents a measure of control and allows them to decide on the balance between the risk of embarrassment and their need for support.

It is very important that you be able to talk freely about sex, alcohol, and other drugs. Bring up sexual issues regularly and informally. Prepare yourself to handle awkward questions with ease and be quite knowledgeable about the prevention and treatment of sexually transmitted diseases. We strongly believe that no teenager should leave the care of a professional nurse today without a thorough assessment of the teen's knowledge about alcohol, other drugs, sexually transmitted disease, pregnancy prevention, and resources for substance abuse and sexual counseling.

Summary

In this chapter we discussed developmental readiness as it affects the client who is a child. We used general systems theory, behavioral, gestalt, and humanistic perspectives as well as the information processing viewpoint to consider how the child's biologic development influences and is influenced by the child's environment, both internal and external. After a brief review of typical characteristics and features at each phase of development, we offered nursing implications, which are summarized in Table 5-1.

TABLE 5-1

Nursing Implications for Various Developmental Stages

Age	Psychosocial (Erikson)	Cognitive (Piaget)	Language	Nursing Implications
Infancy	*Trust vs. mistrust.* 5-6 weeks: responsive smile to families' faces & voices. Emotionally symbiotic with main caretaker. Individual temperament emerges in earliest weeks of life. Needs balance of rest, exercise, nutrition, love, strokes. Cuddliness varies.	Sensorimotor: Basic reflex habits (i.e., sucking nipple within 2 wks). Higher levels later: 2-3 mos. looks for sounds. 8-9 mos. object permanence. Thinks in pictures.	*6-7 weeks* Prelanguage sounds. Inner language: recognizes objects. Audioreceptive: recognizes spoken words.	Teach parents/caregivers. Calibrate for their anxiety when child is very ill. Anticipatory guidance re: growth and development, Safety, and Stimulation (talk & touch).
Early Childhood 2-3 years	*Autonomy vs. shame and doubt.* "No!" Frustrated by personal and external limits. Egocentric. Needs: to explore safely, to succeed.	Sensorimotor: still thinks in pictures. Starts development of object formation, representation, extension.	Single, 3-word sentences; nouns, verbs & adjectives: "ball, carry, soft." Age 3, time: "yesterday."	Needs: Safe play space, love, security. Find out routines, special words. Comfort toy. Give positive simple command. Read or make up relevant picture books with tape. Most teaching through parent.
3-6 years	*Initiative vs. guilt.* Fears: unknown, separation, strangers, disapproval, pain, punishment, own aggression. Roles: male, female.	Sensorimotor, expanding imagination and concepts.	Rapid growth. By 5 years has usual speech patterns.	Encourage play. Use it to diagnose child and to teach. Give simple explanations: "You will smell icky perfume." See . . . hear . . . . feel . . . Make tape & picture books, objects. Use timing: tell child soon enough to allow processing but not to get panicky. Allow only one stall. Positive commands: "You hold Bandaid."
Late Childhood 6-12 years	*Industry vs. inferiority.* Makes things. Peer influence is important.	Concrete operations. Inductive reasoning. Memory.	Good command of language: can use it to tell stories, ask questions, argue, tease.	Assess child's reading ability. Likes mechanical explanations.

—Continued next page

TABLE 5-1

Nursing Implications for Various Developmental Stages—*cont'd*

Age	Psychosocial (Erikson)	Cognitive (Piaget)	Language	Nursing Implications
Continued Late Childhood 6-12 years	Developing parent & ego states.	Considered teachable in many cultures.		Help child gain control by participating in his/her own care & procedures. Can pay attention to teaching. Can do own hygiene, choose good food, recognize signs of illness.
Adolescence	*Identity vs. role confusion.* New & more mature relationships. Sexual identity. Changing body. Becoming emotionally independent from parents. Preparing for adult responsibilities: career, love. Workable value system. Social responsibilities. Mood swings & ambivalence. Fears "loss of face."	Formal operations. "One's thinking takes wings." (Piaget)	Depends on IQ, culture, socioeconomic group. Slang.	Ask for meaning of slang. Use peers to teach & persuade. Protect "face," privacy. Expect mood swings. Be honest & straightforward. Try to read between the lines of what teenager is trying to say or does not say.

ASSESSMENT OF THE CHILD CLIENT

Purposes:

- Practice application of the theory contained in this chapter
- Deepen sensitivity to child clients and their families
- Try out a variety of strategies for teaching children and their families

Directions:

- Divide into study groups and select one or more of the following exercises.
- Rehearse so that you can present it to the rest of your peers.
- Assume the roles of nurses and children as necessary.

1. You are teaching a health education class to a group of preschoolers. Compose a health promotion song with gestures, using the tune of a popular nursery song. For example, "Safety the Snowman" (to the tune of "Frosty the Snowman"). Use any props you find nearby. Teach it to the rest of your peers.

2. Role play a Baby Doll Clinic. Involve a nurse, some children, and their dolls. Have the "mothers" come and see the nurse on "walk-in" or make an appointment over the phone. Voice your concerns for the doll's health, ask what the mother wants, such as a well-doll checkup, or ask about the doll's fever or upcoming surgery. Ask a health or safety question about the doll. Instruct mother to bring in a girlfriend to introduce her to the clinic and nurse. Prompt her on what to ask. Have the nurse find out what the mothers want done for their dolls and give the appropriate examinations, treatments, and advice. If you suspect an underlying problem, make a return appointment. Use the real equipment you can find and pretend equipment from your imagination.

3. Be a group of fifth or sixth graders with a nurse leader discussing a topic of your choice: refusal skills, drugs, sex, and/or any other hot topic. Have the nurse lead the kids in role playing and discussing a difficult situation.

4. Be a group of children who have stress-related diseases. Have the nurse tell the children to lie on the floor in order to teach them how to relax using their imagination (breathing, putting their troubles in floating balloons, floating up in rocket ships, clouds, or rainbows). Have kids travel to and decorate favorite places of their choice in their imagination. Have them discuss when and how they could do this in their families.

5. Be a group of junior high students and play a card game about feelings. Make up the cards and the rules. Have each student write one card asking a question about feelings and collect all the cards. Talk about what might be appropriate things to write on a card, and then give them some ideas about rules: If you don't want to answer, you can pass, or you can trade with someone.

6. Describe a child with a long-term chronic illness. Include information, such as age, developmental needs, amount of regression, and how the illness interferes with normal developmental tasks. Design substitute experiences that would enhance the child's chances for meeting appropriate developmental needs.

References

Anderson, G.C. (1989). Skin to skin: Kangaroo care in western Europe. *American Journal of Nursing,* 89(5), 662-666.

Berne, A.S., Dato, C., Mason, D.J. & Rafferty, M. (1990). A nursing model for addressing the health needs of homeless families. *IMAGE: Journal of Nursing Scholarship,* 22(1), 8-13.

Bingham, R. (Writer, Director). (1987). *The Sexual Brain* [Videorecording]. Princeton NJ: Films for the Humanities & Sciences.

Brophy, C.J. & Mitchell, M.E. (1989). Children with chronic illness: A structured strategic family approach. *Journal of Psychotherapy & the Family,* 6(34), 129.

Cain, E. (1988). *Fulfilled Parents.* Brighton CO: Nanel Unlimited.

Coppens, N. (1990). Parental responses to children in unsafe situations. *Pediatric Nursing,* 16(6), 571-574.

Crowe, C. (1986). Innovations in family and community health. *Family and Community Health,* 9(1), 82-85.

Curran, D. (1985). *Stress and the healthy family.* Minneapolis: Winston.

Donar, M.E. (1988). Community care: Pediatric home mechanical ventilation. *Holistic Nursing Practice,* 2(2), 68-80.

Donnelly, G.F. (1988). Imaginative play and the physically disabled child. *Holistic Nursing Practice,* 2(2), 81-88.

Erikson, E.H. (1963) *Childhood and society* (2nd ed.). New York: W.W. Norton.

Erikson, E.H. (1968). *Identity: Youth and crisis.* New York: W.W. Norton.

Fernald, A. & Kuhl, P. (1987). Acoustic determinants of infant preference for motherese speech. *Infant Behavioral Development,* 10: 279-293.

Fisher, N.L. (1992). Ethnocultural approaches to genetics. *The Pediatric Clinics of North America,* 39(1), 55.

Flavell, J.H. (1985). *Cognitive development* (2nd ed.). Englewood Cliffs NJ: Prentice-Hall.

Flavell, J.H., Green, F.L. & Flavell, E.R. (1986). *Development of knowledge about the appearance-reality distinction.* Chicago: Society for Research in Child Development.

Frey, M.S. & Denyes, M.J. (1989). Health and illness self care in adolescents with IDDM: A test of orem's theory. *Advances in Nursing Science,* 12(1), 67-75.

Fulghum, R. (1988). *All I really need to know I learned in kindergarten.* New York: Ivy Books.

Garcia-Coll, C., Halpern, L.F., Vohr, B.R., Seifer, R., & Oh, W. (1992). Stability and correlates of change of early temperament in preterm and full term infants. *Infant Behavior & Development,* 15(2), 137.

Ginsburg, H. & Oper, S. (1979). *Piaget's theory of intellectual development* (2nd ed.). Englewood Cliffs NJ: Prentice Hall.

Harter, S. & Chao, C. (1992). The role of competence in children's creation of imaginary friends. *Merrill-Palmer Quarterly,* 38(3), 350.

Ingalls, A.J. (1991). *Maternal and child health nursing.* St. Louis: Mosby.

Johnson, J.S. & Newport, E.L. (1989). Critical period effects on second language learning: The influence of maturational state on the acquisition of English as a second language. *Cognitive Psychology,* 21: 60-99.

Kaluger, G. & Kaluger, M.F. (1984). *Human development The span of life* (3rd ed.). St. Louis: Mosby.

Keepers, T. & Babcock, D. (1986). *Raising kids o.k. Human growth and development throughout the life span* (2nd ed.). Menlo Park CA: Menalto Press.

MacGregor, S.N., Keith, L.G., Chasnoff, I.J., Rosner, M.A., Chisum, G.M., Shaw, P. & Minogue, J.P. (1987). Cocaine use during pregnancy: Adverse perinatal outcome. *American Journal of Obstetrics and Gynecology,* 157: 686-690.

Meltzoff, A.N. & Moore, M.K. (1989). Imitation in newborn infants: Exploring the range of gestures imitated and the underlying mechanisms. *Developmental Psychology,* 25(6), 954-962.

National Commission to Prevent Infant Mortality (1988). *Indirect costs of infant mortality and low birth weight.* Washington DC: The Commission.

Pidgeon, V. (1989). Compliance with chronic illness regiments: School aged children and adolescents. *Journal of Pediatric Nursing,* 4(1), 36.

Poulson, C.L., Kymissis, E. & Reeve, K.F. (1991). Generalized vocal imitation in infants. *Journal of Experimental Child Psychology,* 51(2), 267.

Reinisch, J.M., Rosenblum, L.A. & Rubin, D.B. (1991). Sex differences in developmental milestones during the first year of life. *Journal of Psychology & Human Sexuality, 4*(2), 19.

Sachs, J.S. & Johnson, M. (1976). Language development in a child of deaf parents. In *Baby Talk and Infant Speech,* W. von Raffler Ergel & Y. le Brun (Eds.). Amsterdam: Swets and Zeitilinger.

Saudino, K.J. & Eaton, W.O. (1991). Infant temperament and genetics: An objective twin study of motor activity level. *Child Development, 62*(5), 1167.

Schuster, C.S. & Ashburn, S.S. (1986). *The process of human development: A holistic life-span approach* (2nd ed.). Boston: Little, Brown & Company.

Slavin, R.E. (1991). *Educational psychology: Theory into practice.* Englewood Cliffs NJ: Prentice-Hall.

Smith, D.P. & Nix, K.S. (Eds.). (1991). *Comprehensive child and family nursing skills.* St. Louis: Mosby.

Smith, M.J., Goodman, J.A. & Ramsey, N.L. (1987). *Child and family: Concepts of nursing practice* (2nd ed.). New York: McGraw-Hill.

Stein, Z. & Kline, J. (1983). Smoking, alcohol and reproduction. *American Journal of Public Health,* 73: 1154-1156.

Stevens, M.S. (1987). Which adolescents breeze through surgery? *American Journal of Nursing,* 87(12), 1564-1565.

Willitt, J.B. (1988). Sticks and stones may break my bones . . . Reasoning about illness causality and body functioning in children who have a chronic illness. *Pediatrics,* 88(3), 608.

When the Learner Is an Adult

There is gradually emerging,
therefore, a conception of
education as a lifelong process
beginning at birth and ending
only in death, a process related
at all points to the life
experiences of the individual

. . .

Leigh, 1930, p. 123.

6

Objectives

Upon completion of this chapter you will be able to:

- Analyze yourself in terms of the three categories of adult learners.
- Identify the two basic elements that motivate adult learners.
- Analyze selected assumptions of andragogy.
- Apply andragogic theory to teaching adult learners.
- Discuss teaching/learning implications for the adult learner.

Key Words

pedagogy	motivation	goal and learning
andragogy	life transitions	orientations to
assumptions	activity	learning
		lifelong learning

Introduction

In this chapter we review briefly the historic context in which adult learning theories have evolved. Selected research on how and why adults learn is followed by discussion of the difference in assumptions about teaching children (pedagogy) and teaching adults (andragogy). We include recommendations for applying the information in this chapter to clients, and we invite you to apply the theories to yourself.

Historic Context

Interest in the adult learner has increased since the publications of Thorndike's monograph, in which he concluded that adults can learn (1928). Less than 70 years ago, the idea that adults can learn and that they learn differently than children was a new discovery.

Lindeman (1926) laid the foundation for a systematic theory about adult learning, which included the following propositions: adult education should be conducted via the route of situations rather than subjects. Teachers and texts should adjust themselves to the needs of the learners rather than vice versa.

An outgrowth of this thinking was the Journal of Adult Education, which was published between February 1929 and October 1941. Knowles was the founding executive director of the Adult Education Association, which was the association responsible for producing the journal. Eventually, adult education became recognized as a new profession (Brunner, Wilder, Kirchner, & Newberry, 1959).

During the last few decades learning has gradually gained recognition as a lifelong process, and not a preparation for life that is completed at some point with formal schooling. Allport (1955) defined learning and growth as a process of becoming. Humanists in general agree with that notion; namely, that the process is more important to the individual than the product (Rogers, 1951, 1961).

Maslow and Rogers had much to say about the learning processes of adults. Maslow claimed that growth is attractive and intrinsically more satisfying than staying with the gratifications with which we have become familiar (Slavin, 1991). Rogers (1951) believed that therapy was mainly a learning process. The following is a list of Rogers' hypotheses about student-centered learning.

1. We cannot teach another person directly; we can only facilitate the individual's learning.
2. A person learns significantly only those things that are perceived as being involved in the maintenance of or enhancement of the structure of self.
3. Perceptions that would lead to a reorganization of self tend to be resisted by denial or distortion. Personal change is easier in a climate of trust and relaxation and is more difficult in a climate of threat.
4. The educational situation that most effectively promotes significant learning is one in which threat to self is reduced while the noting of differences in other people and their ideas is facilitated.

Houle (1961, 1980) at the University of Chicago began a course of investigation that was extended by Tough at the Ontario Institute for Studies in Education. Through in-depth interviews, researchers at the university surveyed a group of 22 people who were identified as adult learners. These researchers studied why adults engage in continuing education. A fortuitous by-product was that researchers also learned something about how adults learn. Houle found that adults continue their education for a variety of reasons. He also conceived three categories that described adults' general orientation to learning.

Orientation to Learning

Goal-Oriented Learners

Goal-oriented learners used their educational endeavors to accomplish fairly clear and identifiable objectives. They did not make any real start on their continuing education until their middle 20s and sometimes much later. Their continuing education activities tended to occur in episodes. Each series began with the realization of a need or the identification of an interest that expands their skills and knowledge. Houle found that there was no even flow to their learning although it was a recurring pattern in their lives. These learners' studies were not restricted to academic settings nor to any one institution or topic. Goal-oriented learners sought courses of instruction or other forms of learning when they became aware of a need. Many people who attend night courses fit this category. When you take workshops that add to your professional expertise, particularly when those courses are taken at your own expense, you fit this category.

Activity-Oriented Learners

Activity-oriented learners selected activities that were likely to meet their need for human contact. Those who fit in this category were "course takers" and "group joiners." The content of the courses or purpose of the organization was secondary to their social needs. These learners began their educational activities when their need to reach out to others became pressing. Divorce adjustment groups attract people attempting to fill specific needs, as do widows who reach out to other widows. A young mother joined a La Leche group to fulfill her need for socialization as well as for support and information to breast-feed successfully, and she took a class in astronomy to "talk to other people about something other than diapers." When you set up health education programs for older learners, assessing their interests via a survey is helpful. Although many may indicate specific interests, a substantial number may just want something to do and may be attending primarily for social reasons.

You should know how to find such groups, and consider this category of learning activities whenever you diagnose social isolation and loneliness as one of your clients' problems. Newspapers periodically carry lists of self-help and special interest groups. You should include such lists in your resource files. We urge you to note when such lists are published and bring them to the attention of your peers.

Learning-Oriented Learners

Learning-oriented individuals seek knowledge for its own sake. They report being engrossed in learning all of their lives and being avid readers since childhood. These learners see themselves as students of life, and they investigate everything that is of interest. In addition, they tend to join groups, classes, and organizations that they anticipate will be educational. For example, such a learner might join a Greater Books discussion group at the library.

Learning-oriented people select media that they believe will be most likely to be educational: the *Christian Science Monitor*, Public Broadcasting Television stations, and radio programs on specific subjects.

When these people travel, they prepare for their trips by engaging in activities that will make the trips more informative. For example, they will read about their destination in books or periodicals, such as the *National Geographic* magazine, or they might take a language course. These people report choosing occupations and making other life decisions in terms of their potential for growth. Figure 6-1 summarizes the three orientations to learning that Houle identified. Most people find that they fit into each of the categories but at different times in their lives. Some people find that they do emphasize one category more often.

Houle concluded that most adults engage in continuing education every year, and that these activities are planned by the learners themselves. He also made the point that people do not have to fit into one category only. His generalizations were meant to clarify motivations rather than to pigeonhole people.

Tough also used a small sample of people to investigate in depth what motivated those people to start a learning project (1979). Below are listed some short-term benefits of learning that the people cited and an example of each benefit. One person was satisfying a curiosity: "What's all the commotion about a paradigm shift?" Enjoying the content itself

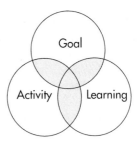

Figure 6-1   Individuals learn for different reasons; three primary orientations to learning are goal, activity, and learning.

was another, "I've always wanted to paint, but I was too busy working for a living." Many find pleasure in the process of learning itself. Some skills, such as wind surfing, are fun even during the learning, "My mouth started hurting, and then I realized I had been smiling the whole way across the lake!"

Teachers and would-be teachers often engage in a learning project so that they will be able to teach it to others. Others take courses so that they will be prepared for some possible situation in the future. For example, some women who took passive roles in their marriages are beginning to notice that they need to participate in important activities such as estate planning and bill paying. Certainly hopes of job promotion, increased salary, and other kinds of status symbols are strong motivators for adults. Tough (1979) summarized all of the benefits he identified into the two basic motivators: pleasure and self-esteem.

There are times when you are convinced that learning something is important to the client's well-being, optimum rehabilitation, or even survival. Not all clients are willing to make the effort or endure the pain of that task. It is hoped that the above information will be useful for you as you search for possible motivators. The information is also useful to anyone who wishes to market a service to adults. The box in the next column summarizes a number of observations about adults that are worth noting and discussing.

Andragogy

Knowles (1990) calls his theory of adult learning *andragogy*. He found the word being used in Europe before he brought it to the United States. *Andragogy* means the art and science of helping adults learn. He noted that the forces that impinge on young children in many schools and other child-oriented groups have more to do with achieving than with learning. He cited passing tests, scoring high on the Scholastic Aptitude Tests (SAT), and getting into college or graduate school as the goals of too much formal education. He also noted that many of the assumptions that underlie the

---

Observations about Adult Learners*

Adults Are People Who Have:

1. A good deal of first-hand experience.
2. Relatively large bodies, subject to gravity.
3. Set habits and strong tastes.
4. A past.
5. Some amount of pride.
6. Very tangible things to lose.
7. A reflex toward authority.
8. A great many preoccupations.
9. A bewildered reaction to options.
10. Preset reactions in groups.
11. Established values and attitudes.
12. Selective stimuli filters.
13. Strong feelings about learning situations.
14. Ideas to contribute.
15. Experience with life crises.
16. An allergy to too many basics.
17. A strong attraction for utility—now.
18. Secret fears about falling behind and being replaced.
19. Need for a vacation.
20. The ability to change.

*Modified from Davis, L.N. (1974). *Planning, conducting and evaluating workshops*, Austin, Tx.: Learning Concepts.

---

teaching methods used on adults were derived from pedagogy—the teaching of children. Knowles popularized a different set of hypotheses. The assumptions that form the foundation of Knowles' theory are presented in the following section with pertinent examples.

Need to Know

Adults in general need to understand why they should learn something before they are willing to learn it. Adults who initiate new learning projects on their own spend considerable time and effort weighing the cost/benefit ratio before they expend large amounts of energy on their projects.

Your opening remarks in any teaching/learning encounter will include making a case for the benefits of the learning that you will market to your clients. Another approach will be to set up a situation in which clients will discover for themselves the likely benefits of their efforts. An equally important endeavor will be to find out what motivates the individuals in your target group. You can do that by asking the following questions.

Example: "Why bother?"
"What do you hope to get from this lesson?"
"What is the best outcome you hope for?"
"What would be the worst possible outcome that might come of our time together?"
"Why have you bothered to come out on this beautiful/awful day?"

Self-Concept

People's need and capacity for self-direction increases steadily through childhood and rapidly during adolescence. Parents and caretakers of adolescents would probably agree easily on the increased need for self-direction. Whether or not the adolescent has the capacity to do so is sometimes an area of conflict between parents and their children. Adults in mainstream United States culture eventually arrive at the self-concept whereby they see themselves as responsible for their own decisions. They have a deep psychologic need to be seen and treated by others as if they are capable of self-direction (Beden & Carrea, 1988).

This need for self-direction often presents a problem for both your client and you because encounters frequently necessitate dependency. In the hospital you will know much more about the acutely ill client's physiologic status than the client and family and will often be in a better position to decide what information would be helpful for them to know. During certain stages of illness the client needs to relinquish control and have faith in your expert caregiving.

The client who values independence and is conscious enough to understand that he or she is dependent may respond with fear, bitterness, and sarcasm. For example, an older gentleman who was used to being the boss, was very nasty to the nurses who cared for him while he was suffering from incontinence. Although one nurse was matter-of-fact and unperturbed while changing the man's soiled bed, he was anything but. He asked her in a sarcastic and angry tone of voice if she had brought a diaper.

Health and illness problems may evoke mixed feelings about earlier unmet dependency needs and patterns in the client, and complementary issues in you, such as the need to control. The following comments by a client in counseling exemplify these mixed feelings.

Example: "I've come to you because I trust you and know that you're a fine professional with a good reputation. I have been to all sorts of therapists and self-help groups since my husband left. I am filled with rage and guilt. In retrospect I have been angry and felt guilty most of my life. I've been trying to find out what to do, but none of them (therapists, therapeutic groups) have been helpful. They don't tell me anything I can use; most of them don't know what they're doing or they don't care. I've received poor quality care. I know more about what's wrong with me and what I should do than they do, and they're the so-called experts! You tell me what I should do."

On the one hand this woman was asking for advice, yet previously she had expressed dissatisfaction with people who gave her advice.

A medical/surgical nurse experienced the dependency problem when dealing with burn clients. "If only they'd do what I say they'd find out that they'd feel and look better in the long run. They don't know what not moving will do to the final results of their burn healing. I know it's easier not to move now, but they won't know the consequences of immobility until it's too late! They better listen to me or they'll be sorry!" This nurse wanted the client to trust her advice and depend on her. In addition, the nurse was adamant about her role and the role she expected of the client.

Role of Learners' Experiences

For children, experience is something that happens to them, but for adults, experience is what defines them. A way to check out this assumption is to ask people of various ages, "Tell me about yourself." You will hear differences in the way children and adults answer.

As people mature they accumulate an expanding reservoir of human experience. These experiences are likely to serve them with useful generalizations in any new learning situation. They are also likely to have a wider base of associations to which they can attach new learning. If adults' experiences are ignored or devalued, they experience rejection that goes beyond their knowledge. They perceive it as rejection of their personhood. We believe this phenomenon is behind the deep resentment adults express when they return to school after years of earning a living and hear or feel treated like they are not professionals.

In general, adults learn better in a workshop environment. We recommend that you function as a facilitator. Speak with clients about their previous experiences and currently perceived learning needs. Present your own perceptions of the possible benefits of the workshop and negotiate with the learners about objectives on which you and they can agree. An important component of the workshop is the co-teacher and co-learner roles that you will adopt along with all members present. Adult clients will learn more easily in two-way communication patterns, ones in which they speak while you listen and vice versa (Brundage, 1980). Another important component is immediate implementation of theories and principles so that clients can discuss how useful the learning is likely to be in their unique situations. As co-consultants they frequently are able to give each other ideas for practical applications of the theories that you will present.

Adult clients will learn better, therefore, when you employ strategies that respect this broader base of knowledge and experience and make use of it in the learning environment. Other strategies, such as discussion, laboratory, simulation, field experience, team projects, and other action-learning techniques, are more conducive to the way adults learn and have strong experiential and integrating components.

On an individual basis you can assume that your client has experience that will affect his or her learning positively or negatively. Assessment of your client's beliefs, assumptions, and related experiences may be crucial to successful learning. Adults' previous experiences can have a negative effect on their gaining the outcomes you hoped they would gain. For example, a nurse felt quite positive about the type of surgery that her client was waiting to have. The nurse knew that the surgical procedure for relieving an enlarged thyroid gland is commonplace and usually produces a very positive result. The man, who had lost several friends or relatives after throat surgery (malignancies perhaps), did not act reassured by the nurse. The nurse needed to back up and address the client's perceptions before deciding on what learning objectives were appropriate.

Readiness to Learn

It is assumed that children are ready to learn according to their developmental (biologic) and academic progress. Developmental readiness is also necessary for adults' learning. Needs of adults, however, are related less to their biologic maturation and more to the developing roles in life that they are choosing or have had thrust upon them. A nurse's first pregnancy is one example. "I had been a good student, and done well in many OB/GYN experiences and state board examinations. Some years later, when I was pregnant and went to child birth education classes, I was amazed at all I did not know. I listened with keener attention, and made many associations, which had not occurred to me when I was learning how to attend the labor and delivery of other women. My increased interest was due to a change in role. It was now I who was entering the role of pregnant woman and expectant parent."

Adults want to learn whatever will help them cope with their present circumstances and evolving social roles. Their developmental tasks are related to their role changes and life's exigencies. Recently, a class entitled "How to Remember" was offered in a setting that attracts retired citizens who have the time, energy, and resources to attend such activities. The enrollment was three times higher than any other class that had been offered by the sponsoring organization. The main reason for such high numbers was the topic—memory. Older people experience difficulty in remembering, and it is a blow to their self-concept. This workshop offered attendees an opportunity to address an important need.

Knowles makes the point that it is not always necessary to wait for readiness to develop. You will foster it through experiences that you will create. You will do this when you expose clients to successful role models. An example is Reach to Recovery, a program for cancer patients and cancer survivors. Having clients role-play might evoke emotional and intellectual anticipation of the problems to come.

Orientation to Learning

Those who teach children usually present subjects in a logical and systematic manner. One of the assumptions behind this technique is that children need to learn how to organize their thoughts and to study using a systematic method. Another assumption is that the teachers know what is best for the children to learn. As they go through school, young people become accustomed to this type of educational pattern and the postponed application this pattern entails. Children hear that they will need the information when they get out in the working world, and adolescents hear that they will need good grades to qualify for certain colleges. Those who are unwilling to take their teachers' and parents' admonitions seriously, find out that certain doors may indeed be closed to them.

Andragogy assumes that adults learn better when life-centered or task-centered problems are the organizing factor. Adults are reluctant to expend their resources (time, money, and energy) to learn attitudes, skills, and information that they do not see as directly relevant to their current lives or problems they anticipate having. When you take a continuing education program and enroll in degree-advancing programs you will want to know, "How can I use this when I go to work tomorrow?" Adult clients will expect you to be knowledgeable and experientially familiar with your topic. People in the working world become impatient with self-styled experts who are no longer in touch with the real challenges of today. Clients quickly separate health educators who really know what they are talking about from those who do not. Adults find lessons easier to grasp when they are presented in a practical life context. When clients say, "Give us an example," they want you to present a real-life example to which they can relate. Another equally valuable approach would be to set up a simulation and have the clients apply the lesson to the situation before them.

Organization is important to learning and to good teaching. There are, however, great differences in which organizational principle is most effective. A good axiom is to teach from the simple to the complex. Clients will appreciate material that is presented from simple to complex and within contexts to which they can relate. Other axioms are to use a logical train of thought and to promote association. There are times when presenting the concept and then following it with more specific applications is the most effective way of teaching. There are other times when experiencing a number of events and then looking for their relationship to one another is more meaningful. The point is worth repeating. Organization is important; the most effective type of organization will vary with the goal, the client, you, and the situation.

Motivation

Adults are more responsive to internal drives to learn—such as self-esteem, quality of life, and job satisfaction—than they are to external motivators—such as better jobs, more money, and promotions—although these have some value. Brundage (1980) also observed that adults seldom need further stimulation in the form of increased pressure or demands from the instructor; rather they need support in the motives they bring with them that have channeled them into the learning situation. Another factor that influences an adult's motivation is the attitude he or she has toward change. Generally, adults have more, stronger, and longer emotional responses to change than do children. Because Knowles' hypotheses have become more widely known and used, he reports that teachers tell him many of his assumptions can be used with younger learners, too. Table 6-1 summarizes the comparison between pedagogy and andragogy.

Tough's research (1982) validated the claims of the humanists in general and Maslow in particular: Adults are motivated to keep growing and developing. Tough (1982) also concluded that barriers, such as negative self-concept, inaccessibility of opportunities or resources, time constraints and programs that violate adult learning principles, all interfere with the growing process. Our own experiences as clinicians working with high- and low-risk populations, as teachers working with people of all ages, and as adults leads us to believe that these principles have very broad application.

Quite frequently when you encounter clients, they are going through transitions: from child at home to school child, from single person to married person, from a childless couple to parents, from independent to dependent (temporarily or permanently), from healthy to sick and/or handicapped, and from married to single. A life transition may force them to make a paradigm shift and endure the process of accommodation described earlier in Chapter 3. A life transition is the process that individuals undergo when their roles change drastically as in death of a significant other, birth, marriage, divorce, moving from a stable environment, and making a radical work change. The individual adapts by relinquishing a reality that no longer fits and by developing a new reality that will allow the individual to function with integrity and with an intact sense of self. During this process the individual often feels discombobulated and confused, in an alien environment, and out of sync. Answers to questions, such as "Who am I?" and "How does this world work?" may no longer be taken for granted. Although counseling is a vital aspect of crisis intervention, teaching is an equally valuable skill that you can offer to clients as they struggle to resolve the uncertainty of their changing lives (Selder, 1989).

In the first part of this book, your enthusiasm was identified as an important variable that facilitates learning. It is just as true in a discussion of motivation and adults. When you act enthusiastic and convinced that the topic under discussion is

TABLE 6-1

A Comparison of Assumptions of Pedagogic and Andragogic Approaches to Learning

Assumptions about Learning	Pedagogy	Andragogy
Need to know	Established by the teacher; accepted by the learner	Must relate to the learners' need to know
Self-Concept	Accepts direction from the teacher	Increasing need for self-direction
Role of experience	Happens to the learner	Integrally involved with self-concept; must be acknowledged
Readiness to learn	Biologic and academic development	Evolving social and life roles
Orientation to learning	Logic and system selected by the teacher	Life-centered and/or task and problem centered
Motivation	External; approval of the teacher	Internal drives and life goals

Modified from Knowles, M. (1990). *The adult learner: A neglected species* (4th ed.). Houston: Gulf.

vital, that attitude has a positive effect on your clients' ability to motivate themselves.

Summary

As we deal with change in our business, personal, and professional lives, we realize with dawning chagrin and/or excitement that learning is a lifelong process. We may learn by ourselves, by observing role models, by reading, by informal teaching, or by formal instruction. Adults' approaches to learning vary. Some like it on general principles, others learn when they feel the need for specific skills or knowledge. Still others engage in learning activities mainly for the social benefits. In any event, adults engage in learning efforts for increased pleasure and/or self-esteem. Several assumptions were offered that increase the likelihood that teacher/learner interactions will be more mutually satisfying. These assumptions include understanding the purpose or value of the learning, treating people as self-directed individuals, respecting client's previous experiences, and tying the learning into role changes and life-centered or task-centered problems.

THE ADULT LEARNER

Purposes:

- Test some of the theoretic notions advanced by noted authors
- Use available theories when communicating with potential clients of different ages

Directions:

1. Identify a child to work with. Determine that child's age.
2. Ask that child the question: "Tell me about yourself."
3. Note the answer. If the child asks you, "What do you mean?" then answer, "Oh, anything you want to tell me."
4. Repeat the above assignment with an adult. If you pick up sensitivity about age, you can ask, "Do you consider yourself a young adult or a mature adult?" If you think that the age question would distract from the spontaneity of your answer, skip the question, and just move onto, "Tell me about yourself."
5. Note differences and similarities between the child's response and the adult's response with regard to Knowles' hypothesis that experience has different meaning for adults than children.
6. Discuss your findings with peers.

ORIENTATION TO LEARNING

Purposes:

- Become more aware of your own orientation to learning according to Houle
- Become more aware of how your orientation to learning affects your motivation, learning strategies, and topics of interest
- Use your own insights as a base from which to assess other learners

Directions:

1. Categorize yourself using Houle's hypothesis.
2. Discuss the implications this has on you as a learner.
3. Describe how this information might be useful with clients.
4. Differentiate between andragogy and pedagogy.
5. Discuss your reflections with your peers.

References

Allport, G. (1955). *Becoming a person.* New Haven: Yale University Press.

Beden, H. & Carrea, N. (Winter, 1988). The effects of andragogical teacher training on adult student attendance and evaluation of their teachers. *Adult Education Quarterly*, 38(2), 75-87.

Brundage, D.H. (1980). *Adult learning principles and their application to program planning.* Ontario: The Ministry of Education.

Brunner, E., Wilder, D.K., Kirchner, D. & Newberry, Jr. J. (1959). *Adult Education*, Chicago IL: Adult Education Association.

Davis, L.N. (1974). *Planning, conducting and evaluating workshops.* Austin TX: Learning Concepts.

Houle, C.O. (1961). *The inquiring mind.* Madison: University of Wisconsin Press.

Houle, C.O. (1980). *Continuing learning in the professions.* San Francisco: Jossey-Bass.

Knowles, M. (1990). *The adult learner: A neglected species.* (4th ed.). Houston: Gulf.

Leigh, R.D. (1930). Comments on education as a lifelong process. *Journal of Adult Education, 2*(2), 123.

Levine, S.L. (1989). *Promoting adult growth in schools: The promise of professional development.* Boston: Allyn and Bacon.

Lindeman, E.C. (1926). *The meaning of adult education.* New York: New Republic.

Rogers, C.R. (1951). *Client-centered therapy.* Boston: Houghton-Mifflin.

Rogers, C.R. (1961). *On becoming a person.* Boston: Houghton-Mifflin.

Selder, F. (1989). Life transition theory: The resolution of uncertainty. *Nursing & Health Care*, 10(8), 437-451.

Slavin, R.E. (1991). Educational psychology: Theory into practice. Englewood Cliffs, NJ: Prentice Hall.

Thorndike, E.L. (1928). *Adult learning.* New York: Macmillan.

Tough, A. (1979). *The adult's learning projects.* Ontario: Institute for Studies in Education.

Tough, A. (1982). *Intentional changes: A fresh approach to helping people change.* Chicago, IL: Follett Publishing.

When the Client Is Older

The setting sun is as beautiful as
the rising sun.

Japanese proverb

Objectives

Upon the completion of this chapter you will be able to:

- Discuss ageism and the subjective experience of the older client
- Describe the psychosocial and physiologic changes that affect learning in the older adult
- Identify common chronic diseases in older clients and the implications these have for teaching
- Analyze the changes in cognitive functioning that are associated with aging
- Describe how you might alter your teaching plans with ethnically diverse older clients
- Discuss teaching/learning implications for the older adult

Key Words

ageism	visual acuity	auditory acuity
developmental tasks	presbyopia	presbycusis
physiologic changes	peripheral vision	cognitive functioning

Introduction

Statistics verify the observation that Americans are living longer. In 1900 the average life expectancy was 47 years. In the past 8 decades it has increased by almost 30 years. It is projected that life expectancy for women will increase from 78.5 years in 1989 to 81.0 years in 2005. Life expectancy for men during this same time span will increase from 71.8 to 74.2 years (U.S. Bureau of the Census, 1991).

You will encounter more older clients because the number of people older than 65 is increasing much faster than the rest of the population. In the past 2 decades, the 65-and-older population grew twice as fast as the rest of the nation. In 1900, 4% of the population was age 65 and older. By 1980 this number had increased to 11.3%. By 2050 the number of people older than 65 is expected to reach 21.7% (U.S. Senate Special Committee, 1989).

This chapter will focus on providing health education to older clients. We will do this by first looking at the concept of ageism. We will also address psychosocial changes, physiologic

—Continued next page

changes, visual and auditory changes, chronic disease, cognitive functioning, the ethnic elderly, and communication with older clients. Our concern is the implications of these factors on health education.

Ageism

Ageism is a term used to denote discrimination against the elderly. Although fascination with youth in the United States has waned, this country still does not have a culture that values everyone regardless of age or ethnic background. It is important that you examine your attitude about aging. How you see older clients wittingly or unwittingly influences how you react and treat them. Personal independence is highly valued in this country. When people can no longer live independently and require some assistance, they are viewed as inferior in some way (Matteson & McConnell, 1988). The elderly remind us of our own mortality. Ebersole and Hess (1990) noted that dying is the "most culturally obscene subject" (p. 11) in the United States. Interestingly, it is the younger, better-educated person who has contact with the well elderly and who has the most positive regard for them.

Psychosocial Development

Maslow's pyramid, discussed in Chapter 3, provides a framework for viewing the importance of individual needs based on a hierarchy. It is a theory of motivation that applies to the elderly. At certain times in the older person's life, basic needs, such as nutrition, may be most important, whereas at another time the same individual may be engaged in self-actualization. Erikson (1963) proposed a theory of personal and social development. He identified eight psychosocial stages through which people move during the life cycle. Critical issues must be resolved in each stage before moving on to the next. Each stage deals with a particular aspect of personality and involves relationships with other people. The developmental task of late adulthood is that of maintaining integrity versus despair, to be through having been and to face not being. During this time,

older people with good self-esteem look back over their lives and find integrity in the accomplishments and failures therein. They realize that their lives have been their own responsibility (Erikson, 1963). Illness may precipitate the need to do a life review. Your part in such a task is to listen and to ask interested questions. Do not worry about historical accuracy; the purpose is to create a meaningful myth and maintain or promote self-esteem. Asking the family to bring in an old photo album may facilitate that process. Newbern (1992) found reminiscence to be a valuable research tool as well as a therapeutic one for the older client. Conducting a life review may help alleviate depression and hopelessness, and promote a person's ability to cope.

Older clients reach the point when they weigh the cost and benefits of medical and/or surgical intervention in terms of energy and effort as well as money. "Will it improve my life? Comfort? Mobility?" The older client may need you as his or her advocate if the family urges the client to submit to "doing everything possible" to prevent death. In other words, the client may be more ready to face death than the family or the medical system. The client may need your advocacy to control his or her last phase of life. This may take the form of overt rehearsal, offering to be there during a meeting with others, asking the right questions, and confronting others on hearing the client. Unless you tell them, the clients may not realize that they have the right to make their wishes known and that they have professionals nearby who will support their choices.

As with clients of all ages, encourage the elderly to participate in the teaching/learning process. They should help you identify what they need to learn and how they can best learn it. When identifying learning goals, select ones that are within reach of each particular client (Weinrich, Boyd, & Nussbaum, 1989).

Physiologic Changes of Aging That Affect Teaching/Learning

The health of the older learner is dependent in part on genetics—that is, what was inherited from the person's parents. Life-style patterns are also important. Attitude, the presence of meaningful relationships, and life's accumulation of happy and unhappy events all affect the older learner physically as well as psychologically. Life-style patterns, such as rest, exercise, nutrition, and non-nutrient substance ingestion, greatly affect the health of every individual. In the older person, the long-term, accumulated effects of these patterns become more obvious. Here we will highlight some physiologic changes and pathophysiologic problems that occur with aging and affect the teaching/learning process.

Atrophy and involution characterize the many changes that occur with aging as all body organs decline in function. These changes occur at different rates in different people. In general, the older person is no longer able to adapt physiologically as she or he did when younger. Gawlinski and Jensen (1991) noted that most organs age according to the 1% rule, which says that body systems deteriorate at the rate of 1% of function per year beginning about age 30. The functional implication of this is that organ performance is unaffected at rest but deficient in the presence of stress. Common stressors are drugs, disease, massive life change, and increased physical demand (Matteson & McConnell, 1988).

The most obvious signs of aging are wrinkling, sagging skin, and thinning, graying hair. Many skin changes are due to exposure to sunlight, an etiology on which much health education is focused today. In the musculoskeletal system there is a progressive loss of height, especially among women. This is attributed to progressive narrowing of the intervertebral discs and loss of height of individual vertebrae, which eventually result in compression of the spinal column (Matteson & McConnell, 1988). The appearance of the body changes as fat and lean body mass alters the contours of earlier years. The amount of lean body mass decreases while the amount of subcutaneous fat increases. The latter becomes redistributed with the fat diminishing from the face and extremities and increasing in the abdomen and hips. The bones become demineralized, or less dense, beginning about age 30, as bone absorption begins to exceed bone formation. By age 70, women have lost about 50% of their skeletal mass to osteoporosis, whereas men 70 to 80 years old have just begun to show evidence of the disease (Matteson & McConnell, 1988; Groer & Shekleton, 1989). Expect your older clients to fatigue more easily than younger ones. Taking more frequent breaks will help compensate for this. Your older clients will also be more comfortable sitting in padded chairs with arms (Weinrich, Boyd, & Nussbaum, 1989).

Cardiovascular changes occur with aging as evidenced by a slowing heart rate, decreased stroke volume, and a decline in cardiac output of 30% to 40% (Seidel & others, 1991). The heart undergoes diffuse thickening of the left atrium endocardium, causing left atrial hypertrophy. Some degree of hypertrophy also occurs within the other chambers of the heart. Collagen in the heart muscle becomes denser and sclerosed, with fine foci of calcification. The valves become thickened and fibrotic, with the mitral valve being most commonly affected by some degree of calcification. Coronary blood flow is decreased significantly as is the number of pacemaker cells and fibers in the bundle of His. The latter results in conduction problems. Calcification is present in the arteries, and arterial wall elasticity and vasomotor tone is diminished. Total peripheral resistance is increased, which results in an increase in blood pressure. Atherosclerosis and arteriosclerosis are common. Factors such as obesity, diet, activity, and habits have been implicated as etiologic factors, all of which have implications for you as a health educator, particularly among younger clients (Groer & Shekleton, 1989; Gawlinski & Jensen, 1991; Seidel and others, 1991). Matteson & McConnell (1988) noted that some of these changes may be more related to a lack of conditioning rather than aging per se. Pascucci (1992) reported that older people are more interested in taking care of their health than younger people and that they report undertaking specific activities for maintaining their health, such as regular medical checkups, reduced salt consumption, and good nutrition. A feeling of well-being was one of the strongest incentives for such activities among the population she studied (Pascucci, 1992).

Decreased function also occurs in the respiratory system. Vital capacity is lost as lung tissues lose elasticity. The number of functional alveoli decrease, resulting in an increase in residual volume (the amount of air remaining after maximum expiration). Muscle strength in the thorax and diaphragm is lost, resulting in a barrel-shaped chest. You detect this by noting the anteroposterior diameter compared with the lateral diameter. The alveoli are less elastic and relatively more fibrous, which decreases the older person's ability to engage in physically taxing activities. Dyspnea may be evident upon little exertion or stress (Seidel & others, 1991; Groer & Shekleton, 1989; Bates, 1991; Andresen, 1989).

The above changes affect the older client's energy level, strength, and speed. Endurance certainly may be affected, but another influential variable is the person's usual activity level. Older people who lead very active lives tend to have remarkable endurance. An older person may be able to do a sustained activity that is familiar to him or her better than a younger individual who has had less practice. Schuster and Ashburn (1986) noted that graduated exercises can improve the strength and endurance of people at all ages, including those who reside in nursing homes. You should take into account the client's current rest and exercise balance when deciding on the best time to initiate teaching. The client will learn better when well oxygenated by an invigorated circulatory system and when rested enough to have the extra energy needed to focus on learning. For the elderly, Weinrich, Boyd, and Nussbaum (1989) recommend low-impact exercises during which their feet do not leave the floor. They also recommend slowing the speed of exercise and increasing the warm-up and cool-down time.

Functional changes in the neurologic system occur with aging. The older person's ability to react quickly to stimuli is slowed. (Matteson & McConnell, 1988). Neuron loss occurs, beginning in the middle 20s. This neuron loss has been suggested as one explanation for the "forgetfulness and the more circumscribed outlook that the aged develop over time" (Ebersole & Hess, 1990, p. 71). Neurotransmitters, which have associative and integrative functions in the nervous system, decrease

with age. The decline in epinephrine and acetylcholine may result in changes in memory storage (Ebersole & Hess, 1990).

Sensory changes may have a great effect on the life-style of older clients. The most important sensory changes are vision and hearing impairments. Diminished functional ability in either or both interferes with the older client's ability to communicate orally or in writing with others. This may lead to social isolation as the client avoids the strain of hearing a muted or indistinguishable conversation, personal embarrassment associated with responding inappropriately to the comments of another, or diminished mobility associated with a loss of vision. All senses may be affected by aging, but vision and hearing are the most important for you to consider as you plan health education (Matteson & McConnell, 1988). Because of this, we will address the functional declines in vision and hearing and how you can use this information to adapt your health education to the abilities of your older clients.

Sensory Changes: Vision

The lens loses its ability to accommodate as it becomes less elastic, larger, and more dense. The increased density plus the accumulation of loosened, degenerated cells on the iris, cornea, and lens capsule result in increased scattering of light and sensitivity to glare. The lens becomes progressively yellowed and opaque, resulting not only in visual acuity difficulties but also in the inability to discriminate blues and greens. This is attributed to the decreased ability of the aging, yellowed lens to filter the short wavelengths of light (violet, blue, green). It is much easier to the older client to distinguish among the warm colors such as yellow, orange, and red (Matteson & McConnell, 1988). Use of these colors in your teaching materials will make it much easier for the older client to distinguish. Color clarity has diminished by 25% in the sixth decade and 50% by the eighth decade (Ebersole & Hess, 1990).

This information needs to be used in conjunction with knowledge about visual discrimination. For example, a color with a longer wavelength, such as yellow printed on a white background, would not be easy for the older eye to see because there is insufficient contrast between the two. A thick black outline surrounding the yellow material would greatly improve readability. Even better, a color that contrasts better as background, such as a light blue, would make deep yellow that is outlined in black stand out.

Other visual difficulties include decreased visual acuity, decreased tolerance of glare, decreased ability to adapt to dark and light, and decreased peripheral vision. These changes are attributed to eye structure changes that affect the quality and intensity of light reaching the retina (Matteson & McConnell, 1988).

Visual Acuity

Virtually everyone will have visual difficulties related to the aging process regardless of sex, race, ethnicity, or socioeconomic status. Watch your older clients for signs of difficulty. Note how your clients read. How close must they hold a book to see? How much reading do they do? Your older clients with presbyopia will hold their reading materials at arm's length in order to focus clearly on the print. Symbols, letters, and objects that are small are more difficult to distinguish from one another. Diminishing ability to discriminate between stimuli is evident to the older person in terms of the size of words and pictures as well as their intensity and their color. Small images, which project shorter light waves into the eye, are harder to distinguish, as are crowded or softly colored images. Larger and more intensely colored print is easier to comprehend. There is enough of the image "getting through" the nerve pathways for the individual to "fill in" the missing parts. Allowing space between each of the letters would also make them easier to distinguish.

This would be harder to read for a person with aged eyes because the print is fine and there is a lot of it.

This print is easier to read.

Glare

Glare is a serious problem for your older clients and may affect their ability to drive at night by leaving them virtually blind in its presence. Glare may come from a variety of sources, such as reflections off of windows and shiny floors. Matteson and McConnell (1988) recommend soft, incandescent lighting rather than fluorescent lighting to minimize glare. A sheer curtain or rugs can also help reduce glare. If you become involved with the production of educational materials, avoid using slick, shiny, white paper, which is more likely to produce glare. If you are arranging lighting for an elderly person, make the light brighter but not glaring.

Environmental lighting during a transaction is one factor that is easily overlooked by caregivers. Conscientious caregivers instinctively know how important it is to watch the client's facial expressions, to "read" the client's condition and comprehension. To do this they may arrange their bodies so that the client's face is well lit.

Watching the client's face is indeed an important feedback technique. However, it is important that you do *not* put your own face in shadow during such maneuvers. Your face must also be well lit so that the client can add all available visual and facial clues to your voice tones.

Dark and Light Adaptation

It takes longer for the eyes of your older clients to adapt to dark and light. It will take more time for their eyes to adjust if you darken the room for a video recording, motion picture, or slide showing. Plan for this extra time as you prepare your teaching module. When you turn the lights back on, you may find that extra lighting is required for some clients. Because pupils become smaller when the lights are turned on, less light is reaching the retina; thus extra lighting is required (Andresen, 1989). Ebersole and Hess (1990) estimated that older clients need three times the amount of light as they did in their second decade. This high-intensity lighting is best placed directly on the teaching object or surface rather than increasing the light in the entire room. Level of intensity, however, needs to be balanced against the avoidance of glare to which older eyes are more sensitive.

Loss of Peripheral Vision

With the loss of peripheral vision, your older client is unaware of people or activities outside of her or his line of central vision. This may interfere with how your clients relate to others in a group setting. They may not be aware of others sitting next to them or of objects located in their peripheral visual fields. As a result they may appear to lack social interaction skills or appear clumsy if they spill something or knock something over.

Stimulus Persistence

Stimulus persistence is a phenomenon that affects all sensory channels. Because sensory stimuli are conducted slower, they are slower to arrive at a level of awareness and slower to leave. Older people experience after-images longer than younger learners. This means that the older person may be experiencing a thought, picture, or sound longer than the nurse who is presenting it. If a nurse goes on to the next stimulus before clients' circuits have cleared, the next thought, picture, or sound becomes confused with the earlier one. This is not a comment on client sensorium; it is a comment on a nurse's lack of experience or impatience (Alford, 1982).

Sensory Changes: Hearing

As with vision, some degree of hearing loss inevitably accompanies the aging process. Presbycusis is associated with aging and is the most common hearing loss. It begins in young adulthood and becomes evident usually after age 50. Initially, high-pitched sounds beyond the range of human speech are lost. Because these have little functional significance, the individual is unaware of the loss. As the client ages, the loss eventually involves the sounds in the middle and lower ranges. It becomes problematic for the client when the upper sounds are missed and only the lower sounds are heard. Words sound distorted and conversations are difficult to understand, especially with background noise present. Presbycusis rarely results in total deafness (Bates, 1991; Matteson & McConnell, 1988). With high tone hearing loss, it is more difficult for your client to discriminate among consonants, such as *s*, *t*, *f*, *g*, *ch*, *sh*, *z*, and *th*, which have high frequencies. Clients with presbycusis will have a difficult time distinguishing among phonetically similar words. Words are distorted and sentences make little sense.

A sentence, such as, "I think he should go to the store," might be interpreted as "I wish we could go to the show." As the hearing loss progresses, explosive consonants, such as *b*, *d*, *k*, *p*, and *t*, also become distorted (Miller, 1990).

Your clients with presbycusis will need more time to process information. Rapid speech will be difficult for older clients to understand. McCroskey and Kasten (1982) found that a speech rate of 125 words per minute was better understood by the elderly between the ages of 65 to 88, living independently and in nursing homes, than was a speech rate of 175 words per minute. If you speak rapidly, you will need to remember to slow down when you teach older clients. Lower your pitch and speak more slowly and somewhat or slightly louder. See Figure 7-1.

An older client in a group setting may not want to participate or answer questions for fear of appearing foolish. Hearing loss affects a client's self-confidence and may lead to social isolation. Uninformed health care providers may assume a hard-of-hearing client is demented. Consider the following example of a woman who was attempting to communicate with her elderly mother-in-law. "My mother-in-law does not pay attention to anything I say. Even if I practically shout at her it does not do any good. But let my husband come in the room and just talk to her in a normal voice, and she hears every word he says."

The nursing student responded with sensitivity to what may be symptoms of family conflict. She explained the facts about sound waves to the woman and explained that a woman's voice is likely to contain higher sound frequencies. If she raises her voice in an effort to be heard, it is quite likely that she will also raise the pitch. Tension also can result in a rise in voice pitch. If the relationship already suffers from tension, it is likely that the voice with which the woman begins to speak is already higher than her relaxed voice. These factors would make her speech less intelligible to an aging person whose hearing is diminishing. The man who "casually" comes into the room is likely to speak in a voice with a much lower pitch, which has a longer wavelength.

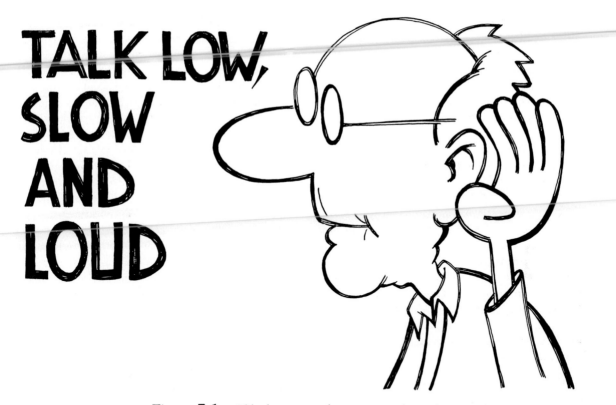

TALK LOW, SLOW AND LOUD

Figure 7-1   Older learners need more time and stimuli.

Suspect a hearing loss if your older client gives an inappropriate response to your question, is unable to follow your oral directions without cues, or frequently asks you to repeat a message. If the client watches you closely, turns his or her ear toward you, gets unusually close to you, does not respond to loud environmental noise, speaks too loudly or inarticulately, speaks in a monotone, or avoids groups settings you should also suspect hearing impairment (Miller, 1990). Remember, however, that not all older clients are hard-of-hearing. It is distressing for older persons to be spoken to as if they are deaf when they are not.

Chronic Disease and Implications for Teaching/Learning

Although Americans older than 65 see physicians only slightly more frequently than do younger people, the increasing number of elderly people means that more elderly are needing services in the health care system. People 65 and older are less likely to have as many acute conditions as younger people; however, they are more apt to have at least one chronic condition for which they are likely to seek assistance. Many have more than one chronic condition (American Association of Retired Persons, 1987; Vander Zanden, 1981).

A holistic view of aging takes into consideration the biologic, psychologic, sociologic, and cultural dimensions of an individual's life. What occurs in one dimension will have an effect on the entire person. Fundamental to the maintenance of good health is a sense of control. Loss of the sense of control, social isolation, and other losses are often associated with ill health in the elderly and most likely mediated via immune system suppression (Rodin, 1986). How these events are perceived by the individual is critical in determining the eventual effect on health.

Common health problems among the elderly include gastrointestinal problems (constipation, diverticulosis, and gallstones), diabetes mellitus, cardiovascular disease (essential hypertension, chronic ischemic heart disease, hypertensive heart disease, and heart failure), respiratory problems (chronic obstructive lung disease, acute upper respiratory infection, bronchitis), cancer, and musculoskeletal problems (arthropathies and osteoporosis) (Matteson & McConnell, 1988). While a nursing student, you will probably see most of these problems among the clients for whom you care. Keep the larger picture in mind. "Only 10% of the elderly population is seriously incapacitated with disease. Being old does not mean being sick, only more fragile and less adaptive" (Groer & Shekleton, 1989, p. 314).

Teaching your older clients how to adapt to chronic disease will be a major theme as you work with them. The causes of chronic disease are multiple and frequently related to life-style. Chronic diseases come on slowly over time. Your older client may not clearly understand her or his illness, especially if it is characterized by exacerbations and remissions. Working with older clients with chronic disease will challenge you as a teacher. You will need to determine how well they understand their diseases and the degree to which they are willing to comply with the prescribed treatment. Clients need to be educated about how to prevent and manage crises, manage the therapeutic regimen, control the symptoms, organize their time, prevent social isolation, adjust to changes in the course of the disease, and have normal life-style and interactions with others despite the disease (Matteson & McConnell, 1988). Refreshing your own memory, by reviewing the nature of a specific chronic disease, will help you prepare to answer questions the older client may have.

Teaching related to general health measures is a fruitful area for older clients. So many of these measures are instrumental in improving health status and helping clients to simply feel better (Pascucci, 1992). Consider teaching about exercising regularly, improving nutritional intake, controlling weight loss or gain, getting adequate rest, managing stress, and cooperating with the medical regimen. We have enjoyed teaching these topics, especially the classes on exercises, to older clients during their noon meal at community lunch sites. The exercises taught were suitable to the age of the clients and involved simple range-of-motion exercises. The clients perked up and began to smile and interact with each other in a way they had not before this activity. Many noted they felt better as a result.

The following experience illustrates how one nursing student made a significant difference in the life of an 87-year-old client, Mrs. Green. She is a widow whose children have also died. When Mrs. Green was younger, she was a supervisor in a large corporation and an avid swimmer with an active social life. She was happily married with two children, both of whom were health care professionals. She has two granddaughters who live in different cities and do not visit her. Through the aging process, she has become even more isolated. She has arthritis, which limits her activity, and cataracts, which limit her sight. These problems, along with a few other physical ailments, have contributed to her becoming a "shut in." At first Mrs. Green was hesitant to let the nursing student come to her home. Previously she had had some unfortunate experiences with physicians and had not been seen by anyone for more than 2 years. Her failing vision had contributed to a fear of strangers and her arthritis had kept her from going out of the house. With some coaxing, and because she was having abdominal pain that she wanted treated, she let the nursing student come to her home.

When the nursing student arrived, Mrs. Green was pleasant but cautious. The student conducted a health history and did a physical assessment. Through a telephone consultation with the clinic physician, Mrs. Green was diagnosed as having a flare up of an old ulcer and appropriate medication was prescribed. The student returned weekly and, within a month, Mrs. Green learned to trust the nurse. Each week, they discussed Mrs. Green's vision and, if it could be improved, how she would be able to continue taking care of herself. At first Mrs.

Green was determined never to see a doctor again, but after a few weeks she made an appointment herself, arranged for a ride, and went to see an eye surgeon. A short time later she had surgery to remove a capsule that had grown over a previously removed cataract. The surgery made a big difference. When the nursing student made her next visit, she found that Mrs. Green seemed like a different person. Instead of spending the whole hour talking about all of her health problems, the nursing student could hardly get Mrs. Green to discuss any of them. Mrs. Green was joyous about the difference the surgery had made in her sight and went on to chat about current events and anything else she could think of. Mrs. Green had gone from being a lonely, fearful person to being outgoing and cheerful. She still is a "shut in" because of her age and arthritis, but she no longer lives in a world of haze. Mrs. Green told the nursing student it was like someone removed the cloud from her eyes and everything became clear again. Mrs. Green is less isolated now. She is safer and will be able to live in her own home longer. The nursing student felt a lot of satisfaction knowing that she had helped improve the quality of Mrs. Green's life.

Cognitive Functioning

Cognitive operations in the older adult have recently become the subject of intense investigation (Poon, Rubin, & Wilson, 1989). In earlier research, intellectual functioning tended to be confused with other variables. Bahrick (1989) pointed out that earlier researchers, in an effort to be more scientific, conducted most of their memory research in the laboratory. One of the observations that came out of that era was that those who measured the intellectual capacity of the aged failed to distinguish the *ability* to do an intellectual operation with the *speed* of response (Charness, 1989). A number of memory tasks were used that were purposely meaningless, in order to eliminate differences that might be connected with prior experience. The information obtained was of limited value to the elderly themselves or to you as a nurse who will care for them. There is a growing trend to now investigate memory problems by using meaningful things, such as grocery lists, rather than just nonsense syllables that are easily controlled in the research lab (Perlmutter & Monty, 1989).

More recent studies (Poon, Rubin, & Wilson, 1989) that differentiated between variables, such as attitude, interest, attention, organization, and pacing, have revealed very hopeful information. Researchers are using the information to offer practical memory training (West, 1989), teaching the elderly how to use mnemonics (Yesavage, Lapp, & Sheikh, 1989), and the use of memory aids in everyday situations (Crovitz, 1989). We have used the information from this research in teaching implications later in this chapter. Intellectual functions, such as IQ, concept formation, problem-solving ability, language production, vocabulary acquisition, organization, and skilled action, tend to last and even increase with advanced age.

> Research findings regarding memory, learning, and creativity are conflicting. Most cross-sectional studies conclude that age-related declines in these abilities exist, but newer, longitudinal studies cast doubt on these findings. Intelligence is a multidimensional concept, and the effects of age versus disease on the various components of intelligence are unclear. Additionally, performance of intelligence tests depends on environmental characteristics, sensory ability, time constraints, motivation, educational level, social expectations, and a variety of other variables that cannot always be adequately controlled. (Matteson & McConnell, 1988, p. 10).

Short-Term Memory

If learning is the process of acquiring new knowledge, then memory is the process of retaining that knowledge over time (Kandel & Hawkins, 1992). In Chapter 3 we pointed out that short-term memory has a limited capacity. Short-term memory seems to be vulnerable to the aging process, although there is disagreement in the research about even this time-honored belief (Poon, Rubin, & Wilson, 1989; Selkoe, 1992). When older clients become aware of memory slippage and stimulus persistence, they frequently come to the conclusion there is something wrong with their brains or that they are losing their minds. The affective response, fear and anxiety, that accompanies such a conclusion can be powerful enough in itself to interfere with the learning process as is seen in Figure 7-2. This increased anxiety can lead to increased memory impairment. Such results can be "evidence" to clients that they are indeed experiencing serious memory loss (Poon, Rubin, & Wilson, 1989). Depression and the expectation of failure can commence a downward spiral and a self-fulfilling prophecy.

Memory in itself is a very complicated process. In the past, memory experts tended to talk about short-term memory and long-term memory as if they were concrete locations in the brain, such as the "temporary file basket" and the longer term "storage cabinets or file drawers (Poon, Fozard, Cermack, Arenberg, & Thompson, 1980)." As technology permits more sophisticated investigation of the working human brain, those ideas are being replaced by a more dynamic theory of the process.

An important variable in memory and learning is the attitude of both the client and you. Your message and the client's internal message both matter. The client may be aware of short-term memory deficits and become discouraged. If you have had little experience with the elderly, you may conclude that the client's memory deficits are insurmountable. It may indeed be true that clients cannot learn as much or as fast as when they were younger. However, older clients can learn when they set the pace of learning to suit their current ability, when they develop the memory aids themselves, and when you and clients

break up the material to be learned into sensible portions delivered at a reasonable pace with adequate space between units. The following is a description of the memory problems experienced by a woman who, at 75, came out of retirement, left her home in Colorado, and went to Alaska to teach children in a completely new and harsh environment. The woman offers nurses the following description and advice. "I go to get some thing in the kitchen, and when I get there, I have forgotten what I needed to get. I forget lists (in my head). Even three items can be troublesome. I cannot recall names of places, people, and things when I need the information, especially if I am in even a very mildly stressful situation. I leave out an item in a familiar recipe. I forget to turn off the stove under cooking pots; a timer is a must. Sequential directions are easily confused or omitted. Did I take my medication or not? Give me short specific instruction. Repeat your directions. Find a way to give me a hands-on demonstration of any procedure."

In addition to the above client's advice, we recommend that you encourage clients to use written lists and reinforce memory compensation devices like the timer on the stove. Color-coding medication with colored dots can help; i.e. put blue dots on the medicine that is taken at breakfast and red dots on the medicine that is taken at both breakfast and supper. A calendar is very helpful for remembering important appointments. Poems help, too. A woman complained to the nurse that she became confused when she stepped off the elevator to go to visit the doctor because elevators on both sides would take her to the correct floor. Once she would step off the elevator, she would forget which way to turn. She finally solved the problem by noting sunlight streaming in one window. She now tells herself, "Turn to the light and then to the right." We recommend that you encourage your older client to make a record of important information in a brightly colored folder: name of doctor, name of insurance, important identification numbers, names of medication, important people's phone numbers. In this folder, older clients should also keep questions that occur between visits to the doctor or to you, the nurse.

Fearful

Forgetful

Figure 7-2 Fearful of forgetting: The self-fulfilling prophecy.

Interest is another important variable: "I remember what I want to remember." In order for clients to invest declining resources into the work of learning, they must be convinced that the effort is worthwhile and is in their own best interest to learn. Help the client find a reason for making the effort. Feeling better is a powerful motivator for the older client (Pascucci, 1992). Fear was the motivator for a 96-year-old gentleman who was learning to walk again after a severe accident. The nurses caring for him remarked on his willpower. He replied: "It is not will power. If I do not keep going, you will put me in one of those places if I do not walk!" He equated a nursing home with a poorhouse, and he wanted no part of one.

Interest is closely related to attention. The questions, "How well do you pay attention? What activities help you pay attention? How do you concentrate?" are important in assessing the client's present level of competence. A good way to pay attention more effectively is to help clients involve several senses. You will find it helpful to establish eye contact with American or Western European clients. Eye contact is an indicator that they are probably listening attentively. Some clients are more assertive or honest than others about hearing deficits. You may find it helpful to give a very brief message and then ask the client to restate the communication. If the client is willing to repeat back the message, you receive several important bits of information. You get some notion of how the client has understood the message, the modality through which the client learns most easily, and the pace that suits the client. "I see what you mean," may indicate that the client is a visual learner. "I get it," may signify a tactile learning style. "I hear you," may be a clue that the client is an auditory learner.

The majority of the population learns more easily and remembers better from visual presentation (Gose & Levi, 1988). That fact helps to explain why so many memory aids make use of vision. To be sure that the visual channel would be helpful to an individual client, ask what visual cues claim the client's attention. You might take the initiative to point out characteristics that may be apparent: "Notice that this little pill is red and round, while that one is long and green." If the pills are violet and blue, they may be indistinguishable to older eyes.

Only a small percentage of the population is made up of people who are auditory learners. If the client is an auditory learner, search for auditory cues to enhance the learning, such as "Let me spell it for you," or "The pill's name is Lanoxin, like Lenox china."

The tactile client can benefit from activities that involve touching or otherwise manipulating the materials. You could give a set of instructions to the client to hold during the teaching session. You may be able to obtain a model (heart) or the actual object (pill) under discussion so that the client may manipulate it.

Other senses, such as taste and smell, may be incorporated as appropriate. If the medicine is a liquid it may have a distinctive odor. If a wound is being dressed or a discharge needs to be monitored, smell can be an important clue to the progression of healing, as well as a warning sign of necrosis or infection. The involvement of several senses raises the likelihood that learning will occur.

One of the challenges that faces some older learners is the fading of their preferred channel of learning. It may take some relearning to capitalize on other available channels. One client, who is left-handed, can no longer hear as well from his left ear. He can hear better out of the right, but he must switch the phone to the other hand. His desk is set up for listening on the left. He could switch the ear he uses, but finds learning this new method an aggravating change.

Memory works through association. Zimmerman (1990) and Yesavage, Rose, and Bower (1983) found that associations that clients design for themselves are more effective than artificially imposed associations. In order to help clients remember a new idea, we suggest that you help them find ways to associate the new idea with ones they already have, and/or help them organize the new information into a gestalt that makes sense for *them* as individuals. Logical connections are helpful but imaginative association is usually stronger. Elderly clients have more success with using associations that make sense to them than younger people, who can be amused by their wild creations, and therefore remember them.

Arousal affects memory. We are more apt to remember events to which we have attached emotions. Events associated with pleasant, aggravating, or frightening emotions all seem to have a higher likelihood of being recalled. You may be able to say or do something really amusing to clients as a way of helping them remember an event or bit of instruction (Nahemow, McCluskey-Fawcett, & McGhee, 1986).

The average person can hold only a limited number of thoughts in the working memory at one time (Poon, Rubin, & Wilson, 1989). Older people need a longer time and more intensity to register a stimulus. This also means that they have more trouble with tasks requiring the division of attention. Those thoughts can get pushed out by a new thought that is persisting or an old thought that is recalled. The person who is able to entertain only a few thoughts at once should be assertive and selective about those on which she or he chooses to focus. The assertive client will say, "I am terribly distracted right now and really cannot pay attention. Can we tend to this other problem, which is more pressing for me?" or "Could we make an appointment for another time when I can concentrate?" It would be nice if all clients were that assertive or even clear about what is running through their minds. Such a scenario is more apt to occur in a mutually trusting relationship. One way to react to a distracted client is to ask questions that might lead to the client's concerns. You can even teach and reinforce the above assertive behavior.

"Do you understand?" is a tricky question as well as a deceptive one. All you will know is whether or not clients act cooperatively. Not all clients are assertive. Many older clients try not to bother you, the busy nurse. When feeling overloaded, clients may hide their feelings of ignorance, smile politely, and agree when asked the above question. This type of response (with a half-hearted "yes" or a smile and a nod) may feel satisfying to you when you are busy, but it can deceive you.

Medication and Cognitive Functioning

When asked, "What medications are you taking?" clients vary in their reliability as historians. Caregivers also vary in the amount of thought they give to the above possibilities and to the skill with which they question clients. Clients may not include the pills they take for headaches, upset stomachs, "regularity," or vitamins in the list of medications. They also may not mention medications obtained from other caregiving systems so that they do not seem dissatisfied with the other caregivers.

Individuals in the older population are more different from each other than individuals among younger populations. (Poon & others, 1980). Each of the elderly clients you encounter may look similar; however the confused, old client you see lying in bed may have been an active community member, as illustrated in Figure 7-3, before experiencing severe trauma.

When working with a confused, elderly client, be sure to consider the medications the client is taking. The client may be receiving a dose that is too high. Another possibility is that multiple medications may be interacting unfavorably. Other considerations are the cumulative effect and side effects of drugs. The elderly need to be taught about how drugs affect them and how to take them safely (Gortner, Dirks, & Wolfe, 1992). One older woman stopped taking all of her medications because "they make my tongue white and take away my appetite." She was indeed on a drug whose side effects include gastrointestinal complications. The nurse finally got the woman to agree to take enough doses of the other medications to control the woman's blood pressure. The nurse taught the client to push on her own ankles to become aware of edema. Knowing the symptoms of high pressure did more to convince the client that she needed at least some medication than did the doctor's displeasure with the woman's blood pressure.

Ethnic Elderly

How old age is defined and how it expresses itself in a society is a function of culture (Reynolds,

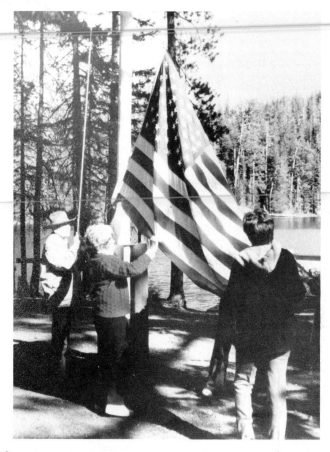

Figure 7-3 The confused, old person you see lying in bed may have been an active community member before experiencing severe trauma. *Photograph by Laura G. Howe. Courtesy American Society on Aging.*

1992). In the United States the dominant culture defines old age as a chronologic event—it occurs at age 65. Beyond this age, a person's social role changes through forced or voluntary retirement with the belief that intellectual, physical, and social capabilities diminish (Leininger, 1978). This is in contrast to other societies in which a person is first defined as old when she or he is unable to work rather than by chronologic age (McKenna, 1989). Aging is a process common to all cultures. See Figure 7-4.

Some ethnic groups may view old age differ-ently than the dominant culture. For example, blacks and Asians may have a positive view of old age and look forward to the respect that it generates among family and friends. Blacks may be more concerned about the ability to function mentally and physically than about chronologic age and may maintain a serene and optimistic outlook about aging. Hispanics' and Native Americans' views on old age are not as well researched. According to the sparse research available Hispanic beliefs flow between feeling old and useless and expecting to be respected and honored. In the former view, aging

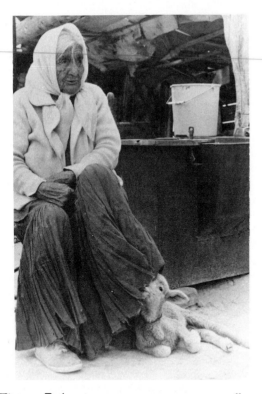

Figure 7-4 Aging is a process common to all cultures. *Photograph by David Lundley. Courtesy of American Society on Aging.*

Clients who are immigrants or first-generation residents in the United States may adhere more strongly to the health beliefs and practices of their primary cultural affiliation. For example, many elderly Asians, Filipinos, and Pacific Rim individuals have recently entered the United States (Ebersole & Hess, 1990). These immigrants, who are coming to this country to join their children, have the unique challenge of relocating to a new culture and language late in life. Other ethnic elderly clients who have lived a lifetime in the United States are more likely to have become assimilated into the American culture, to have had some experiences with the nation's health care system, and to have better knowledge of its health practices. By assessing health beliefs, values, and practices, you can tailor your health teaching to the individual client.

Language may be a barrier in communicating with the ethnic elderly. It may be that the client speaks little or no English. If the latter is the case, find an interpreter to assist you. Family members may serve more effectively as interpreters for the elderly because they know the client and are more likely familiar with the client's mode of self-expression.

In providing health education, be sure that your message is realistic in terms of the client's living situation, support network, educational background, and financial resources. For example, teaching an elderly Hispanic woman about the importance of a daily intake of fresh fruit and vegetables was meaningless because of the client's very limited financial resources. Her situation was compounded because she could not drive and her family lived far away. The client was dependent on neighbors for transportation, which was irregular and unpredictable at best. In another example, an elderly black woman had been on medication for hypertension for several years. The clinic nurse noted that the client's blood pressure had been elevated during the past 6 months. After a lengthy discussion with the client, the nursing student learned that the client had not been taking the medication. Because of her limited financial resources, the client had to make a choice between food and medicine. She had discontinued the medication and waited to see if the nurses and

began at or before age 60 with individuals reporting feeling useless, unable to work, or both. The traditional Native American view of aging is a time of wisdom acquired over a lifetime. Old age occurs when the individual is no longer able to be productive rather than at any particular chronologic age (Evaneshko, 1984).

As with any age group, there is great diversity of beliefs and values among the elderly both across different ethnic groups and within any one particular ethnic group. It is essential that you conduct a thorough cultural assessment in order to identify the health beliefs and values of the older client, family, or group that you will be educating. Your cultural assessment will identify the health practices of the client and the degree to which the client believes in and adheres to folk practices and Western health care practices.

doctors would notice the difference.

If the elderly client is under treatment for a current health problem, inquire about what she or he is doing to treat it. The client may be engaging in a folk practice designed to ameliorate the condition. Listen carefully to the client's self-care practices and determine if these practices are helpful, neutral, or harmful. Unless the practice is harmful, be supportive of the practice and view it as an adjunct to your nursing and medical interventions. Remember that the mind has a profound influence on health and healing, and we do not yet fully understand the extent of the mind's influence. If clients' practices provide them with meaning and give them a sense of participation in healing, then the practices deserve our respect, not disdain.

Gender Differences and Aging

That men are biologically weaker than women is suggested by mortality rates from the moment of conception through the life span (Cowling & Campbell, 1986). A 1989 study concluded that white women have a life expectancy of 79.1 years compared with 72.6 for white men. This ratio is expected to remain the same through the year 2005 (U.S. Bureau of the Census, 1991). McElmurry and LiBrizzi (1986) predicted that in the year 2000, 35 million people will be older than 65 years of age; 20 million of this number will be women. These numbers suggest that aging is primarily a woman's issue. Less is known about women's health because women have been underrepresented in research. Women generally have fewer financial resources, which make it difficult to obtain adequate health care. Even so, women are more likely than men to seek health care, both medical and dental.

The short life span for men has been attributed to a number of factors. For example, men have a high incidence of automobile accidents, use of weapons, use of alcohol, suicide, involvement in hazardous activities, arteriosclerotic heart disease, and coronary-prone behaviors. Some of these factors are associated with traditional male behavioral expectations in the United States. Traditional male behaviors—aggressiveness, impatience, unwilling-

ness or inability to express oneself, and a driving need to control one's life—run parallel to what has been identified as a type A personality. These type A personality traits have been associated with cardiovascular disease. Men's disinclination to seek routine preventive health care compounds these health hazards (Cowling & Campbell, 1986).

Your older clients may be grappling psychosocially with a retirement that has already occurred. Retirement is a major life-style rearrangement for both men and women. For those who have identified themselves by their work without developing strong interests in other areas, retirement may be particularly difficult. These people may experience feelings of dependency, powerlessness, and helplessness that develop as a result of decremental changes in health status and retirement (Cowling & Campbell, 1986). Women may have a broader social network than men upon which to depend as they enter retirement.

As the health educator, you need to be tuned in to your client's changing social roles. If your client is about to retire or is having difficulty adjusting to retirement, encourage him or her to gradually disengage from the work role. Help him or her identify other areas of interest and activities she or he can pursue. Do not overlook the effect on the spouse when one marriage partner retires. Many people have complained to us about the adjustments they have to make when their spouses retired and began following them around the house all day.

You may find some older men engaging in risky behavior. Examples of these behaviors are smoking, caffeine use, and alcohol consumption. Discuss these habits with clients, as appropriate, and let them know that changing these practices can have a positive effect on their lives. Teach your clients about the importance of preventive health care. Many problems can be treated effectively if caught early (Cowling & Campbell, 1986).

Women may present different challenges to you in your role as health educator. Health concerns of older women cited by McElmurry and LiBrizzi (1986) were lack of knowledge about medications, especially common side effects; unsatisfactory self-medication habits; insufficient intake of milk products; poor Pap smear and breast self-exam habits; blurred vision, nocturia; and dry skin. All of these concerns offer a rich array for health education opportunities.

Social support networks are important for both genders. People who maintain relationships with others, and remain active and involved with group activities fare better in terms of health. Your role as a teacher is to foster these support networks.

Finally, never assume that older men and women are not interested in sex. Many individuals continue to be sexually active beyond the expectations and imagination of their younger counterparts. Health education about sexuality in the later years will generate more interest than you anticipate (Steinke, 1988). Consider the example of a 70-year-old female client seen in an outpatient clinic. She came in for her routine checkup and renewal of her prescription for Premarin (estrogen). She exercised regularly, ate nutritious meals, and maintained a long-standing sexual relationship with a 50-year-old man.

Communication

When working with older learners, stop and think about your priorities. When you are busy, sitting down and slowing down to actually find out what the client knows and wants does indeed take time. When pressed for time with many other crucial issues, you may be tempted to present the important information and think that you have fulfilled the teaching obligation. But if you present information to an unreceptive client, you waste your own precious time and the client's energy. There must be better ways that you can use the little time that is available. Perhaps reflective listening would be appropriate and would lead to the client's taking more responsibility for the problem that is currently bothering him or her. The following is an example of the results of communication errors involving a client who is unreceptive in some respects. The example shows what one nursing student did to help.

An elderly lady went to a doctor to see if anything could be done for her scratchy voice. The consulting surgeon was very optimistic and promised quick and easy results. After the surgery and some speech therapy, the woman's voice was no better. She turned down several invitations to social engagements and was reluctant to have company because of the way she sounded. This woman was intelligent and alert but hard of hearing. What she perceived during the therapeutic speech encounters is unknown; what she heard from the surgeon is also not completely clear. Her attitude (do not complain) and her pride in not calling attention to her defective speech or raising doubts about her intelligence, all impinged on her behavior (asking questions) and the clarity of two-way communications. She was hurt by the doctor's accusation that she was causing the scratchiness to persist, and she demonstrated to the nursing student that she could still sing and that she experienced no scratchiness in her voice at that time. Her perception, because the surgeon did not produce the correction he had promised so blithely, was that something more serious was going on. She concluded that she must have throat cancer. She had not told her family, the doctor, or the speech therapist of that perception.

During the assessment phase the nursing student was able to discover this conclusion by listening, speaking loudly, and sitting face to face with the woman. The nursing student also discovered that the client had recently enjoyed a trip to a special exhibit in the art museum. She expressed delight at using one of the audio, self-guided-tour machines: "I could hear him just as if he were standing next to me." The nursing student also noted that the client's younger sister insisted on keeping the radio and the television at a volume that "won't bother the neighbors" in their two-story apartment. The elderly client told the nursing student that she was very appreciative of all that the speech therapist had tried to do but was not willing to return. "She's just so busy with all of her other, more important duties."

The nurse then made the following interventions. She gave the woman some information about vocal chords with written explanations and pictures in order to reduce the likelihood of error. The nursing student also recommended that the client obtain a personal stereo cassette player and sing with the radio and tapes of familiar and favorite songs.

The nursing student explained that the head-phones would allow the woman to adjust the volume for herself and would keep the music from bothering the neighbors. Because several other senior residents of the apartment complex owned similar devices, it might even have had a bit of status value as a new toy.

The nursing student knew that singing would exercise the vocal chords at longer intervals than speech and at the higher registers of vocalization, which the speech therapist had recommended exercising. The nursing student hoped the musical device would stimulate the client to practice singing and to exercise her vocal chords in the privacy of her own home and at her own pace. The nursing student also recommended that the client have a second examination by another ear, nose, and throat specialist. The client was satisfied with the "very thorough going over" that this physician provided. "He said he found no sign of anything wrong, and all it will take is some more time. So that's that." The woman expressed relief at the doctor's finding of nothing more serious.

The above story illustrates how a nursing student took a holistic approach to the elderly client's learning needs, energy resources, life experiences, and orientation to learning. By recognizing the generation the client is from, the nursing student was able to offer the woman comfortable options for coping with the scratchy voice.

Nutrition

Nutrition affects memory. The body is dependent on the presence of many nutrients to manufacture the neurotransmitters that are essential to any learning. The B vitamins are essential ingredients in this process. Iron is essential for the transmission of oxygen to the brain, and water is vital to every metabolic process in the body.

Many Americans do not consume enough liquid daily. This phenomenon is more evident in the elderly because of other physiologic changes. One of the organs that tends to shrink with age is the bladder. Some older people, in an effort to avoid the inconvenience or embarrassment of needing to

empty their bladders more often, tend to drink less. This problem of self-imposed dehydration may be exacerbated by a subculture of the older generation that considers bodily functions or attention to them as taboo. If your client is not properly hydrated, his or her ability to learn will be impaired.

It is unlikely that individuals of that group would mention bladder shrinkage or their solution. The nurse could raise the subject by saying, "I have an older friend/relative who . . ." and explain the cost and benefits of rehydration.

Although more Americans are valuing fitness, many elderly may not see the connection between exercise, effective cardiorespiratory functioning, and an oxygenated, nourished brain. Give clients the information and choose a time to teach when they are more invigorated, such as when the client is rested enough to have the energy to learn but stimulated enough to pay attention.

Memory

Wilson (1989) established that memory can be improved. Learning anything or changing any habit invigorates the brain. Nerve cells, which are stimulated by any change, generate electricity and manufacture chemicals. The more vigorously a neuron fires, the more ribonucleic acid (RNA) it produces. Therefore older humans who maintain an active life in stimulating circumstances are likely to remember better. Individual neurons are able to form new circuits. The brain sends a pattern, "Change your connections."

Understanding enhances memory, both retention and recall. An example of this phenomenon is a client who has received some information about his diagnoses. He reflects with a comment, such as "Oh, so that's why I've been feeling dizzy for the last year or so." The client may have not mentioned dizziness during previous medical encounters because the client did not understand the significance of the symptom. Older people often make the assumption that their changes are due to old age, rather than symptoms of correctable processes.

Repetition is another strategy that has proved helpful in capturing and retaining learning with every age category. Each time a particular word, concept, or experience is repeated, it is processed by many pathways in the brain. As these pathways are activated, neurochemical-electrical deposits are established in the brain. Events, words, and other things are more likely to be learned when these pathways are activated.

Repetition, however, can become routine and boring. People invest less energy in an idea or other activity that is too repetitious. Doing something imaginative or amusing with the material to be learned is one way of increasing the likelihood that it will be retained.

Summary

Older clients are different from younger and middle-aged clients in ways that significantly affect how you will plan and implement your health education. Significant variables include psychosocial development and physiologic changes associated with aging.

Each client must be assessed to identify his or her particular characteristics and to plan health education that meets his or her needs. Chronic disease is present in many older clients and will also affect your teaching plans. Many clients simply need more information about the nature of their chronic disease and how they can lessen its effect and work cooperatively with the physician to implement the treatment regimen.

Although researchers are not in agreement about the causes and the extent of memory changes, many older individuals and their associates are aware of problems with short-term memory. Fortunately, a number of promising and tested remedies are available to the interested older individual. The caregiver who is helping an older client learn information, skills, attitudinal changes, or all three to promote health can make use of the research. You can adapt learning theories and principles to enhance the older client's chances of success.

HELPING CLIENTS HEAR

Purpose:

- Experiment with other ways to reach a hearing-impaired client without shouting

Directions:

1. Pick a partner.
2. Decide who is "nurse" and who is "client."
3. Move your chairs so that you are facing each other knees to knees.
4. Nurse: Make a health statement to the client in a normal voice.
5. Client: Note volume and intelligibility of nurse's words and meaning.
6. Nurse: Reach out to the client and cup your hands behind the client's ears. Repeat the sentence you said before in your normal voice.
7. Client: Report the difference.
8. Switch roles.
9. Discuss your experiences with each other.
10. Repeat the above exercise using the stethoscope instead of cupping your hands.
11. Speak normally. Then put the ear pieces in the client's ears while holding the bell and speaking into it in the same tone that you would use on a microphone.
12. Discuss your experiences with each other.

AGEISM

- Debate the following: Ageism is an outdated issue.

- Divide into two groups and take opposing sides of the issue. Each side will have 15 minutes to prepare for debate.

References

Alford, D.M. (1982). Tips for teaching older adults. *Nursing Life,* September/October: 60-64.

American Association of Retired Persons. (1987). *A Profile of Older Americans.* Washington DC: Author.

Andresen, G.P. (1989). A fresh look at assessing the elderly. *RN,* June, 28-39.

Bates, B. (1991). *A Guide of Physical Examination and History Taking* (5th ed). Philadelphia: J.B. Lippincott.

Bahrick, H.P. (1989). The laboratory and ecology: Supplementary sources of data for memory research. In L.W. Poon, D.C. Rubin, & B.A. Wilson (Eds.), *Everyday cognition in adulthood and late life* (pp. 73-83). Cambridge: Cambridge University Press.

Charness, N. (1989). Age and expertise: Responding to Talland's challenge. In L.W. Poon, D.C. Rubin, & B.A. Wilson (Eds.), *Everyday cognition in adulthood and late life* (pp. 437-456). Cambridge: Cambridge University Press.

Cowling, W.R. & Campbell, V.G. (1986). Health concerns of aging men. *The Nursing Clinics of North America,* March. Philadelphia: W.B. Saunders.

Crovitz, H.F. (1989). Memory retraining: Everyday needs and future prospects. In L.W. Poon, D.C. Rubin, & B.A. Wilson (Eds.), *Everyday cognition in adulthood and late life* (pp. 681-691). Cambridge: Cambridge University Press.

Ebersole, P. & Hess, P. (1990). *Toward Healthy Aging. Human Needs and Nursing Response* (3rd ed.). St. Louis: Mosby.

Erikson, E. (1963). *Childhood and society* (2nd ed.). New York: W.W. Norton.

Evaneshko, V. (1984). Ethnic and cultural considerations. In Steffl, B.M. (ed.). *Handbook of gerontological nursing.* New York: Van Nostrand Reinhold.

Gawlinski, A. & Jensen, G.A. (1991). The complications of cardiovascular aging. *American Journal of Nursing, 91*(11), 26-30.

Gortner, S.R., Dirks, J. & Wolfe, M.M. (1992). Elders after CABG. *American Journal of Nursing, 92*(8), 44-49.

Gose, K. & Levi, G. (1988). *Dealing with memory changes as you grow older.* Toronto: Bantam Books.

Groer, M.W., and Shekleton, M.E. (1989). *Basic Pathophysiology* (3rd ed.). St. Louis: Mosby.

Kandel, E.R. & Hawkins, R.D. (1992). The biological basis of learning and individuality. *Scientific American, 267*(3), 79-86.

Leininger, M. (1978). *Transcultural nursing: Concepts, theories, and practices.* New York: John Wiley & Sons.

Matteson, M.A. & McConnell, E.S. (1988). *Gerontological Nursing: Concepts and Practice.* Philadelphia: W.B. Saunders.

McCroskey, R. & Kasten, R. (1982). Temporal factors and the aging auditory system. *Ear Hear, 3,* 124-127.

McElmurry, B.J. & LiBrizzi, S.J. (1986). The health of older women. *The Nursing Clinics of North America,* March. Philadelphia: W.B. Saunders.

McKenna, M.A. (1989). Transcultural perspectives in the nursing care of the elderly. In J.S. Boyle & M.M. Andrews, *Transcultural concepts in nursing care.* Boston: Scott, Foresman.

Miller, C.A. (1990). *Nursing Care of Older Adults.* Glenview, Il: Scott, Foresman/Little, Brown Higher Education.

Nahemow, L., McCluskey-Fawcett, K. & McGhee, P. (1986). *Humor and Aging.* London: Academic Press.

Newbern, V.B. (1992). Sharing the memories: The value of reminiscence as a research tool. *Journal of*

Gerontological Nursing. 18(5), 13-18.

Pascucci, M.A. (1992). Measuring incentives to health promotion in older adults. *Journal of Gerontological Nursing.* 18(30), 16-23.

Perlmutter, L.C. & Monty, R.A. (1989). Motivation and aging. In L.W. Poon, D.C. Rubin, & B.A. Wilson (Eds.), *Everyday cognition in adulthood and late life* (pp. 373-393).

Poon, L.W., Rubin, D.C., & Wilson, B.A. (Eds.). (1989). *Everyday cognition in adulthood and late life.* Cambridge: Cambridge University Press.

Poon, L.W., Fozard, J.L., Cermack, L.S., Arenberg, D., & Thompson, L.W. (Eds.) (1980). *New Directions in Memory and Aging*—Proceedings of the George A. Talland Memorial Conference. Hillsdale NJ: Lawrence Erlbaum Associates.

Reynolds, C. (1992). An administrative program to facilitate culturally appropriate care for the elderly. *Holistic Nursing Practice, 6*(3), 34-42.

Rodin, J. (1986). Aging and health: Effects of the sense of control. *Science, 233,* 1271-1276.

Schuster, C.S. & Ashburn, S.S. (1986). *The process of human development.* Boston: Little Brown & Co.

Seidel, H.M., Ball, J.W., Dains, J.E., & Benedict, G.W. (1991). *Mosby's Guide to Physical Examination* (2nd ed.). St. Louis: Mosby.

Selkoe, D.J. (1992). Aging brain, aging mind. *Scientific American, 267*(3), 135-142.

Steinke, E.E. (1988). Older adults knowledge and attitudes about sexuality and aging. *IMAGE: Journal of Nursing Scholarship.* 20(2), 93-95.

U.S. Bureau of the Census. (1991). *Statistical abstract of the United States: 1991* (111th ed.), Washington DC: Author.

U.S. Senate Special Committee on aging in conjunction with the American Association of Retired Persons. (1989). *Aging America: Trends and Projections,* Washington DC: Authors.

Vander Zanden, J.W. (1981). *Human development* (2nd ed.). New York: Knopf.

Weinrich, S.P., Boyd, M. & Nussbaum, J. (1989). Continuing education: Adapting strategies to teach the elderly. *Journal of Gerontological Nursing,* 15(11), 17-21.

West, R.L. (1989). Planning practical memory training for the aged. In L.W. Poon, D.C. Rubin, & B.A. Wilson (Eds.), *Everyday cognition in adulthood and late life* (pp. 573-591). Cambridge:

Cambridge University Press.

Wilson, B.A. (1989). Designing memory-therapy programs. In L.W. Poon, D.C. Rubin, & B.A. Wilson (Eds.), *Everyday cognition in adulthood and late life* (pp. 615-637). Cambridge: Cambridge University Press.

Yesavage, J.A., Lapp, D., & Sheikh, J.I. (1989). In L.W. Poon, D.C. Rubin, & B.A. Wilson (Eds.), *Everyday cognition in adulthood and late life*

(pp. 598-611). Cambridge: Cambridge University Press.

Yesavage, J.A., Rose, T.L., & Bower, G.G. (1983). Interactive imaging and judgments improve face-name learning in the elderly. Journal of Gerontology, 29, 197-203.

Zimmerman, B.J. (1990). Self-regulated learning and academic achievement: An overview. *Educational Psychologist, 25*(1), 3-17.

Assessing Culturally Diverse Clients

It is clearly recognized that of all
health care professionals, nurses
have the greatest contact with
clients. Through this contact,
nurses see similarities and
differences across and within
groups, become acutely aware of
the influence of culture on
health care, and strategically
plan to incorporate cultural
factors into the care.

Capers, 1992, p. 20.

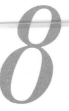

Objectives

Upon the completion of this chapter you will be able to:

- Use an assessment tool to identify the health education needs of culturally diverse clients.
- Adapt your personal and interpersonal skills to effectively communicate with culturally diverse clients.
- Describe verbal and nonverbal communication patterns of culturally diverse clients and the implications of these for health education.
- Adapt your health education objectives, content, and teaching strategies to meet the health care needs of culturally diverse clients, groups, families, and communities.
- Describe the alternative forms of health care that might be used by culturally diverse individuals, groups, families, and communities and how they may affect health education.
- Develop sensitivity to culturally diverse clients in order to adapt health education to the personal belief system and circumstances of individuals, groups, families, and communities.

Key Words

culture	values	illness
transcultural nursing	ethnocentrism	disease
ethnic	stereotype	folk medicine

Introduction

In addition to clients' psychosocial adaptations to their level of wellness, cultural heritage shapes clients' responses to health and illness. Thus culture becomes important during the assessment phase of teaching/learning. To be most effective the professional nurse/teacher considers the influence of culture on how clients define health, their role in preserving it and their responsibilities in recovering from illness.

Teaching Culturally Diverse Clients

Culture and Transcultural Nursing

Culture has many different meanings. Basically it is the sum total of the way of living by a group of people that is transmitted from one generation to another. Included in this definition are the ideas, customs, skills, and arts of a people or group (Neufeldt, 1991). Others note that culture is characterized by beliefs, values, moral principles, habits, dress, language, rules of behavior, economics, politics, dietary practices, and health care (Germain, 1992; Leininger, 1978; Capers, 1992). Culture permeates our lives continuously. Each of us can attribute our beliefs, values, and customs to cultural factors and all of us are being affected by the culture of nursing and the health delivery system. Transcultural nursing is culturally sensitive nursing care that bridges the differences between the cultural belief systems of the nurse and the client. Leininger (1978) defined transcultural nursing as the following:

> Transcultural nursing is a subfield of nursing which focuses upon a comparative study and analysis of different cultures and subcultures in the world with respect to their caring behavior, nursing care, and health-illness values, beliefs, and patterns of behavior with the goal of developing a scientific and humanistic body of knowledge in order to provide culture-specific and culture-universal nursing care practices. (p. 8)

Transcultural nursing blends the disciplines of anthropology, sociology, and biology and applies them to the nursing profession.

Cultural Diversity

A study of cultural diversity covers a broad range of themes and encompasses more than just ethnic background by examining diversity among groups, religious practices, socioeconomic status, gender preferences, and aging (Capers, 1992). Culture can refer to the life-style of those belonging to a specific group, such as the drug culture, youth culture, hippie culture, and the culture of poverty. Caucasians share certain biologic characteristics, such as fair skin, but culturally they may be very distinct. The Irish and Germans, for example, are quite different from each other, as are Italians, French, Russians, and other Caucasian European groups. Religious affiliation, whether Protestant, Catholic, Islamic, or Jewish provides another basis for examining diversity among people. Keep in mind that diversity exists within these groups. For example, the term *Protestant* could refer to Methodists, Mormons, or Southern Baptists. People of the Jewish faith can be described as either Orthodox, Conservative, or Reform (Charnes & Moore, 1992).

Socioeconomic status provides another basis for understanding people. Those who live in poverty grow up with significantly different beliefs and values than those with more substantive financial resources. Blacks, Hispanics, and whites living in poverty are quite different from their counterparts in the middle and upper socioeconomic class. The AIDS and human rights issues have brought attention to gender preference as another dimension to our concept of diversity within the United States. Homosexuality cuts across all ethnic, religious, and socioeconomic groups. Gays and lesbians have formed a subculture united by common concerns. Geography also creates diversity. Rural communities are distinct from urban ones, and urban communities are distinct from suburban ones.

Common to all of these dimensions of diversity is the aging process, and yet aging itself is a basis for diversity. A community may be characterized based on its composition of young, middle-aged, and elderly citizens. Health-education programs directed toward the elderly will be substantially different from programs created for teenagers. Elderly white Poles will hold beliefs and values quite different from elderly Hispanics who immigrated from Mexico. More information about elderly learners may be found in Chapter 7.

All groups of people have beliefs about how to maintain health, prevent illness, treat disease, and care for the dying (Germain, 1992). The key to success in working with any client is conducting a thorough nursing assessment. Asking good questions is fundamental in planning effective health education.

Example: "What do you believe caused you to become sick?"

"How have you treated this in the past?"

"What do you believe will help you get better?"

Ethnicity

Ethnicity is a designation given to a population subgroup having a common cultural heritage as distinguished by customs, characteristics, language, and common history. Being a member of an ethnic group usually refers to being a minority within a larger society (Neufeldt, 1991). In this chapter, we examine four ethnic groups with the highest representation in the population of the United States: Black Americans, Hispanic Americans, Native Americans, and Asian Americans. We will look at cultural beliefs about health and illness, cultural assessment, communication patterns, family relationships, nutritional habits, and how this information is useful to you in providing culturally appropriate health education.

Every region in the United States has a culturally diverse population. The United States continues to accept many people from around the world who are looking for freedom and a better place to live. Examine your own community and the ethnic groups served by the health delivery institution(s). You should learn as much as you can about the beliefs and values of the various groups. (See Figure 8-1.) Within each group, marked variations exist related to educational preparation, social class, degree of acculturation, and length of stay in the United States. For example, a Hispanic banker who has spent most of his or her life in the United States will hold beliefs that are considerably different from the Hispanic migrant worker who has recently moved into this country. By the same token, the black computer specialist's views and values will be significantly different from the black day laborer's views.

These ethnic groups reside in the midst of the dominant cultural group in the United States, which is white, primarily middle-class, and Protestant. To set the stage for a discussion of cultural diversity, let us reflect a moment on the meaning of beliefs and values and examine examples of the same among members of the dominant white culture.

Ethnic Group Descriptors

In our experience, the way a particular group would like to be identified has changed over time and continues to change. Increasing cultural awareness among members of ethnic groups, changing leadership within groups, emerging generations who view life differently from their elders, and changing political climates have all contributed to the changing terminology used to identify particular ethnic groups. For example, at one time black Americans were called *colored, high yellow,* and *negro.* Today, some members of this group would prefer to be called *African Americans* or *Afro-Americans* while others prefer to be called black. The meaning of high yellow is similar to the term *mulatto.* It refers to a person of mixed black and white ancestry. Black Americans may come from African or Caribbean countries.

A similar example can be given for Spanish-speaking individuals. Spanish-speaking individuals may come from many countries such as Mexico, Spain, Puerto Rico, Cuba, and throughout Central and South America. Those from Texas may prefer to be called Latin American or Latino; those from New Mexico may prefer Spanish American; those from California may prefer Mexican American; and activists may prefer Chicano (Evaneshko, 1984). Others prefer to be identified as Hispanic. Murillo-Rohde (1981) noted that Chicano describes those Spanish-surnamed citizens in the West and Southwest sections of the United States who never immigrated here. They are of Mexican descent "whose land was taken over from them by the United States and who suddenly found themselves to be a minority in their own land" (Murillo-Rohde, 1981, p. 225). There is a great deal of sensitivity and controversy among Spanish-speaking people as to how they want to be identified.

Native Americans comprise many tribes. More than 500 federally recognized American Indian tribes exist in the United States today (Heckler,

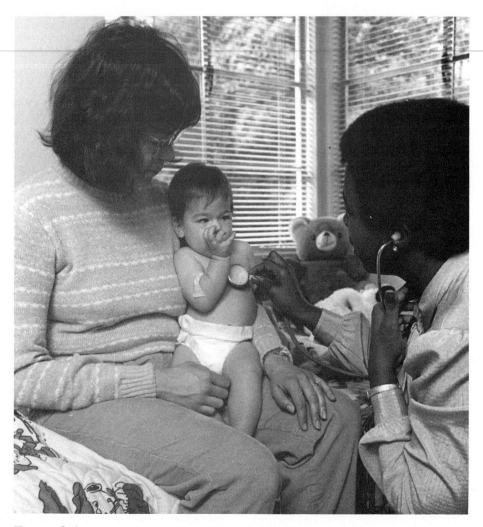

Figure 8-1   The nurse should learn about the beliefs and values of various ethnic groups.
From Bullough, B. and Bullough, V. Nursing in the Community, ed 1, St. Louis, Mosby, 1990.

1985), of which the Navajo tribe is the largest (Hanley, 1991). Other tribes are Sioux, Apache, Cherokee, Ute, Chippewa, Yakima, Hopi, and Zuni. Eskimos and Aleuts are also Native Americans.

As with the other groups discussed, the term *Asian American* includes many groups, the largest of which is Chinese American. Other Asian American cultural groups residing in the United States include Japanese, Filipino, Korean, Vietnamese, and Laotian.

To achieve a more thorough understanding of each of these groups, you will need to do some library research and further reading. Our purpose here is to summarize some of the common beliefs of each group so that you can know how these beliefs may affect the health education you provide. Remember that although cultural values and beliefs may characterize an ethnic group, it is not safe to assume every member of the ethnic groups holds these values and beliefs. An individual is a unique blend of many influences. To know what any one person believes and values, you must observe, ask, and listen carefully.

Values and Beliefs

Values are beliefs and practices that are very important to a group and provide a way by which a group is characterized and understood. Leininger (1970) identified the following as some common American values: optimal health for all people, a belief in democracy, respect for individual rights, achievement, cleanliness, and the wise use of time. The dominant culture also values education, individuality, hard work, material wealth, comfort, humanitarianism, physical beauty, democracy, science, the legal system, achievement, free enterprise, rationality, independence, respectability, self-discipline, effort, and progress (Herberg, 1989). Health practitioners within the Western health delivery system value punctuality, honest and open communication, cleanliness, and compliance with health care directives. Western health care practitioners in the United States generally believe the biomedical model of health care is superior and, despite its faults, is the best in the world.

How closely do the above-mentioned values and beliefs represent your own? What values and beliefs can you add to these? How well do you know the values and beliefs of your classmates? What are your own personal health and illness beliefs and practices? If what you do differs from what you espouse, why? When you are knowledgeable only about your own values, beliefs, and sociocultural system to the exclusion of all others, you are ethnocentric. Ethnocentrism assumes that your culture provides the right way, the best way, and the only way to live. In short, ethnocentrism assumes that your way of viewing the world is superior to others (Leininger, 1978). Ethnocentrism is a barrier to critical thinking because it devalues the beliefs and values of people from other cultures. Ethnocentrism contributes to many social ills embodied in the practice of prejudice, discrimination, and racism.

When you work with clients from different cultures, it is easy to stereotype, or label, them. Stereotyping creates a standardized mental picture that does not allow for individuality or critical judgment (Neufeldt, 1991). Someone once said that stereotyping is an exercise of a lazy mind. Certainly it is something many have done. Stereotyping is a way of grouping information when you do not have the time, energy, or desire to understand it more thoroughly. The tendency to stereotype is greatest when you know very little about something.

The United States is changing from what was once described as the great melting pot, in which immigrants gave up their own traditions in order to become Americans, to a new pride and appreciation of the various cultural groups that reside within the United States. The new, preferred analogy is a tossed salad. More than ever before, while blending and taking on American values, different groups are also celebrating their own heritage, values, and traditions (Tiedt & Tiedt, 1990). Many are proud of the contributions ethnic groups have made to the development of this great nation.

Professionals within the health delivery system are recognizing that changes need to be made if they are to meet the health care needs of the culturally diverse groups that they serve. Although not disavowing belief in the biomedical model, health professionals recognize that clients have their own explanations of what causes disease and what maintains health. To adequately serve these clients, health care providers are recognizing the importance of accommodating other paradigms or health belief systems. This is what the delivery of culturally appropriate health education is about.

Belief Systems about Health and Illness

Each of us has a set of beliefs about what maintains health and what causes illness. These beliefs have been modified somewhat with exposure to the biomedical model through your nursing education. For example, some may believe that a vitamin a day will make up for any deficiency unwittingly experienced in the daily diet. This is particularly true for those who have a hectic life-style and do not consider eating three square meals a priority. This vitamin-a-day belief is also promoted by the pharmaceutical industry. Others will argue that this practice has no substantive effect on maintaining health and is largely a waste of money. Another example is the use of vitamin C to prevent illness. To prevent or mollify a cold, some believe in the efficacy of large doses of vitamin C. Others argue that vitamin C, although not harmful, is not effective for this purpose. Consider your own beliefs. In what activities do you engage that you believe will keep you healthy or prevent illness?

Let us distinguish between illness and disease as descriptors of human conditions. Many use these terms interchangeably, but there is a difference. Disease refers to pathology experienced in the body or mind that is identified by symptoms, classified diagnostically, and treated according to medical protocol. Flaskerud (1989) distinguished between illness and disease. When a person first becomes aware of being sick, he or she is experiencing illness. The person begins to identify and label the symptoms and a healer is sought. Once the person seeks help from a practitioner, the symptoms become part of a diagnostic picture that results in a diagnostic classification. At this point the illness becomes known as a disease and specific treatment is then outlined. A person may have an illness, a disease, or both. For example, a person may believe him or herself to be ill as a result of a spell or hex or because of a stressful interpersonal relationship. No organic pathology is present, but the person experiences symptoms. Another client may have a health problem, such as endometriosis, and not consider herself to be ill.

Within the construct of Western medicine, or the biomedical model, many variations abound among individual beliefs about the best way to maintain health and prevent illness. Although many beliefs are held in common, individual nuances are present. As we look at other belief systems, also called paradigms, keep in mind that they provide the larger context within which to view health and illness. To become meaningful in providing culturally appropriate health education, you will need to explore the values and beliefs held by the individual client.

Albers (Herberg, 1989) identifies three major

world views through which people explain life events. They are the magico-religious, scientific, and holistic paradigms. To some degree components of all three may be found in all cultures; however, one is usually dominant. These paradigms will help you understand a cultural group in the largest sense. On an individual level, performing a thorough cultural assessment will help you discover the beliefs of a particular client.

Magico-Religious Paradigm

The magico-religious health paradigm views the fate of the world and its occupants as being under the control of supernatural forces. God, gods, or other supernatural forces for good or evil are in control while humans are at the mercy of these forces. Adherents believe that charms and religious articles ward off these forces. Human behavior may or may not be a relevant factor, such as the belief that punishment is a result of transgressions. In this paradigm

> illness is initiated by a supernatural agent with or without justification, or by another person who engages the services of a sorcerer or practices sorcery himself. The cause-effect relationship is not an organic one; rather, the cause of health or illness is mystical. Health is seen as a gift or reward given as a sign of God's blessing and good will. Illness may be seen as a sign of God's special favor, insofar as it gives the affected person the opportunity to resign himself to God's will, or it may be seen as a sign of God's possession or as a punishment. (Herberg, 1989, p. 27).

Another aspect of this belief system is that one individual may "directly or indirectly influence the health or illness of another person. This sense of community is virtually absent from the other paradigms" (Herberg, p. 28).

This belief system may be found among Hispanic people who attribute illness to things, such as possession by evil spirits, breaching a taboo, and supernatural forces (sorcery, witchcraft). For example, *mal de ojo* is a Mexican American belief that is also known as the evil eye. It is thought to result from the intrusion of a disease-causing spirit and affects infants and children. It occurs voluntarily or

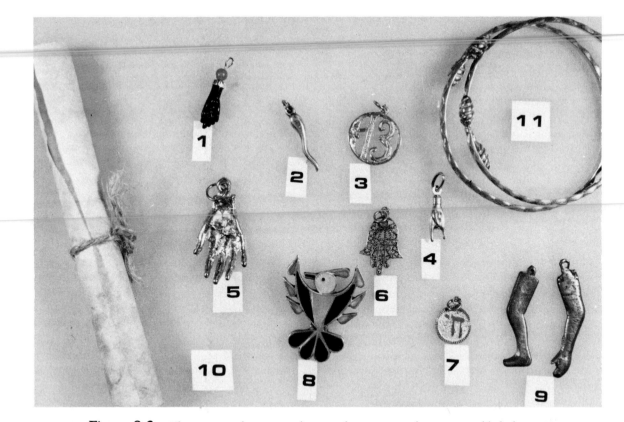

Figure 8-2 The magico-religious paradigm emphasizes magical, supernatural beliefs as symbolized by these objects, which are used to prevent illness. They are (1) *Azabache*, or *mano negro*—blackhand, (2) *Corno*, or goat's horn, (3) Lucky 13, (4) *Mano cornuta*, (5) *Mano milagroso*, (6) Hand of God, (7) *Chat*, (8) Thunderbird, (9) *Milagros*, (10) Talisman, (11) Bangles. *From the private collection of Rachel Spector, Boston College, photographed by Rob Schadt. Used with permission.*

involuntarily when someone who has been born with *vista fuerte* (strong vision) looks admiringly at a child but does not touch the child. Crying, fever, vomiting, and loss of appetite might result. The spell is broken when the child is touched by whomever cast the spell. The person should add, "God bless you," or some similar phrase. Likewise, touch is effective in preventing the illness (Kuipers, 1991; Baca, 1978; Foster, 1981). A nurse admiring a Mexican American baby, therefore, must be sure to touch the baby to avoid causing the disease.

Aire or *mal aire* (air or bad air) is perhaps the most frequent cause of illness among Spanish Americans according to Foster (1981). It is thought to occur when a person goes from a closed room

into the fresh air and is struck by a current of air or a breeze. For example, a postsurgical client was experiencing severe gas and abdominal distention. The client attributed the cause to air that entered through an abdominal incision (Baca, 1978). Others see *mal aire* as evil spirits that inhabit the air. These spirits may enter a person and cause illness and, perhaps, paralysis.

Many Hispanics have a fatalistic view of life. Many believe that the individual is subject to outside influences, particularly the divine will, and that little can be done to influence surrounding circumstances. Good health is viewed as a matter of chance—the result of good luck or God's reward for good behavior (Kuipers, 1991). Baca (1978) noted that microorganisms have no place as causative agents in this belief system.

Magico-religious beliefs, though not culturally dominant, are also found among whites. For example, in talking with cancer clients and encouraging them to share their innermost thoughts, we discovered that some have wondered if their cancer was possibly a punishment from God. This relationship is heard much less frequently from clients with other types of health problems, such as heart disease.

Black Americans may hold similar views. God may be conceptualized as a stern but loving parent who keeps close tabs on the behavior of His children. God may be punishing transgressions by causing illness to befall the sinner. Furthermore, the sins of the parents may be visited upon innocent infants and children resulting in deformity, seizure disorders, or retardation. Just as God punishes, He also heals (Snow, 1983). In times of illness and difficulty, many black Americans may draw upon their strongly held religious beliefs. Many may believe that God loves them and will take care of them in difficult times. The saying, "If you trust in Him, He will take care of you" epitomizes this belief.

In this belief system events and illnesses may be seen as either natural or unnatural. Natural events are in line with the intentions of God, whereas unnatural events upset the harmony of nature and are counter to God's plan. In the extreme, unnatural events represent evil and the work of the devil. Examples of natural events include cold air and impurities in the air, food, and water, which may enter the body and cause illness. Natural events may result from failure to take care of the body. Blacks and Mexican Americans may see natural illnesses as divine punishment for sin. Examples of unnatural events leading to illness issue from a belief in demons and evil spirits. These evil spirits await entry into an unprotected person. Among Hispanic Americans, these evil spirits are referred to as *malas influencias*. In this belief system the most common cause of unnatural illnesses is witchcraft. Blacks who hold similar beliefs may use terms such as roots, rootwork, witchcraft, voodoo, hoodoo, fix, hex, or mojo to indicate that such a curse has been "put on" them. Hispanics will describe this unnatural illness as *mal de ojo, mal artificial, brujeria, hechiceria,* or *enfermedad endanada*. The type of practitioner sought depends on how the illness is categorized. The physician will be perceived as able to handle natural illnesses but incapable of dealing with the more complex problems associated with unnatural illnesses, which result from divine punishment or from witchcraft activity. Physicians cannot subdue the devil with drugs (Snow, 1981).

Within the context of natural illnesses, illness can be due to a variety of causes, such as cold, dirt, improper diet, and improper behavior. Blood and cold are related concepts in that blood is thought to be thicker during the winter to serve a protective function against problems associated with cold and thinner during the warmer months. Cold is seen as the cause of arthritis. Dirt and a failure to bathe are causes of illness as are irregular bowel movements and sexual excesses. In this belief system, it follows that the body must be cleaned. Some black Americans may be particularly concerned with gastrointestinal functioning and may abuse laxatives in an effort to maintain health. Menstruation is also viewed as ridding the body of dirty and excess blood. Preventing illnesses associated with dirt involves bathing, using laxatives, avoiding behaviors that would inhibit menstruation, and sexual moderation (Snow, 1983).

Table 8-1 provides an overview of common folk illnesses, along with the cause, signs and symptoms, practitioner, and treatment of black and Hispanic Americans. It will be helpful to you if you work with clients who hold these beliefs.

Scientific or Biomedical Paradigm

The second paradigm is the scientific or biomedical health paradigm. It is the paradigm of the American health delivery system.

> According to this world view, life is controlled by a series of physical and biochemical processes that can be studied and manipulated by humans. The scientific paradigm is characterized by several specific forms of symbolic thought processes. The first is

Folk Illnesses

Culture	Folk Illness	Etiology	Signs/Symptoms	Practitioner	Treatment
Hispanic	*Susto* (fright)	An individual experiences a stressful event at some time prior to the onset of symptoms. The stressor may vary from death of a significant person to a child's nightmare, to inability to adequately fulfill social role responsibility. Children are more susceptible to **susto.** *It is believed that the soul or spirit leaves the body.*	Restlessness during sleep Anorexia Depression Listlessness Disinterest in personal appearance	*Curandero* or *Espiritualista (Espiritista)*	A ceremony is performed using branches from a sweet pepper tree and a candle. Motions by the ill person and the curer are performed that form a cross. Three *Ave Marias,* or *credos* (Apostles' Creed) are said.
	Empacho	Bolus of undigested food adheres to the stomach or wall of intestine. The cause may be the food itself, or due to eating when one is not hungry, or when one is stressed.	Stomach pain Diarrhea Vomiting Anorexia	Family Member *Sabador Curandera*	Massage of the stomach or back until a popping sound is heard. A laxative may be given.
	Caida de la Mollera (Fallen fontanel)	Trauma—a fall or blow to the head or the rapid dislodging of a nipple from an infant's mouth causes the fontanel to be sucked into the palate.	Inability to suckle Irritability Vomiting Diarrhea Sunken fontanel	Family Member *Curandero*	One or more these: Insert a finger into the child's mouth and push the palate back into place. Hold the child by the ankles with the top of the head just touching a pan of tepid water for a moment or two. Apply a poultice of soap shavings to the fontanel. Administer herb tea.
	Mal de ojo (evil eye)	A disease of magical origin cast by a person who is jealous or envious of another person or something the person owns. The evil eye is cast by	Fever Diarrhea Vomiting Crying without apparent cause.	*Curandero Brujo*	Passing an unbroken egg over the body or rubbing the body with an egg to draw the heat (fever) from the body. Prayers such as the Our Father or

—Continued next page

Culture	Folk Illness	Etiology	Signs/Symptoms	Practitioner	Treatment
	Mal de ojo Continued	the envious person's vision upon the subject thereby heating the blood and producing symptoms. Usually a beautiful child is envied or admired but is not touched by the admirer and the evil eye can be inflicted. The admirer may not be aware of the damage done. If the child is admired and then touched by that person the evil eye is not inflicted.			Hail Mary may be said simultaneously with the passing of the egg. The egg is then broken in a bowl, placed under the head of the bed and left there all night. By morning if the egg is almost cooked by the heat from the body this is a sign that the sick person had *mal de ojo*.
	Mal Puesto (evil)	Illness caused by a **brujo,** witch, or **curandero,** or other person knowledgeable about witchcraft.	Vary considerably Strange behavior changes Labile emotions Convulsions	*Curandero* *Brujo*	Varies, depending on the hex.
Black	High Blood (too much blood)	Diet very high in red meat and rich food. Belief that high blood causes stroke.	Weakness Paralysis Vertigo or other signs/symptoms related to a stroke.	Family member or friend or Spiritualist or self. The later does this after referring to a Zodiac almanac.	Take internally lemon juice, vinegar, epsom salts, or other astringent food to sweat out the excess blood. Treatment varies depending on what is appropriate for each person according to the Zodiac almanac.
	Low Blood (not enough blood—anemia is conceptualized)	Too many astringent foods, too harsh a treatment for high blood. Remaining on high blood pressure medication for too long.	Fatigue Weakness	Same as for high blood	Eat rich red meat, live beets. Stop taking treatment for high blood. Consult the Zodiac almanac.
	Thin Blood (Predisposition to illness)	Occurs in women, children, and old people. Blood is thin until puberty, and remains so until old age except for women.	Greater susceptibility to illness.	Individual	Individual should exercise caution in cold weather by wearing warm clothing or by staying indoors.
	Rash appearing on a child after birth.	Impurities within the body coming out.	Rash anywhere on the body, may be	Family member	Catnip tea as a laxative or other

—Continued next page

Folk Illnesses—cont'd

Culture	Folk Illness	Etiology	Signs/Symptoms	Practitioner	Treatment
	Rash appearing on a child after birth. *Continued.* No specific disease name— the concept is that of body defilement.	The body is always being defiled and will therefore produce skin rashes.	accompanied by fever. commercial laxative. The quantity and kind depend on the age of the individual.		
	Diseases of witchcraft, "hex" or conjuring.	Envy and sexual conflict are the most frequent causes of having someone hex another person.	Unusual behavior that is not normal for the person. Sudden death Symptoms related to poisoning, i.e., foul taste, falling off (weight loss). Nausea. Vomiting. A crawling sensation on the skin or in the stomach. Psychotic behavior.	Voodoo Priest(ess) Spiritualist	*Conja* is the help given the conjured person. Treatment varies depending on the spell cast.

Reprinted with permission. © *The Nurse Practitioner: The American Journal of Primary Health Care, 1979,* (4) 23–34.

determinism, which states that a cause-and-effect relationship exists for all natural phenomena. The second, *mechanism*, relates life to the structure and function of machines; according to mechanism, it is possible to control life processes through mechanical and other engineered interventions. The third form is *reductionism*, according to which all life can be reduced or divided into smaller parts; study of the unique characteristics of these isolated parts is thought to reveal aspects or properties of the whole. One of the ideas of reductionism is *Cartesian dualism*, the idea that the mind and the body can be separated into two distinct entities. The final thought process is *objective materialism*, according to which what is real can be observed and measured. There is a further distinction between subjective and objective realities in this paradigm.

The scientific paradigm disavows the metaphysical. It usually ignores the holistic forces of the universe as well, unless explanations for such forces fit into the symbolic forms discussed above. Members of most Western cultures, including the dominant American cultural group, espouse this paradigm. When the scientific paradigm is applied to matters of health, it is often referred to as the 'biomedical model.' (Herberg, 1989, p. 28)

This belief system views all disease as having a cause that is known or unknown and is illustrated in Figure 8-3. Such causes may be related to "wear and tear (stress), external trauma (injury or accident), external invasion (pathogens), or internal damages (fluid and chemical imbalances or structural changes)" (Herberg, 1989, p. 29). If the cause is known, the next step is to institute a plan for its treatment and eradication from the body. Treatments consist of physical acts, such as dressing changes, exercise programs, inhalation therapy, and administration of medications. If the cause is unknown, then it may become the focal point of scientists who conduct scientific studies and search for it. The assumption is that a physical or chemical cause exists and that the condition could be treated,

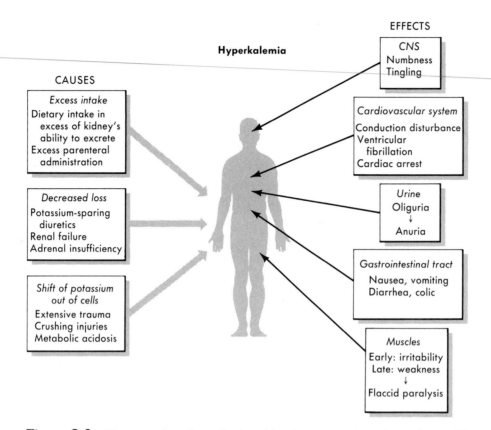

Figure 8-3 The scientific or biomedical model isolates a specific etiology. This model characterizes Western health care. *From P.G. Beare/J.L. Myers,* Principles and Practices of Adult Health Nursing, *ed 1, St. Louis, Mosby, 1990.*

if only the cause were known. This conceptualization of disease is supported by the federal government and many voluntary health agencies in the United States, which commit vast amounts of money to research endeavors.

Even psychologic processes are thought to have a basis in biochemistry. For example, schizophrenia and depression are thought to be caused by chemical imbalances (Andraesen, 1984). With this explanation, there is little room to accommodate other explanations for disease such as psychologic stress within families or at work.

The scientific or biomedical paradigm is the dominant belief system of white Americans. Belief in and use of the scientific method by researchers has led to new knowledge, knowledge that has

lengthened the life span of individuals with diseases, such as AIDS, cancer, Alzheimer's, multiple sclerosis, and infections.

Holistic Paradigm

The third paradigm for viewing health and illness is the holistic health paradigm. This paradigm is best described using the concepts of harmony and natural balance.

> Human life is only one aspect of nature and a part of the general order of the cosmos. Everything in the universe has a place and a role to perform according to natural laws that maintain order. Disturbing these laws creates imbalance, chaos, and disease. (Herberg, 1989, p. 29)

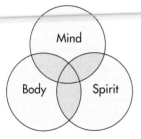

Figure 8-4 The holistic paradigm integrates body, mind, and spirit.

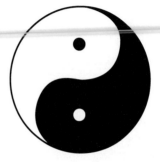

Figure 8-5 Yin Yang symbolizes forces in nature which are balanced to maintain harmony.

This paradigm views the totality of the person within the context of the total environment and represents unity among the body, mind, and spirit (see Figure 8-4). Within this framework, environment, behavior, and sociocultural factors are influential in the maintenance of health and the prevention of disease. This view may be found among Native Americans and Asian Americans. Components of it may be found among blacks, Hispanics, and whites.

➤ Three metaphors found in the holistic paradigm are yin/yang, hot/cold, and harmony/disharmony. Maintaining and restoring a balance among the three forces—yin/yang, hot/cold, and harmony/disharmony—is important to health. If imbalance occurs and persists, disease results and restoration is necessary.

Yin and Yang

Yin and yang represent forces in nature that regulate both the universe and the body. When they are in balance, there is harmony. The yin yang symbol is seen in Figure 8-5. Yin is the female force and characterized as negative, inactive, dark, cold, and empty. Yang is the male force and characterized as positive, active, full, light, and warm. Body organs and health states are categorized as yin and yang. The liver, heart, spleen, lungs, and kidneys are yin, whereas the gallbladder, stomach, large intestine, small intestine, bladder, and lymphatic system are yang. Cancer, lactation, menstruation, postpartum period, pregnancy, shivering, and wasting are yin

health conditions. Constipation, hangover, hypertension, infection, sore throat, toothache, upset stomach, and venereal disease are yang health conditions. An imbalance between yin and yang will result in illnesses, whereas a balance enhances health. Although this appears to be sufficiently straightforward, different cultures have different perceptions of what is classified as yin and yang. It is therefore best to work directly with a particular client's beliefs (Chang, 1991; Herberg, 1989; Ludman & Newman, 1984; Campbell & Chang, 1981).

Hautman (1979) uses the analogy of the interactive relationship between the sympathetic and parasympathetic nervous systems to understand yin and yang. "The yang forces protect the body in much the same way as the sympathetic system mobilizes the body for defense. The yin force is restorative and conserves body energy like that of the parasympathetic system (Hautman, 1979, p. 26)." Excessive yin forces cause colds, nervousness, and apprehension, and predisposes one to gastric disorders (Campbell & Chang, 1981), cancer, postpartum psychoses, menstruation, lactation (Chang, 1991), pregnancy, shivering, and wasting (Ludman & Newman, 1984). Excessive yang forces cause fever, dehydration, irritability, tenseness (Campbell & Chang, 1981), infections, hypertension, sore throat, toothache (Chang, 1991), constipation, hangover, upset stomach, and venereal disease (Ludman & Newman, 1984).

Yin and yang are also thought of as cold and

hot forces. Yin is cold and yang is hot. This conceptualization does not always relate to their physical characteristics (Hautman, 1979). For example, foods are categorized as yin and yang. These forces are thought to be either the cause or treatment of illness. If diseases or conditions with excessive yin forces are present, they are treated with yang foods such as beef, chicken, eggs, fried foods, spicy foods, hot foods, vinegar, and wine. If diseases or conditions with excessive yang forces are present, they are treated with yin foods such as bean curds, honey, carrots, turnips, green vegetables, fruits, cold foods, and duck (Ludman & Newman, 1984). Ginger root, considered to be hot, is used to strengthen the heart, which is a yang organ; ginger root is also given to treat nausea and dyspepsia, which are yin conditions (Campbell & Chang, 1981).

Hautman (1979) noted there is no master list of yin and yang illnesses, conditions, and foods. The health educator should discuss the situation with the client and assess the degree to which this particular client believes in yin and yang forces as etiologic agents and therefore appropriate treatments for his or her condition. From this base, culturally appropriate nursing interventions and health education can be planned. Respect for the client's beliefs will encourage compliance with the treatment regimen.

Hot and Cold

As noted above, the cause of illness may also be attributed to hot and cold imbalance. Asian and Hispanic clients are those most likely to believe in this conceptualization. The hot and cold imbalance is based on the Greek concept of the four body humors, which are yellow bile, black bile, phlegm, and blood. In a healthy individual, these humors are in balance, whereas they are in a state of imbalance in disease. In states of imbalance, the goal is to restore by adding or subtracting substances that affect the humors. If a hot substance caused the disease, then to restore balance, the treatment would be the application of the opposite quality. Hot or cold refers to qualities possessed by air, food, beverages, medicines, herbs, and body organs. The terminology is misleading in the sense that hot or cold classification is not necessarily based on temperature or spiciness. For example, conditions considered hot are fever, infections, diarrhea, kidney problems, rashes, sore throat, liver problems, ulcers, and constipation. Examples of cold conditions are cancer, pneumonia, malaria, joint pain, menstrual periods, teething, earache, rheumatism, tuberculosis, colds, headache, paralysis, and stomach cramps. Examples of hot medicine or herbs include anise, castor oil, cod liver oil, iron tablets, penicillin, tobacco, garlic, cinnamon, vitamins, and aspirin. Examples of cold medicine or herbs are Linden flowers, mannitol, nightshade, orange flower water, sage, milk of magnesia, and bicarbonate of soda. How foods, beverages, and medicines are classified varies across cultural groups and may not be the same from group to group (Kuipers, 1991; Herberg, 1989; Murillo-Rohde, 1981; Andrews, 1989).

Harmony and Disharmony

Black Americans might hold beliefs related to the concept of harmony and balance. One common belief is that illness is a natural occurrence that results from disharmony and conflict in some aspect of one's life. Another related belief is based on the concept of opposites. For example, for every birth there must be a death; for every marriage there must be a divorce; and for every occurrence of illness, there must be a recovery. Although health is viewed to be a gift from God, illness is seen as God's punishment for sin (Snow, 1983).

Native Americans may believe in living in harmony with nature and in the wholeness of the person. According to this belief, one should not separate the body and the mind. To be sick is to be out of harmony with nature. Although Native Americans may recognize the value of Western medicine, they may continue to value the medicine man or woman and folk practices, such as ceremonies, singing, rituals, and chants (Primeaux & Henderson, 1981).

The holistic health paradigm is gaining favor in the United States. Concepts related to this world view are found in some nursing programs today. Although this view is not replacing belief in the biomedical model, the holistic paradigm broadens the view of the nature of health and disease. Through the holistic paradigm, other factors are considered as important as the biomedical approach to the achievement of the fullness of health. The holistic paradigm includes biologic, mental, emotional, spiritual, sociologic, cultural, and environmental factors as well as relationships and lifestyle choices. This paradigm allows for the presence of wholeness during high-level wellness and during the process of dying or coping with chronic disease. Many nurses are no longer willing to ignore healing forces that they perceive as powerful and effective even if these forces cannot be explained by the re-

ductionistic and mechanistic paradigms.

As you contemplate these paradigms, remember that they are quite logical to the believer. What may not make sense to you may make a lot of sense to someone else. These paradigms are not a disparate collection of misinformation and superstition. They are systems of belief that have been years in the making and have worked for past believers (Maduro, 1983).

Vestiges of all of these paradigms can be found in the belief systems among whites. For example, the concept of moderation in all things is commonly found among whites, particularly those with

---

T A B L E   8 - 2

Summary of Belief Systems About Health and Illness*

	Magico-Religious	Scientific/Biomedical	Holistic
World view	Fate of world is under control of supernatural forces. God(s) or other supernatural forces for good or evil are in control while humans are at the mercy of natural forces.	Life is controlled by physical and biochemical processes that can be studied and manipulated by humans.	Harmony, natural balance. Human life is only one aspect of nature and part of the general order of the cosmos. Everything in universe has a place and role according to laws that maintain order.
Illness/disease	Initiated by supernatural agent with or without justification, via sorcery. Cause of health or illness is not organic, rather it's mystical. Causes: possession by evil spirits, breaching a taboo, supernatural forces (sorcery, witchcraft).	Wear and tear, accident, injury, pathogens, and fluid and chemical imbalance. Cause/effect relationship exists for natural events. Life related to structure and functions like machines. Life can be reduced or divided into smaller parts. Mind and body two distinct entities. Cause exists, if only it were known.	Disease, imbalance, and chaos result when these laws are disturbed.
Health	Gift or reward given as a sign of God's blessing and good will.	Illness prevention activities; restoration through exercise, medication, treatments, and other means.	Environment, behavior, and sociocultural factors are influential in maintenance of health and prevention of disease. Maintaining and restoring balance are important to health.
Ethnic group	Hispanic Americans, black Americans; components found in other groups.	White Americans.	Native Americans, Asian Americans; components found in other groups.
Other concepts			Yin/yang Hot/cold Harmony/disharmony

*Modified from Albers cited in Herberg, P. (1989). Theoretical foundations of transcultural nursing. In Boyle, J.S. & Andrews, M.M. *Transcultural concepts in nursing care*. Boston: Scott, Foresman.

strong Christian influences. Moderation in food intake, work, play, and family relationships is stressed within this framework. The maxim, "All work and no play makes Johnny a dull lad," conveys this message. The concept of moderation parallels that of harmony and balance (holistic paradigm). The concept of holistic health is a relatively new concept in health care. It is being embraced by a greater number of nurses, but it has yet to find its way into mainstream thinking in the nursing profession.

Another belief held by many whites is that disease is a punishment for sin. Beseeching God for relief is common. In part, this helps explain the role of the clergy in American hospitals. Although whites might not admit to holding a strong belief in the mystical and spiritual world, many would not consider beginning the day without reading their horoscope. During the Reagan presidency, such beliefs were alleged to be a factor in managing the affairs of this country (magico-religious paradigm).

It is inaccurate to conceptualize the biomedical model as free of superstitions or untrue beliefs. Much of what Western health practitioners do is not supported by research. Practitioners engage in certain practices because they believe them to be in the best interest of clients. A good example of this is a recent study, which found that deeply anesthetized infants undergoing cardiac surgery had a significantly lower mortality rate than did infants receiving light anesthesia (Anand & Hickey, 1992). The deeply anesthetized infants also had a lower incidence of sepsis, metabolic acidosis, and disseminated intravascular coagulation. This research conflicts with the present practice of operating on babies while using very light anesthesia. Light anesthesia has been preferred because doctors believed it to be less toxic for babies, not because they had a scientific base for the belief (scientific or biomedical paradigm). A summary of the three belief systems about health and illness is given in Table 8-2.

Folk Medicine and Folk Practitioners

Folk medicine encompasses a variety of popular remedies that are designed to maintain health, re-store health, or prevent disease. Common treatment modalities include chicken soup, herbs, poultices, and religious practices and rituals. Treatments may be self-administered, administered by close friends or family, or administered by a folk practitioner.

Identification and training of folk practitioners is the local or indigenous way in which a cultural group provides health care for its members. Folk practitioners have developed and refined their skills over many generations and continue to be active in many communities, satisfactorily serving clients (Leininger, 1978). Each paradigm has its own unique health practitioner.

You can expect that some clients will be seeking help from their respective folk practitioners at the same time they are seeking help from Western health practitioners. Do not try to stop this activity because it will create needless problems in your relationship with the client. Such attempts might even create a crisis of confidence, and you might never see the client again. A better approach would be to learn to operate within the client's belief system as well as the biomedical system. Inquire about the folk practitioner the client is seeing and consider how the two treatment plans can be blended to create the best treatment plan for the client.

Individuals of various ethnic groups often view Western medicine as effective for certain problems and folk practitioners more effective for others. For example, some Chinese Americans believe tuberculosis is best treated by Western medical practitioners, whereas skin diseases and blood disorders are best left to folk practitioners (Campbell & Chang, 1981).

Let us focus briefly on the various folk practitioners sought out by the different ethnic groups. A widely consulted Hispanic folk practitioner is a curandero (male) or curandera (female). Another Hispanic practitioner may be a family member, an espiritualista or a spiritualist, a yerbero, or a sabador. Native Americans may be served by the medicine man or woman, also known as a shaman. An "Old Lady," a spiritualist, and a voodoo priest or priestess are types of folk practitioners that might be used by black Americans. Asian Americans might see an herbal specialist (Hautman, 1979). Refer to Table 8-3.

The curandero or curandera is the traditional Hispanic healer. This practitioner treats most of the traditional illnesses. We have had the privilege of working with a curandera who was hired by the city-supported health care facility, Denver Health and Hospitals. The curandera described her role as a link between the Mexican American belief system and the white health delivery system. The curandera provided a listening ear and cultural understanding to the client while linking the client with health care services the client needed. In addition, the curandera could provide culturally appropriate treatments. The espiritualista or spiritualist's role is to prevent illness or bewitchment by using medals, prayers, and amulets, whereas the yerbero's role is prevention and cure using herbs. The sabador's role is similar to that of the chiropractor (Hautman, 1979).

For the black American, the church may play an important role in maintaining cultural traditions. The most important person to serve this client is the minister (Smith, 1976). A black folk practitioner may be an older woman, a spiritualist, or the voodoo priest or priestess. The older woman commonly uses spices, herbs, and roots to treat diseases, whereas the spiritualist combines rituals, spiritual beliefs, and herbal medicines to bring about a cure. The voodoo priest is knowledgeable about the herbs and the interpretation of signs and omens. This practitioner also treats illness caused by voodoo. Some Mexican Americans and Native Americans might also seek out the voodoo priest (Jordan, 1979; Hautman, 1979).

Black American voodoo has three major components (Jordan, 1979). The first deals with spells and spirits, the magical component; the second component deals with psychologic support for the client; and the third component is herbal and folk medicine. Spiritualists may be excellent therapists in that they listen and offer counsel to clients with various kinds of anxieties and neuroses, thereby helping clients cope with life's events more effectively.

Navajos have their medicine men and women who serve in a variety of roles, such as diagnostician of the cause of disharmony. These practitioners perform and direct healing ceremonies; they also treat illnesses through the use of herbs (Hanley, 1991).

The Chinese American may go to an acupuncturist, an herb pharmacist, or an herbalist, all of whom provide similar treatments. The herbalist examines the client and then prescribes herbs that the herbalist or an herb pharmacist provides. The client may approach the herb pharmacist for advice and treatment recommendations. The acupuncturist will also examine the client but his or her treatment is different because it consists of inserting fine needles into various parts of the body (Campbell & Chang, 1981).

Ask your client about the advice given by the folk practitioner and any treatment prescribed to determine if these practices are helpful, neutral, or harmful from the biomedical perspective. If you determine that the practice is harmless and valued by the client, it is best to reinforce and support the practice or, at the least, let the information and treatment go unchallenged.

If the advice or treatment is harmful to the client, then the nurse should carefully explain why this is so. It will be helpful for others in the client's support network to hear your explanation. Sometimes when clients are under stress, they may not remember what you have said, or the client may have misunderstood your message. Misperceptions may also occur, particularly if you and the client do not share the same primary language. If the client is older, it may be helpful for a younger member of the client's support network to hear your message. The younger person may be more familiar with or less frightened by Western health care practices. This person may be a positive force in ensuring the client's compliance with your health teaching.

There are times when adding a new practice works better than forbidding an entrenched practice. For example, a medical practitioner said that he was unsuccessful at getting the midwives in a South American community to stop sealing off umbilical cord stubs with dung (animal manure). "Finally we decided to teach the midwives to give

Folk Practitioner for Various Ethnic Groups

Culture	Folk Practitioner	Preparation	Scope of Practice
Hispanic	Family member	Possesses knowledge of folk medicine	Common illnesses of a mild nature that may or may not be recognized by modern medicine.
	Curandero/Curandera	May receive training in an apprenticeship. They may receive a "gift from God" that enables them to cure. Knowledgeable in use of herbs, diet, massage, and rituals.	Treats almost all of the traditional illnesses. Some may not treat illness caused by witchcraft for fear of being accused of possessing evil powers. Usually admired by members of the community.
	Espiritualista or Spiritualist	Born with the special gifts of being able to analyze dreams and foretell future events. May serve an apprenticeship with an older practitioner.	Emphasis on prevention of illness or bewitchment through use of medals, prayers, amulets. May also be sought for cure of existing illness.
	Yerbero	No formal training. Knowledgeable in growing and prescribing herbs.	Consulted for preventative and curative use of herbs for both traditional illnesses and Western illnesses.
	Sabador (may refer to a chiropractor by this title)	Knowledgeable in massage and manipulation of bones and muscles.*	Treats many of the traditional illnesses particularly those affecting the musculo-skeletal system. May also treat non-traditional illnesses.
Black	"Old Lady"	Usually an older woman who has successfully raised her own family. Knowledgeable in child care and folk remedies.	Consulted about common ailments and for advice on child care. Found in rural and urban communities.
	Spiritualist	Called by God to help others. No formal training. Usually associated with a fundamentalist Christian church.	Assists with problems that are financial, personal, spiritual, or physical. Predominantly found in urban communities.
	Voodoo Priest(ess) or *Hougan*	May be trained by other Priests(esses). In the U.S. the eldest son of a priest becomes a priest. A daughter of a priest(ess) becomes a priestess if she is born with a veil (amniotic sac) over her face.	Knowledgeable in properties of herbs, interpretation of signs and omens. Able to cure illness caused by Voodoo. Uses communication techniques to establish a therapeutic milieu like a psychiatrist. Treats blacks, Mexican-Americans, and Indians.
Chinese	Herbalist	Knowledgeable in diagnosis of illness and herbal remedies.	Both diagnostic and therapeutic. Diagnostic techniques include interviewing, inspection, auscultation, and assessment of pulses.

*Preparation is for *Sabador*, not Chiropractor.
Reprinted with permission. © *The Nurse Practitioner: The American Journal of Primary Health Care, 1979,* 4(4), 23–34.

tetanus shots to newborns. This added to their status and gave them another skill, which was also useful in vaccinating the population at large" (personal communication).

As you contemplate the role of ethnic folk practitioners, remember that you yourself do not see a physician every time you become ill. There are many problems you treat by yourself, such as colds, backaches, stomachaches, headaches, diarrhea, and constipation. As a nursing student, you probably have noticed that your family and friends have consulted you about health matters. They see you as possessing special knowledge and skill that, when shared, may restore them to health. This is essentially the role of a folk practitioner.

Applications to Health Education

Information on various cultures will help you to understand the needs of clients from other cultural backgrounds as you fulfill your role as a health educator. In providing health education, your goals are to communicate the message, to see that it is understood within the context of the client's belief system, and to encourage compliance. To achieve these goals, we will now look at cultural assessment, communication, locus of decision-making, and nutritional habits that affect health education. We will also examine an application to a specific health problem.

Cultural Assessment

The following guidelines will help you when conducting a cultural assessment of a client who has a health problem and needs health education. When asking questions, it is important that you consider the client's vocabulary and level of comfort (Tripp-Reimer, Brink, & Saunders, 1984).

Before beginning your questions, establish rapport with the client by giving something of yourself. Introduce yourself and let the client know your role and how long you will be around. When appropriate, address the client's physical condition.

Example: "The other nurse told me you have been in this country for 2 months now. How is it going for you?" or
"I see that you are pale and look worried."

Early in the interview, ask the client how long she or he has been in this country. This information, along with the client's age, will give you a rough estimate of the client's position along the continuum of acculturation. Refer to the box on p. 144 for questions related to cultural assessment. We recommend that you use the questions as a guide for areas to explore. It is crucial that you couch your questions in metaphors and language that will be understandable to your clients.

Communication

Effective communication is a lifelong challenge. Communication style and patterns are established early in life and are reinforced within the culture. Even when cultural heritage and family upbringing is common to a group of individuals, misunderstandings are a daily occurrence. It is frequently necessary to clarify the meaning of messages. It is not difficult to imagine how the challenge of effective communication is compounded when individuals come from different cultural backgrounds. Communication is further complicated by the technical nature of Western health-related messages that must be sent and received.

We will now turn our attention to communication styles among the various ethnic groups. It will help you to contrast these styles with the culturally dominant white style of communication in which people are expected to speak up and let others know what they are thinking. Generally, whites value assertiveness in communications, whether in the work setting, family, community, or political arenas. Whites might expect others to identify their needs, ask questions when a meaning is unclear, and express their feelings. Within families, whites often expect open communication and resolution of problems. Indeed, family therapy models are based on this expectation. For the most part, the white

1. Can you tell me about your problem? How can I help you today?
2. What do you think has caused your problem?
3. Why do you think it started when it did?
4. What does your sickness do to you? How does it work?
5. How severe is your sickness? Do you think it will have a long or short duration?
6. What kind of treatment do you think you should receive?
7. What are the most important results you hope to receive from this treatment?
8. What are the chief problems your sickness has caused you?
9. What do you fear about your sickness?
10. What does this condition mean to you?
11. Is it a hot or cold condition? What foods or other conditions do you need to aid your recovery? What do you need to avoid?
12. What have you been doing for your sickness in the past? What are you doing for it now?
13. What do you plan to do about this condition?
14. How should a person with this condition act?
15. How should one with this condition be treated by the family?
16. What can be done to help? What should not be done?
17. Who in your family gives advice on how to stay well or get better?
18. Does this condition affect your spiritual health?
19. What would be helpful to you in restoring your spiritual health?
20. Would you like me to pray with you? (Offer only if you, the nurse, would feel comfortable with this suggestion.)

culture is a vocal one. Figure 8-6 illustrates the basic importance of communication to health education.

Verbal Communication

In working within a culturally diverse community, listen carefully to the words a client uses to describe his or her condition. How is the condition de-

scribed? How sophisticated is the language the client uses? What words are used repeatedly? This will provide some direction for you as you begin to establish rapport with the client.

As you converse, come to an understanding of what key words mean. For example, the black client may use the term *high blood* to mean there is too much blood in the body or that blood has suddenly shot up into the head (Snow, 1983), whereas you may call this condition hypertension. Other terms the black client may use are *miseries* to mean pain; *low* or *tired blood* to mean anemia; *locked bowels* to mean constipation; and *running off* or *grip* to mean diarrhea (Cherry & Giger, 1991).

Some clients might be reluctant to share personal information. For example, Latin Americans might believe it is inappropriate to reveal personal circumstances or family information to others. Murillo-Rohde (1981) noted that many Hispanics believe that personal or family information should never be revealed to strangers or even friends if the situation does not involve these people. Family matters are private and best kept within the family. Many Native Americans hold similar beliefs. Those who hold these beliefs might value individual rights and feel that each person has the right to speak only for himself or herself. No other member of the family has the right to speak for another person. For this reason, it might be difficult to obtain information from family members about your Native American client (Primeaux & Henderson, 1981). Both of these examples are in contrast to whites, who are more open and willing to share personal and family information.

As you converse, use words that are simple and appropriate to the client's characteristics. This means that you will need to constantly translate medical jargon into language suitable for your client. This will be necessary for virtually all clients unfamiliar with Western health care. Black clients who are used to speaking black English might take offense if you attempt to use the same pronunciation or phraseology. They might perceive this as mimicking them. The nurse should also avoid chiding or correcting the client's speech. It is important for the nurse to realize that black English is considered

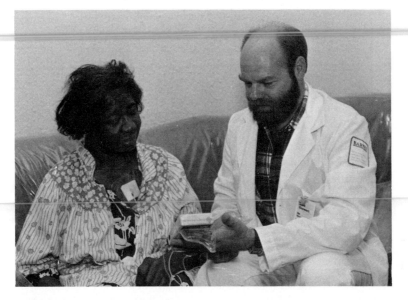

Figure 8-6   The ability to communicate with clients from different cultures is fundamental to effective health education. *Photo by Greg Blumenfeld from R. Rice,* Home Health Nursing Practice: Concepts and Application, *Mosby, St. Louis, 1992. Used with permission.*

neither substandard nor ungrammatic (Cherry & Giger, 1991; Thomas, 1981). We have noted black English being spoken by some black professionals with whom we work. They speak it most frequently when they are with other blacks and feeling comfortable in their surroundings. They commonly use Standard English when conversing with whites.

Asians might also be very reluctant to express themselves verbally. They might prefer to communicate indirectly, which will take some effort on your part to identify their concerns. In conversing with Chinese Americans, avoid using a negative when asking questions. Such questions might not make sense to them grammatically and might leave them in a quandary about how to reply.

Example: "Haven't you taken your medication today?"

This question might be difficult for them because the question is difficult to answer. Is the correct reply, "Yes, I haven't taken them?" or "No, I have taken them?" Clients might feel embarrassment and shame regarding their perceived inadequate linguistic skills (Chang, 1991).

Nonverbal Communication

Nonverbal communication is important in dealing with culturally diverse clients. As you seek feedback from clients about their understanding of your message, you might expect a polite, positive response, perhaps with some nodding and other gracious nonverbal behaviors. Many clients of Hispanic, black, and Asian heritage will frequently exhibit these behaviors as a sign of courtesy and respect for the health educator. It does not necessarily indicate that the clients understand what you are saying and agree with it. It may just be their way of dealing with health care providers. For example, during the teaching of a Hispanic American with newly diagnosed diabetes mellitus, the essential highlights of the disease, the need for daily insulin injections, the proper injection technique, and injection site rotation were carefully explained. Throughout the presentation, the young male client listened and nodded appropriately. Although verbal communication was limited, nonverbal client feedback indicated he was grasping the information. When asked to demonstrate the injection procedure on a model, the client could not do so and was terribly embarrassed that he had not grasped what was taught.

Eye contact is an important variable in nonverbal communication. Whites tend to value eye contact and interpret it as being fully attentive to the speaker. Other cultural groups do not share this interpretation. Navajos might avoid eye contact, because direct eye contact is viewed as a sign of disrespect. To Native Americans, looking into another's eyes is to look into his or her soul, and might even cause the loss of the soul (Primeaux & Henderson, 1981). Asian Americans might also avoid direct eye contact. Making direct eye contact is a sign of rudeness; avoidance of eye contact does not indicate inattention (Chang, 1991).

The Chinese tend to value silence and harmonious relationships, which translates into avoidance of disagreements and criticism. Harmony is valued so highly that the Chinese might decline to openly disagree with one another. Even raising the voice might be viewed as a loss of control. The word "no" is seldom heard; rather, expressing the negative is more subtle. For example, facial expressions, tensions, movements, the speed of interaction, and the location of interaction communicate meaning (Chang, 1991). Asians are very sensitive to nonverbal behaviors. This style of communication is in contrast to that of Latin Americans, who are more emotional and freely use hand gestures while communicating.

In contrast with many Latin Americans, most Chinese Americans do not value touching while conversing. It is important for you to remember that it might be inappropriate to touch the head of Chinese Americans, especially babies. The head of an Asian baby is considered very delicate, and patting it on the head can be quite dangerous. To touch someone while arguing indicates a shameful loss of self-control (Chang, 1991).

Sketches and body language such as pantomime can be quite useful and amusing. A nurse's willingness to appear "foolish" reduced tension with one Asian family, and the use of stick drawings enhanced communication, both verbal and nonverbal. The family members laughed and then used gestures and pictures of their own to make their messages quite clear.

Communication Challenges

Other communication challenges might be encountered. Thomas (1981) helps us understand the range of behaviors some blacks might exhibit. These behaviors may include submission, outward aggression and anger, and/or paranoia. These behaviors have their roots in the history of racial prejudice. Some black Americans have adopted defensive behaviors in response to the hostile environment created by multiple discriminatory experiences, which have been a daily occurrence in this country.

> In a crowded environment, where high unemployment is the norm, where the primary cause of death among black men between the ages of 21 and 25 is homicide, and where at each critical point the black man's normal masculine development is thwarted, hostility is bound to prevail. Certainly hostility is a means of survival for individuals living in this type of environment. (Thomas, 1981, p. 215)

In communicating with black Americans who display the above-mentioned behaviors, recognize that you are not being personally attacked. Recognize the behavior as a style of communication developed over time. It serves no purpose if you are drawn into defensive behaviors and respond in kind. It will be much more effective if you reflect back the emotions the person is communicating.

> *Example:* "I can see you are angry. What do we need to do, so we can communicate more effectively?"

Once this has been addressed, it may be possible to continue with your health education.

Your professional communication serves as the means by which your clients gain a greater understanding of their health status and achieve some degree of control over it. Adequate communications are fundamental to achieving this. In working with culturally diverse groups, you will find yourself focusing more on communication to ensure that your clients are understanding your message. It is important that you learn to communicate as effectively as you can in order to fully serve your culturally diverse clients.

Teaching/Learning Context

Within the teaching/learning situation, the teacher is viewed as an authority. Some clients, especially Asians, will be reluctant to ask questions or to provide the feedback you need as a teacher to let you know that your message needs to be adapted to fit their particular circumstances. You will need to make an extra effort to provide a comfortable learning environment and to draw clients out. Many Asians are reluctant to ask questions. To do so is to challenge the teacher's knowledge. Let your clients know that their questions are welcome and that you expect them to ask some. Give them every opportunity to ask questions and clarify misunderstandings. You can do this by ensuring that the teaching situation is relaxed and unhurried. You can also provide more time for clients to formulate their questions and gather the courage to verbalize their concerns. Ask only one question at a time and then give them time to think about it. This may mean that the periods of silence will be longer than whites find comfortable. Invite the Asian clients to see you in private if they continue to be reluctant. Another important factor is to remember to be friendly and not condescending. In the long run, these approaches may be effective in engaging your clients.

Some clients may have a poor command of English or may not speak it at all. When teaching these clients, you must identify the most important messages to communicate. Distinguish between that which is essential from that which is nonessential. Identify what needs to be communicated right away from that which could wait until another visit. Once you have identified the appropriate health education content, then communicate one point at a time. Focus on that message until you are confident that the client understands it before you go on to the next point. Such thoroughness is difficult when you are very busy, but it is best to have fewer points fully communicated than to review many items, none of which are fully understood by the client. Jumbling messages together might only ensure that none of them will be understood.

If you work in an area with a large number of people who speak no English, you might consider learning their language. At minimum, you could learn some key words and phrases associated with the most commonly seen health problems for which health education is essential. This outreach gesture on your part would demonstrate your caring and concern for the clients you serve.

Use of Interpreters

It may be necessary to use an interpreter when the client does not speak English. Many Hispanic Americans and Native Americans are bilingual, but some first-generation Hispanics and Native Americans speak only their native tongue and are dependent upon family and others to translate for them. This might also be true for your Asian American clients, particularly those who are recent immigrants from Southeast Asia.

Interpreters can be wonderful, depending on their bilingual, bicultural skills and their rapport with the health teacher and the client. If you find it necessary to work through an interpreter, Putsch (1985) and Nidorf and Morgan (1987) have made a number of helpful questions to consider. Is the person you are considering for the role of interpreter employed in the health care institution? If so, is interpreting the person's primary, full-time job? If the person uses interpreting as a part-time, secondary job, then the interpreter might be hurried and might not fully appreciate the need for a complete investigation into the client's health background and problem. The result may be brief, inadequate answers. How much medical background does the interpreter have? Is he or she knowledgeable about medical jargon and procedures? Does the client trust the interpreter? Interpreters who are employees of the health care institution might be influential members of the ethnic community and might be someone the client knows socially. How comfortable is the client sharing personal information in these circumstances? If the interpreter is a member of the family, will an adolescent who wants birth control education feel at ease? It is best not to have a member of the family serving in this role unless it is clearly the client's choice.

Once you have determined that an interpreter is essential to providing health education, the next step is to take some time and establish rapport with this person. Let him or her know what you expect during the teaching/learning encounter. Position yourself so that you face your client. Then, speak directly to the client, not to the interpreter. It is, in fact, the client with whom you are communicating, who is the focus of your professional efforts, not the interpreter. As the interpreter translates for both parties, observe the client's nonverbal communication. What is this communication telling you? Are there nuances about which you should seek further information? Does the client's body language match the interpreter's message?

As you are conversing, keep in mind that there may be no equivalent word between English and another language. For example, the words bacteria, allergies, and depression simply do not exist in the Navajo language. It will be necessary to use other terminology to communicate some messages. Your health message should be simple. Present only one point at a time until you have communicated all essential points, and keep your information on a concrete level by avoiding the abstract. Abstract conceptualizations do not readily translate and will only serve to confuse the client (Putsch, 1985).

Convey your message in short phrases. Allow the interpreter to convey each part before continuing. Be alert to the length of transactions. Many times an expert interpreter will speak a long paragraph of context before giving advice or asking for the information you seek. If the interpreter's message is shorter than yours, it may be that the interpreter is not fully understanding and/or communicating your point. A knowledgeable and skillful interpreter may need to give the client a long paragraph of context before he or she can convey your question in a way that will be intelligible to the client. You might need to speak with the interpreter for a while to find out what you can meaningfully convey. If the interpreter's message is much shorter than the client's verbalizations, assume the client's message did not get back to you. It might be that

the client is complaining and the interpreter is sparing your feelings.

Sometimes an interpreter is simply not available when you need help communicating with a client. Modern technology can be helpful under these circumstances. One creative nurse found a skilled interpreter who was willing to help interpret but had a very busy life and could not be physically present with the client. This interpreter handled interpretation over the phone by speaking alternately with the nurse and client. While not ideal, this solution proved effective in this situation.

If you and the client must continue your interchange without an interpreter, be patient and supportive of the client's attempts to communicate. One client, who grew up in a household that spoke only Spanish, said that when she went to school she knew nothing about English. The other children laughed at her and called her a dummy. When she tried to speak English at home her family ridiculed her, so she decided to stop speaking. Sharing these experiences helped the client begin relating differently to white professionals.

The client who does not speak English, like the person who cannot see, hear, or speak, does not benefit from English shouted louder. Flash cards are often quite helpful. These can be simple pictures of common activities or objects needed by the hospitalized person. By speaking to the client in normal English and gesturing freely, you can convey a surprising amount of information. Pantomime also helps. Your efforts to convey a message or ask a question through the use of dramatic gestures can be amusing and help reduce tension. This in itself will improve communication efforts.

Decision-Making in Families

You might expect clients you teach to make health-related decisions on their own; after all, their lives are directly affected. Such behavior is characteristic of many white Americans who value individuality and the assumption of responsibility for decisions. However, if you persist with this expectation, you might find some surprises as you work with individuals from other cultures. Other ethnic groups involve the entire family in the decision-making process. To provide effective, culturally appropriate health education, the nurse must consider the client's family. The family provides the "social context within which illness occurs and is resolved, and within which health promotion and maintenance as well as treatment are defined and promulgated" (Boyle, 1989, p. 231).

Family is very important to all the ethnic groups presented here—Hispanics, Native Americans, black Americans, and Asian Americans. Although most whites emphasize the nuclear family—consisting of mother, father, and children—other groups might include the extended family. When extra support is needed, whites tend to look to individuals and groups outside the family. Hispanic Americans might include grandparents, aunts, and uncles in the definition of family. It is upon these relatives that Mexican Americans will probably depend and from whom they will seek help if it is needed (Kuipers, 1991). Boyle (1989) stated:

> Because of the strong family orientation of Latin families, the family plays a significant role in all aspects of the ill member's life, including either rejection or reinforcement of health lifestyle changes. It is therefore crucial that the family be involved in the plan of care from the beginning (p. 232).

Within the black family, the wife or mother might be assigned the responsibility for the health of family members, including assisting others in maintaining good health and determining treatment if a person becomes ill (Cherry & Giger, 1991). The dominant family figure in most black families is the mother or the oldest female in the household (Boyle, 1989).

This is in contrast to some Hispanic American families in which the husband or father is dominant and serves as principal decision-maker. In these families the mother is expected to be submissive. Such roles are grounded in behaviors, such as *machismo* (manliness). The "Mexican culture prescribes that the men are stronger, more reliable, and more intelligent than women. Machismo dictates that the man will show a high degree of individuality outside

the family. Weakness in male behavior is looked down on" (Henderson & Primeaux, 1981, p. 71). Identifying the primary decision-maker is important because this person must be included in your health teaching and in generating support for the health education goals of your client.

In general, the Navajo family is matriarchal in structure. Mother is responsible for the needs of the family within the home, whereas the father's focus is on responsibilities outside of the home (Hanley, 1991). The concept of family extends beyond the nuclear family to include grandparents, aunts, uncles, cousins, and even nonblood relatives who are members of the same tribe. These extended members may even live together at various times; this practice may be seen among families who have relocated to urban settings. Navajos value family so much that "to be poor in the Indian world is to be without relatives" (Primeaux & Henderson, 1981, p. 242). Family members are a source of security, strength, and emotional support during times of crisis and may all, including the children, be involved in the decision-making process (Boyle & Andrews, 1989).

Many Asian families are hierarchic in structure. In such families, elders and ancestors are respected and revered, and children are expected to submit and show deference to their elders and other authority figures. Family communications are one-way, from parent to child. Failure to adhere to these expectations brings on feelings of shame and guilt. Strong feelings are rarely verbalized, but when they are, this action demonstrates a lack of self-control and poor socialization. Asians are taught to avoid calling attention to themselves and are therefore likely to be silent during any group health education activity (Henderson & Primeaux, 1981).

Nutritional Habits and Patterns

Food habits and patterns are a function of many variables. Our first exposure to food patterns comes from our earliest moments, the circumstances surrounding our birth and upbringing. We are nourished by foods selected by our caretakers according to their preferences. Food choices are a function of the availability of foods in a particular region of the country, economic circumstances, ethnic factors, and religious influences. Over time, we expand our exposure to foods and develop our own preferences. We also establish daily dietary habits, such as the time we eat, the number of meals, the size of our meals, and preferred ways of food preparation. The meal itself becomes an event with greater or lesser significance in each of our lives.

Western health care emphasizes the importance of nutrition in the maintenance of good health and prevention of disease. Good nutrition is important in every developmental phase of life—from birth, through the growth years, pregnancy, and old age. Proper nutrition is also an important factor in recovery from disease. It is a treatment modality for a number of diseases, such as hypertension, diabetes mellitus, and gastrointestinal problems.

In making a judgment about culturally appropriate health teaching about nutrition, first perform a thorough assessment of the client. You will want to know about the client's usual nutritional patterns.

> *Example:* What foods are usually eaten?
> In what quantities are specific foods eaten?
> How are the foods usually prepared?
> How many meals are eaten per day?
> How frequently are meals eaten at home?
> Away from home?
> How regular are the meals?
> Does the weekend pattern differ from the weekday pattern?

In evaluating the data, determine whether the client's nutrition practices are beneficial, neutral, or harmful (Andrews, 1989). If the practice is beneficial or neutral, then no nursing interventions are needed other than reinforcing the client's choices. If it is harmful, then you will want to develop a teaching plan to help the client change it. Incorporate into your teaching plan food that the client and family usually eat. Make this the point of departure for starting your discussions. From here, culturally acceptable foods may be added or deleted as necessitated by the health problem.

When a client must change a dietary practice

in response to disease, major adjustments might be necessary. For your nutritional education to be effective, it must be appropriate to the cultural context of the client. This might require you to make some adaptation in your usual health teaching and in the teaching materials you use to illustrate your message. Working with clients to change dietary habits may be quite frustrating. Andrews (1989) reminds us that of all the cultural practices modified during the process of acculturation, dietary habits are the most enduring.

Ethnic-Specific Nutritional Information

In discussing ethnic-specific nutritional information, it is pointless to generalize about specific dietary practices or deficiencies. The dietary practices of ethnic groups vary widely because of geographic areas, economic factors, knowledge of nutrition, food preferences, and food preparation practices. To determine whether a client is nutritionally deficient, it is best to perform a thorough assessment. Only general ethnic nutritional information will be included here.

Black Americans

The nutritional patterns of black Americans are very similar to those of non-blacks living in the same geographic region (Cherry & Giger, 1991). Blacks in the lower socioeconomic class are more prone to have dietary deficiencies. Heckler (1985) noted that there is no characteristic dietary pattern for blacks. Other variations, such as urban or rural, southern or nonsouthern, native born or foreign born, and religious affiliation, affect eating patterns.

Among blacks, common health problems related to nutrition are hypertension, obesity, and lactose intolerance. Soul foods, such as collard greens, chitterlings, and dandelion greens are all heavily seasoned with salt and spices. Salt contributes to water retention, which is problematic in the management of hypertension. Greens are rich sources of vitamins A and C and calcium.

The majority of American blacks, Hispanics, Native Americans, and Asians are lactose intolerant. This is a condition in which the body is lactase deficient. Lactase is an enzyme that breaks down lactose, which is found in milk. The client may develop flatus, abdominal pain, and perhaps vomiting and diarrhea as a result of ingesting milk (Andrews, 1989). Milk products, such as buttermilk, yogurt, fermented cheese, and small quantities of milk, might be tolerable.

Some black Americans believe in "high blood," which means there is excess blood in the body. Strokes are believed to result from high blood and are attributed to eating too much rich food, red meat, or pork. According to this belief, pregnant women are particularly susceptible to high blood. Women may avoid this condition by not eating meats and high-calorie foods and by increasing the consumption of sodium-rich foods. The treatment for high blood is the "use of astringent and acidic foods, such as vinegar, lemons, pickles, and Epsom salts to open the pores and let excessive sweat escape" (Andrews, 1989, p. 339).

Dietary adjustments might be difficult for diabetic clients who are black and who are in the lower socioeconomic strata. Many of the foods on the exchange lists are not within economic reach of clients, and foods that are on the lists might not be palatable to them (Thomas, 1981). This results in poor control of the disease process. When teaching such clients, determine the client's usual dietary patterns and food choices. From this assessment, you might be able to provide guidance and/or negotiate a compromise. One nurse, for instance, got an elderly client to lift her collards and dandelions out of the fluid flavored with salt pork before the client ate the greens.

Hispanic Americans

The diet of Hispanics is generally adequate to meet daily dietary requirements. Consumption of sodium and carbohydrates is high in many diets (Heckler, 1985). Food staples vary with the region of the country. Examples of commonly consumed foods are beans, tortillas, eggs, chicken, lard, chili peppers, onions, tomatoes, squash, potatoes, bread, carbonated beverages, herb teas, canned fruits, gelatin, sweets, and sweetened, packaged breakfast cereals. In the Southwest more chili, chili con carne, enchiladas, tamales, tostadas, chicken mole, and nopalitos are eaten. Migrant workers in California eat refried beans, tacos, tortillas, and some hamburgers, macaroni and cheese, and hot dogs (Andrews, 1989).

For Hispanic clients who believe in the hot and cold theory for the treatment of disease, special dietary practices might be undertaken. For example, a client may increase the intake of a hot food to relieve the body imbalance caused by a cold. As long as there is no contraindication regarding the choice of the hot food, the practice should be viewed as harmless and supported. One nurse was consulting with a pregnant woman (hot condition), who was reluctant to take vitamins (hot food). The nurse asked for a list of cold foods to counterbalance the vitamins. Together they agreed upon orange juice.

Native Americans

Dietary practices are different among the various American Indian tribes. Food availability, preference for nonminority food, and place of residence (urban or reservation) affect choices. In general, diets are high in refined carbohydrates, fat, and sodium and low in meat, eggs, cheese, and milk (Heckler, 1985). Nutritional problems may be attributed to food scarcity and insufficient variety among foods. Fresh fruits, vegetables, and meats are expensive and frequently not available. Corn, beans, and squash are common foods. Chili pepper is widely used as a spice. The diet of most Native American tribes tends to be high in carbohydrates and fats and deficient in protein, calcium, essential vitamins (C and A), and minerals (Hanley, 1991; Andrews, 1989).

Asian Americans

Asian Americans favor rice as the primary source of calories, along with vegetables, fruits, fish, and shellfish. Because dairy products are infrequently used, calcium is obtained from soybean curd (when it is set with calcium), sardines, and green leafy vegetables (Heckler, 1985). Common dietary choices of Chinese Americans include rice, pork, chicken, vegetables, eggs, various soy preparations, and tea. Foods are cooked briefly thereby retaining vitamins.

Sodium intake is high, whereas fat intake is usually low. Vietnamese Americans favor fish, rice, vegetables, and tea (Andrews, 1989).

Soy sauce, commonly used by Chinese Americans, is high in sodium and therefore presents problems to clients on sodium restricted diets. Campbell and Chang (1981) noted that it is useless to instruct the client to stop using soy sauce. A better approach is to have the client limit the amount of soy sauce used while cooking. Some companies now offer low-sodium soy sauce, which might work as an alternative.

Health Education for Clients with Specific Health Problems

We will now focus on information that may be helpful to you as you teach clients about hypertension. We use hypertension as an example because it is common across ethnic groups and provides countless opportunities for health education.

One common assumption you might make is that clients view health and illness as you do. You might also assume they understand what has caused their illness and will see logic in the steps they must take to get well and to prevent future problems. To be successful in working with culturally diverse clients, you will need to recognize that these are faulty assumptions. Even when you recognize the major differences among the belief systems across various cultural groups, you might still have a tendency to assume that all clients from a single cultural group hold similar beliefs. This assumption is also faulty. Just as there is tremendous variety in the belief, attitudes, and behaviors among whites, there is also great individual diversity among non-whites. Problems arise when you fail to recognize these differences and fail to take them into consideration when providing health education.

Hypertension is a silent disease with few subjective symptoms. Clients frequently become aware of it during health screening activities. Because they experience no symptoms, clients might find it difficult to believe that the condition requires treatment. Once treatment for hypertension begins, it might be difficult to get the client to sustain the medication regimen because the medication might

have some negative side effects, such as sexual impotence. Some clients might suspect that the physician is simply making money by unnecessarily urging medications to treat a condition that is not creating any perceivable problems.

The word *hypertension* means different things to different people. Although Western medicine defines hypertension as blood pressure in excess of 140 over 90 (American Heart Association, 1991), others confuse it with psychologic tension and stress. Black Americans might equate your references to hypertension to a natural folk illness referred to as "high blood." High blood means either there is excess blood in the body or that the blood has shifted its location, which occurs when there is believed to be increased flow to the brain. Both of these events are related to diet and emotions and may result in a stroke (Snow, 1981; 1983). Some blacks confuse hypertension with nervousness and stress. Similar misunderstandings were found among Mexican Americans (Ailinger, 1982) of whom only 28% knew the correct definition of hypertension. Incorrect definitions were bad circulation, rapid heart rate, tension or nervousness, and feeling hot.

Treatment for hypertension is a lifelong activity. It requires daily medications and subsequent monitoring of the medication regimen. Usually, hypertension requires a client to change dietary habits by reducing the amount of sodium consumed and by losing excess weight. If the client smokes, giving up this habit is advised. Other life-style changes might be in order, such as how the client copes with the stresses of daily living. Black Americans (Snow, 1981, 1983) might use astringent foods, such as vinegar, lemon juice, and pickles, to treat hypertension. You will need to teach the client to avoid salty foods.

Mexican Americans might have difficulty with the concept of long-term treatment of hypertension because their primary concern is with the relief of symptoms, and they are not as interested in the long term (Kub, 1986). While Kub noted they expect a cure with short-term therapy, Ailinger (1982) documented a surprisingly high level of knowledge regarding treatments. Ailinger found that 92% believed medicines would relieve hypertension, 89% were aware that a low-sodium diet was a treatment modality, and 85% were aware that exercise was effective in relieving hypertension. Continuance of treatment even after a normal blood pressure is obtained was known by 95% of the respondents. How will you address these health education issues with culturally diverse clients? Begin with the assumption that you share responsibility with the client for maintaining control of the client's hypertension (Kub, 1986). This creates a relationship whereby changes in attitudes and behaviors can be facilitated.

Consider targeting children for health education. Wheeler and colleagues (1983) found statistically significantly higher systolic and diastolic blood pressures among black children. Because health behaviors and habits are established early in life, you might be more effective with your health education by focusing on the younger age groups. By establishing health patterns early in life, you might be able to reduce the number of health problems seen in later life.

Special Problems in Health Education

Intergenerational Value Conflicts

Intergenerational value conflicts might be a problem that you will need to take into consideration (Rawl, 1992). Conflict might exist between immigrant parents and their children. The younger generation might be caught between the values and beliefs of their parents and the desire to become Americanized and be like their American counterparts. For example, Asian parents value respect for authority and expect this from their children. This means the children are expected to accept the parent's position and not question it. Yet these same children are exposed to American children who are taught to verbalize their feelings, behavior that Asian parents view as disrespectful. Conflict within the Asian family results. An example of intergenerational conflict is found in Figure 8-7.

Intergenerational conflict might cause considerable strain within the family. "Migrant youngsters, particularly, often view their parents as old-fashioned, rigid, and adhering too staunchly to what

they perceive as backward customs and traditions. More than other adolescents, these youngsters may perceive parental constraints and pressures as unfair and unrealistic" (Nidorf & Morgan, 1987, p. 76).

Consider the situation of 18-year-old Amy, who came into a street clinic for abortion counseling. Amy was Hispanic, approximately 7 weeks pregnant, and terrified of having a baby. She had just graduated from high school and was looking forward to college. She did not want to spend the rest of her life in the neighborhood where she was raised and saw education as her way out of it. She felt she was too young to begin a family and was not ready to marry. In short, she wanted an abortion but was terrified of her family's reaction, particularly her father's. She was very anxious, embarrassed about her situation, and deeply concerned about confidentiality. Upon being assured of confidentiality, Amy shared her concerns. Having an abortion would go against the family's religious beliefs as well as her parent's expectation that she remain a virgin until she marries. She could not tolerate the thought of seeing the disappointment in their eyes. But equally strong were Amy's feelings that she was simply too young to begin a family. Her plans were to continue with her education, become financially independent, and then consider marriage and family, the same plan shared by two of her close, influential friends. The nurse presented to Amy the choices regarding her pregnancy. Because Amy had already made up her mind about having an abortion, a referral was made to the city health facility. Amy had the abortion done the next week and everything went well. Four weeks later she returned for birth control counseling.

Another type of intergenerational conflict is occurring among children who have lived in this country for 10 to 15 years and who are now bringing their elderly parents to the United States. This is the situation of many Vietnamese families. The parents are expecting to find their children adhering to the beliefs and values they were taught, but instead they find that their children have become Americanized.

In assessing intergenerational conflict, ask about the client's social contacts outside of the home.

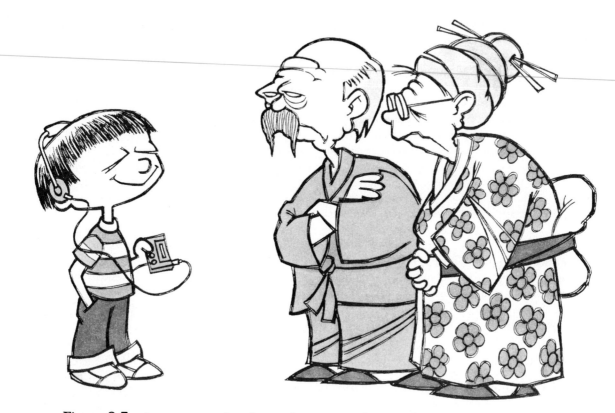

Figure 8-7 Intergenerational conflict is a factor to consider in teaching culturally diverse families.

Example: How involved is the client in the community?

Is he or she employed?

Doe he or she participate in a church?

How often is he or she out of the house?

How influenced has the client been by the American culture?

Your teaching approach will differ depending on whether the clients have few or many contacts outside of their ethnic communities.

Cultural Differences Between Client and Nurse

All people have cultural needs just as they have physical and psychologic needs. Recognizing and meeting cultural needs is less problematic when you and the client share the same cultural heritage. It is more problematic when you and the client are from different cultural backgrounds (Boyle & Andrews, 1989). It is important for you to recognize when differences exist and to take them into consideration when planning health education.

In the coming years, it is expected that the nursing profession will become more effective in recruiting and retaining nurses from culturally diverse backgrounds. It is important that nurses from all ethnic backgrounds recognize cultural differences between themselves and clients. Because most nurses belong to the dominant cultural group, it is easy to assume they are the ones who will need the most cultural sensitivity training. However, all nurses, regardless of cultural heritage, need to develop this sensitivity. For example, an Asian nurse will need to learn to be sensitive to the beliefs and touch needs of the elderly Hispanic client. Hispanic nurses will need to learn the health beliefs and practices of black clients. Black nurses will need to learn how to work with Native American folk practitioners to achieve culturally appropriate goals. This is the nature of the world in which we live.

Being sensitive to the needs of culturally diverse clients means several things, according to Boyle and Andrews (1989). It includes:

(1) identifying cultural needs,
(2) understanding the cultural context of the client and family, (3) using culturally sensitive nursing strategies to meet mutual goals,
(4) having the skills to use the resources of a variety of cultural subsystems within a community, and (5) having the ability to learn from and respond to culturally diverse situations (p. 67).

This is a challenge for all who aspire to become professional nurses.

Approaches to Health Education

How can you communicate your health message to culturally diverse populations? How can you most effectively reach the many special populations that are at risk and need to be educated? The Secretary's Task Force on Black and Minority Health (Heckler, 1985), recommended continued efforts in disseminating health information, education materials, and program strategies specifically designed for minority sectors of the population. These efforts should be directed to the major health problems, which are cancer; cardiovascular disease; chemical dependency; diabetes; homicide, suicide, and unintentional injuries; and infant mortality. We will now direct our attention to some of the ways in which you can educate culturally diverse communities.

No single medium is effective in reaching all population groups. Television, however, comes the closest. Putnam and colleagues (1982) found that mass media approaches, such as television and radio spots, were more effective awareness-raising vehicles than primary educational tools, such as printed

material in teaching Hawaiians about the dangers of excessive sun exposure. Television was the primary source of information, followed by their doctors, magazines, newspapers, and family or friends. Whites and Filipinos received their information primarily from television and their doctors. The primary source of information for the Chinese and Japanese was the newspaper. The Hawaiian's primary source was television and family or friends.

In a similar study of white, black and Mexican Americans, Corell (1984) found that television was the primary source of information for all three groups. Following television whites turned to magazines, then family members for information. Blacks turned to physicians followed by pamphlets, and Mexican Americans turned to magazines and then to radio.

Health information and education materials must be developed that are developed for a specific cultural group. Such materials must be attractive to the target group and written at an appropriate readability level. These materials will be more effective if they are compatible with the cultural beliefs of that group. If you are participating in the development of these materials, you might find it helpful to form an advisory group composed of members who are representative of the various target groups, both clients and professionals, who can offer valuable insights (Heckler, 1985).

Other, more novel approaches might prove effective and need further study. For example, telephone information numbers are advertised as part of a media blitz for raising community awareness of a particular health problem. The fact that use of these numbers dramatically increases during the blitz does not answer the question of who uses them. Some theorize that this helpline strategy is more effective among the white, middle class, urban, and suburban populations.

In this electronic age, videotapes might prove an effective medium for health education. McAvoy and Raza (1991) found videotaped health messages more effective than leaflets or fact sheets in persuading Asian women to be tested for cervical cancer. Leaving the videotape for the woman to watch at her leisure was more effective than watching it at a set time with the health educator. The effectiveness of the leaflets and fact sheets increased when they were reviewed with clients by the health educator.

Many pamphlets, leaflets, and fact sheets are printed in the language of the target cultural group. Remember that all of the information about readability level and attractiveness is as applicable to culturally diverse groups as the dominant culture. Ideally, written materials should be culture specific, but this may not always be possible. Even if materials are available in a client's primary language, remember that the client might be illiterate.

Other community-wide approaches might be effective. For example, in one small community with a large population of Mexican American, migrant farm workers, health educators organized a family social/health fair. Word about the fair circulated among the workers and many attended. Lively games and activities appropriate for all age groups were available. Also available were booths where blood pressures were taken, nutritional counseling given, and specific health education provided. Health providers and educators thus attempted to become a part of the cultural group they serve. It was an effective means of developing trust.

In providing health education for a particular cultural group, consider holding it in a setting where people will feel most comfortable. The social/health fair just described was held at the local school children attended during the day. Other suitable settings for you to consider are churches, community centers, and places of employment. Perhaps someone would be willing to have a small group meet in his or her home. It might enhance your credibility if you are willing to teach in the client's preferred setting rather than your own.

Summary

A cultural assessment for health education involves collecting information about the client's ethnic heritage, health beliefs and practices, religious beliefs, dietary practices, family relationships, daily lifestyle pattern, and sick-role behavior. If your assessment reveals that a knowledge deficit exists, then determine the direction for your health education effort.

Example: What needs to be communicated the most?
What can you reasonably achieve?

Then discuss this with your client and together establish appropriate education goals. Include the family to the degree that it is culturally appropriate for this particular client. Consent and cooperation of the client is fundamental to any effective health education effort and expectation for long-term compliance. Community education efforts might be even more effective if they are conducted within the cultural expectations of the target population.

However sophisticated and enthusiastic your teaching methods might be, you might "miss the boat" if you fail to assess your clients' health beliefs. These beliefs affect clients' adherence to lifestyle changes. It is important that you look beyond your own beliefs to investigate the beliefs of your clients.

It is equally ineffective to take the few bits of information you acquire about cultures other than your own and apply these generalizations as facts, rather than as guidelines for individualized investigation. Generalizations, thus, can be barriers to knowledge when they become stereotypes unaccompanied by observation and critical thinking. Learn to use generalizations as a place to begin while you conduct a thorough assessment of your client.

CROSS-CULTURAL COMMUNICATION

Purposes:

- Develop your skills in the area of cultural assessment
- Apply anthropologic principles to client teaching
- Deepen your awareness of the differences among cultural definitions of health, illness, trust, and self-responsibility

Directions:

- Interview someone whose cultural heritage is different from your own.
- Use the following questions as an interview guide. You may develop your own questions as well.

1. In your family, what does "good health" mean?
2. How can you tell if someone is healthy or sick?
3. What can you do to keep your family well? What did your mother do to keep the family well?
4. What home remedies do you use? What home remedies did your mother use when anyone in the family was sick?
5. Did you ever go to someone for advice when you were sick?
6. Who did you go to?
7. What kind of advice did this person give to help you recover?
8. What causes sickness?
9. What can you do to avoid the major kinds of sickness?
10. What do you feel is important to you in life?
11. What do you do to maintain your religious health?
12. Describe three things you value most in life.

MULTICULTURAL LEARNING

Purposes:

- Become more aware of cultural differences among your colleagues
- Strive for an attitude of respect for cultural differences

Directions:

1. Find out which nurses in the class grew up in rural communities, in very traditional homes, in first-generation immigrant homes and/or with elderly relatives.
2. Divide into groups. The groups should be homogeneous according to one of the variables mentioned in No. 1.
3. In your group decide what you could teach your colleagues from your intuitive and first-hand knowledge of your culture and upbringing.

References

Ailinger, R.L. (1982). Hypertension knowledge in a Hispanic community. *Nursing Research, 31*(4), 207-210.

American Heart Association. (1991). *1991 Heart and Stroke Facts.* Dallas: Author.

Anand, K.J.S. & Hickey, P.R. (1992). Halothane-morphine compared with high-dose sufentanil for anesthesia and postoperative analgesia in neonatal cardiac surgery. *New England Journal of Medicine, 326*(1), 1-9.

Andraesen, N.C. (1984). *The broken brain.* New York: Harper & Row.

Andrews, M.M. (1989). Culture and nutrition. In J.S. Boyle & M.M. Andrews, *Transcultural concepts in nursing care* (pp. 333-355). Boston: Scott, Foresman.

Baca, J.E. (1978). Some health beliefs of the Spanish speaking. In R.A. Martinez, (Ed.). *Hispanic culture and health care* (pp. 92-98). St. Louis: Mosby.

Boyle, J.S. (1989). Alterations in lifestyle: Transcultural concepts in chronic illness. In J.S. Boyle and M.M. Andrews, *Transcultural concepts in nursing care* (pp. 223-241). Boston: Scott, Foresman.

Boyle, J.S. & Andrews, M.M. (1989). Transcultural perspectives in the nursing process. In J.S. Boyle & M.M. Andrews, *Transcultural concepts in nursing care* (pp. 67-92). Boston: Scott, Foresman.

Campbell, T. & Chang, B. (1981). Health care of the Chinese in America. In G. Henderson & M. Primeaux, (Eds.) *Transcultural health care* (pp. 162-171). Menlo Park CA: Addison-Wesley.

Capers, C.F. (1992). Teaching cultural content: A nursing education imperative. *Holistic Nursing Practice, 6*(3), 19-28.

Chang, K. (1991). Chinese Americans. In J.N. Giger & R.E. Davidhizar, *Transcultural nursing assessment and intervention* (pp. 359-377). St. Louis: Mosby.

Charnes, L.S. & Moore, P.S. (1992). Meeting patients' spiritual needs: The Jewish perspective. *Holistic Nursing Practice, 6*(3), 64-72.

Cherry, B. & Giger, J.N. (1991). Black Americans. In J.N. Giger & R.E. Davidhizar, *Transcultural nursing assessment and intervention* (pp. 147-182). St. Louis: Mosby.

Corell, J. (1984). Ethnicity and cancer prevention in a tri-ethnic urban community. *Journal of the National Medical Association, 76*(10), 1013-1019.

Evaneshko, V. (1984). Ethnic and cultural considerations. In B.M. Steffl, (Ed.). *Handbook of gerontological nursing.* New York: Van Nostrand Reinhold.

Flaskerud, J.H. (1989). Transcultural concepts in mental health nursing. In J.S. Boyle & M.M. Andrews, *Transcultural concepts in nursing care* (pp. 243-269). Boston: Scott, Foresman.

Foster, G.M. (1981). Relationships between Spanish and Spanish-American folk medicine. In G. Henderson & M. Primeaux, (Eds.) *Transcultural health care* (pp. 115-135). Menlo Park CA: Addison-Wesley.

Germain, C.P. (1992). Cultural care: A bridge between sickness, illness, and disease. *Holistic Nursing Practice 6*(3), 1-9.

Hanley, C.E. (1991). Navajo Indians. In J.N. Giger & R.E. Davidhizar, *Transcultural nursing assessment and intervention* (pp. 215-238). St. Louis: Mosby.

Hautman, M.A. (1979). Folk health and illness beliefs. *The Nurse Practitioner: The American Journal of Primary Health Care, 4*(4), 23-34.

Heckler, M. (1985). *Report of the Secretary's Task Force on Black and Minority Health,* U.S. Dept of Health and Human Services, 1985.

Henderson, G. & Primeaux, M. (1981). The importance of folk medicine. In G. Henderson & M. Primeaux, (Eds.). *Transcultural health care* (pp. 59-77). Menlo Park CA: Addison-Wesley.

Herberg, P. (1989). Theoretical foundations of transcultural nursing. In J.S. Boyle & M.M. Andrews, *Transcultural concepts in nursing care* (pp. 3-65). Boston: Scott, Foresman.

Jordan, W.C. (1979). The roots and practice of voodoo medicine in America. *Urban Health, 8*(10), 38-48.

Kub, J.P. (1986). Ethnicity: An important factor for nurses to consider in caring for hypertensive individuals. *Western Journal of Nursing Research, 18*(4):445-456.

Kuipers, J. (1991). Mexican Americans. In J.N. Giger & R.E. Davidhizar, *Transcultural nursing assessment and intervention* (pp. 185-212). St. Louis: Mosby.

Leininger, M. (1978). *Transcultural nursing: Concepts, theories and practices.* New York: John Wiley & Sons.

Leininger, M. (1970). *Nursing and anthropology: Two worlds to blend*. New York: John Wiley & Sons.

Ludman, E.K. & Newman, J.M. (1984). Yin and Yang in the health-related food practices of three Chinese groups. *Journal of Nutrition Education*, 16(1), 3-5.

McAvoy, B.R. & Raza, R. (1991). Can health education increase uptake of cervical smear testing among Asian women? *British Medical Journal*, 302(6780), 833-836.

Maduro, R. (1983). Curanderismo and Latino views of disease and curing. *Western Journal of Medicine*, 139(6), 868-874.

Murillo-Rohde, I. (1981). Hispanic American patient care. In G. Henderson & M. Primeaux, (Eds.). *Transcultural health care* (pp. 224-238). Menlo Park CA: Addison-Wesley.

Neufeldt, V. (Ed.) (1991). *Webster's New World Dictionary* (3rd ed.). Cleveland: Webster's New World.

Nidorf, J.F. & Morgan, M.C. (1987). Cross cultural issues in adolescent medicine. *Primary Care*, 14(1), 69-83.

Primeaux, M. & Henderson, G. (1981). American Indian patient care. In G. Henderson & M. Primeaux, (Eds.). *Transcultural health care* (pp. 239-254). Menlo Park CA: Addison-Wesley.

Putnam, G.L., Brannon, B. & Yanagisako, K.L. (1982). Multimedia public/professional skin cancer education in a multiethnic setting. *Issues in cancer screening and communications*. New York: Alan R. Liss.

Putsch, R.W. (1985). Cross-cultural communication: The special case of interpreters in health care.

Journal of the American Medical Association, 254, 3344-3348.

Rawl, S.M. (1992). Perspectives on Nursing Care of Chinese Americans. *Journal of Holistic Nursing*, 10(1), 6-17.

Smith, J.A. (1976). The role of the Black clergy as allied health care professionals in working with Black patients. In Luckraft, D. (Ed.). *Black Awareness: Implications for Black Patient Care*. New York: The American Journal of Nursing.

Snow, L.F. (1981). Folk medical beliefs and their implications for the care of patients: A review based on studies among Black Americans. In G. Henderson & M. Primeaux, (Eds.). *Transcultural health care* (pp. 78-101). Menlo Park CA: Addison-Wesley.

Snow, L. (1983). Traditional health beliefs and practice among lower class Black Americans. *Western Journal of Medicine*, 139(6):820-828.

Thomas, D.N. (1981). Black American patient care. In G. Henderson & M. Primeaux, (Eds.). *Transcultural health care* (pp. 209-223). Menlo Park CA: Addison-Wesley.

Tiedt, P.L. & Tiedt, I.M. (1990). *Multicultural Teaching*. Boston: Allyn and Bacon.

Tripp-Reimer, T., Brink, P.J., & Saunders, J.M. (1984). Cultural assessment: Context and process. *Nursing Outlook, 32*, 78-82.

Wheeler, R.C., Marcus, A.C., Cullen, J.W., & Konugres, E. (1983). Baseline chronic disease risk factors in a racially heterogeneous elementary school population: The "know your body" program, Los Angeles. *Preventive Medicine, 12*, 569-587.

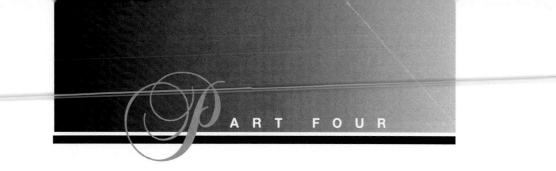

PART FOUR

Preparing the Teaching Module

Analyzing Assessment Data

. . . If you are not sure where
you are going, you may end up
someplace else!

Inspired by Mager (1984).

Objectives

Upon completion of this chapter you will be able to:

- Identify three purposes for stating learning objectives.
- Discuss the use of at least five factors that need to be considered in establishing learning objectives.
- Describe how the selection of content is affected by time constraints.
- Differentiate between words commonly used in writing behavioral objectives that have few interpretations and words that have many interpretations.
- Formulate learning objectives in each of the three domains.
- Select the appropriate hierarchical order of complexity (taxonomy of learning objectives) in each of the domains in a given situation.
- State the rationale for selection of content in a given teaching/learning situation.

Key Words

learning objectives   levels of complexity   conditions
content   performance   criteria
learning taxonomies

Introduction

In the previous chapters, we examined input into the teaching/learning system and addressed the assessment step of the nursing process. Now we deal with the question: So what? How will all that data you collected help you decide what to teach your clients? You will analyze the data you collected during the assessment phase of the teaching/learning process. To select the appropriate content you will decide what clients need to learn.

As a result of the assessment phase, you will have identified those deficiencies and/or potentials in the clients' knowledge, attitudes, or skills that you realistically can alter. Do clients desire information that you can supply? Do their attitudes suggest a potential for even better health? Do their attitudes interfere with their healing and/or sustaining health? Do they lack skills that would promote their recovery or prevent further deterioration of health? Are they interested in acquiring skills that would promote optimum health? Analyzing clients' needs leads to formation of the objectives of nurse/client teaching. Because analysis of clients' needs appears to be the

—Continued next page

163

most difficult component of the nursing process to learn (Andersen & Briggs, 1988; Kim, McFarland & McLane, 1989), we have included some examples in Appendix D. In Appendix D you will find brief vignettes, nursing diagnoses, and learning objectives and our rationale for choosing these objectives. At the end of this chapter, we have included an exercise designed to help you integrate nursing diagnosis with selection of behavioral objectives; for example, outcomes for client teaching. Nursing diagnosis as a rational model of thinking is well-suited to the development of learning objectives with and for clients (McFarland & McFarlane, 1989).

General Considerations

Content selection should be based on what clients need rather than what you find easiest or least threatening to teach. Certainly you will have the authority to teach much content in the areas of health promotion and maintenance, prevention of illness, recovery from disease, and reduction of the aftermath of accidents and other forms of dysfunction. To stay current you will educate yourself regarding the current research in any field you teach so that you can remain informed of current knowledge.

You can also teach some aspects of related disciplines. You will be qualified to give basic information on the pyramid. For example you could help a client understand that butter is *not* a member of the milk, yogurt, and cheese group, even though it *is* a dairy product and a derivative of milk. From the perspective of the pyramid, butter is a member of the fats, oils, and sweets group, which should be used sparingly. It does not have the protein and calcium that foods in the milk, yogurt, and cheese group have. The food groups have been reevaluated to emphasize the importance of complex carbohydrates and to decrease the intake of fat (Hamilton, Whitney, & Sizer, 1991).

It has been our experience that nurses in general assume clients know more than they do. Kleoppel and Henry (1987) reported that clients understand much less than medical personnel think

they do. Clients are also much less clear about concepts that medical personnel believe they have conveyed quite well. You will learn to reach a balance between assuming clients know more about health related matters than they do and failing to find out what clients already know. Many people today are indeed taking more responsibility for their own health and recovery; however, they are by no means the majority of clients whom you will encounter.

Establishing Learning Objectives

The definition of an objective is a goal, something worked toward or striven for (Neufeldt, 1991). Goals are frequently called objectives in the educational literature, which contains much of the research on learning and planning.

The main purpose of stating objectives is to guide planning, implementation, and evaluation of the desired learning. Teaching is the helping relationship in which the outcome of the relationship is most clearly spelled out (Litwack, Linc, & Bower, 1985). Objectives help you make clear, to yourself and to your clients, exactly what is to be accomplished. These objectives serve as guides for planning action, and they indicate what needs to be measured and evaluated to determine the success of the teaching effort. Another important purpose of stating objectives is to help clients organize their own personal style of approaching and focusing on the learning tasks (Mager, 1984).

Objectives function as advance organizers. An advance organizer is a statement, activity, or object that helps your audience develop a mind set most conducive to meeting the intended learning objective(s). Advance organizers vary according to your characteristics, those of the client, and those of the situation. Advance organizers may address cognitive, affective, and/or psychomotor objectives. The following is an advance organizer for the cognitive domain.

Example: "You have already learned to give yourself insulin; today we're going to focus on why you need to take it and how it works in your body."

In the affective area of learning, you might say the following.

> *Example:* "You say that you are now aware that your anger is harmful to yourself and you want to find ways to be less angry. Let's explore three methods and hope that at least one of them suits you and is worth pursuing further."

In the area of psychomotor learning you might say the following to clients.

> *Example:* "By the time we're done today, you'll be able to give yourself your own shot."

Factors to Consider When Establishing Objectives

In addition to determining the domains in which clients are deficient, you need to take into account: your own educational philosophy, the philosophy of the client's physician and the hospital or other caregiving system.

> *Example:* How much should clients know?
> How much independence should clients be allowed?
> How much independence should the client be required to exhibit?

A related concern is the institution's educational policies. It is important that you become aware of nursing service standards relative to client education. You should also know the standards published by the American Hospital Association.

Knowing who determines what clients should be taught is also important. In many institutions with strong nursing leadership, nurses establish their own professional areas of responsibility. In some private institutions, however, physicians retain control of all educational decisions.

It is also important to identify what clients want to learn. Attitudes among the general public as well as the medical professions are changing. It is no longer considered ethical or effective to discount this consideration (Bandman & Bandman, 1988). In addition to what they want to learn, you will con-

sider clients' developmental, emotional, and experiential readiness. For example, clients in denial are less likely to benefit from teaching efforts than those who are facing their health challenges. An example of experiential readiness is the level of literacy. If the client cannot read, then you will need to choose strategies that do not depend on reading ability.

In these days of diagnostic related groups (DRG) and Medicare restrictions, you will need to give careful attention to time factors. You will also need to consider time factors in prioritizing, teaching, and collaborating with other colleagues who may teach on other shifts or after discharge. Many lessons take time to be learned. You will establish priorities, select intermediate objectives, make sequential arrangements, and provide for continuity of care. For example, this might include stating clearly how far the client has progressed in learning and what remains to be learned. Forms for continuity of care are very important in facilitating this process.

Another reality that affects the establishment of objectives is the environment in which the learning will take place. This includes the physical environment as well as the psychologic atmosphere.

> *Example:* What is the physical environment like?
> Is functional audiovisual equipment available?
> Are sufficient pamphlets, posters, and books available?
> Is the learning atmosphere unhurried?
> Is there sufficient time to learn?
> Is it a nonthreatening atmosphere where clients feel free to learn?

Clear communication is a prerequisite for establishing objectives and evaluating learning. To be clear, you will need to use words with precise meanings. Use clear language when writing objectives, particularly when choosing the verb that identifies the action the client is to take. Mager (1984) differentiated verbs that are open to many interpretations from verbs that are open to fewer interpretations. Verbs that are open to many interpretations are more vague and describe internal events that cannot be seen or measured. Verbs that

Verbs with Vague or Specific Meanings	
Vague Verbs	**Specific Verbs**
know	write
understand	recite
really understand	identify
have faith in	contrast

are open to fewer interpretations are more specific and concrete. They are more apt to be behaviors or indicators that you and the client can see. Verbs that are more precise describe external events that are measurable. In the box above, we have provided a sample list of vague and specific words.

Components of Clear Objectives

Purpose

Mager (1984) discussed the importance of defining objectives precisely in substantial detail. In addition to explaining the importance of specific words, he used a three-part method of writing objectives, which has been found to be quite useful. Although the method is not flawless, it does help with clarity. Mager's three-point method for writing objectives follows.

Performance

Performance is any activity in which the client is to engage, such as any activities the client will be able to do. The activity can be a visible one, such as writing or repairing, or invisible, such as adding, solving, or identifying.

Conditions

If there are important conditions under which the performance is expected to occur, then these conditions should be spelled out.

> *Example:* What will the client be allowed to use?

What equipment is the client expected to use?
Under what time constraints is the learning to occur?

The statement of conditions is not always necessary to the clear statement of objectives, but it should be included when pertinent. Conditions might be stated with the following phrases.

> *Example:* "Given a list of. . . ."
> "Given an injection kit. . . ."
> "Given a urine sample. . . ."

Criteria

The quality or level of performance that will be considered acceptable should be specified. How well must the client perform for the learning to be considered successful? The criteria might include concepts, such as *amount*. For instance, clients may be considered successful if they are able to slow their pulse during relaxation training by 5 beats per minute. *Accuracy* would be an important criterion when a client is preparing an insulin injection. Others might be: *without any verbal guidance* or *from memory*.

Together with the client, the doctor, and the institution, you have looked at the factors that must be considered when you determine what the client is to learn. You have considered the importance of wording your objectives so that you will be able to communicate the goals to clients and colleagues. You also considered a three-part framework for the clear statement of an objective.

In nursing you are usually concerned with wanting clients to think, feel, or do something differently that will positively affect their health. The learning domains related to these goals have been identified as the cognitive, the affective, and the psychomotor domains. In addition to determining the domain in which learning will be concentrated, you will think about the level of complexity and the depth you believe clients should achieve. One purpose for this selectiveness is the need to be precise. There is quite a difference between the level of knowledge needed to answer the question, "Why is the IV in the top of your hand?" and the question "What did the IV pyelogram show regarding the functioning of your kidneys?" Another purpose for specificity is to help you identify the target level that is appropriate to the task. There is a difference between the client's giving his or her own insulin and doing his or her own dialysis. Learning how to write behavioral objectives will prepare you for the future. As education becomes an increasingly large part of health and sickness care, you must be knowledgeable about recognized structures for establishing and measuring learning objectives. Finally, you must be able to communicate to colleagues who will continue the client teaching you have started. They may do this on subsequent shifts, classes, clinic visits, or in the home.

Historical Context

A great deal of thinking and research about the stating of objectives has occurred in the field of education, particularly among specialists in the field of testing and evaluation. The following section of this chapter introduces the subject and outlines some of the concepts that have been borrowed from that field.

In 1948, at an informal meeting of college examiners attending the 1948 American Psychological Association Convention in Boston, a desire to improve the reliability of evaluation emerged. Several attendees wanted to develop a theoretic framework that could be used to facilitate consistent evaluation. They believed that such a framework could do much to promote the exchange of test materials and ideas about testing.

It was obvious to the group that they were attempting to classify phenomena that could not be observed—namely thinking and conceptualizing. The questions were raised: What does the phrase *really understand* mean? What does *internalize knowledge* mean? They decided that there must be a way to describe clues to these internal gains.

Those at the convention wanted to classify various academic achievements according to educational outcomes. They called their classification system a *taxonomy* of learning objectives. Tax-

onomy refers to the science, laws, or principles of classification. You are probably most familiar with some of the taxonomies of nature: animal, cordate, mammalia, primate, hominid, and *homo sapiens,* all of which describe the classification for the human being.

The learning categories that those educational evaluators chose were cognitive, affective, and psychomotor domains. They further differentiated those domains according to increasing levels of complexity and depth. Some of the members worried that the taxonomy might lead to fragmentation and loss of the real goals of education. In spite of such drawbacks, their taxonomy has received wide recognition in many education-related fields. Since the pioneering work of those educators, many other authors have built on their work. The material on the following pages makes use of their taxonomy as published in a series of handbooks (Bloom & others, 1956; Krathwohl, Bloom, & Masia, 1964; Harrow, 1972; Simpson, 1972).

The Taxonomy of Learning Objectives

In the following section of this chapter, we state objectives in the cognitive, affective, and psychomotor domains. The first group we list are objectives related to the cognitive domain, such as increased knowledge about a subject and increasing ability to make use of that information. The examples we use in the following explanations are phrased as questions that the client should be able to answer. We chose the medical diagnosis of arthritis. Each of the levels of knowledge that you might wish the client to achieve are stated as questions posed to the client.

Cognitive Domain
Knowledge

The first level of the cognitive domain is concerned with memory and simple recall. The client can recall terminology and demonstrate knowledge of specific facts. Recall of trends and sequences can be demonstrated. Learning at this level can be demonstrated by sorting through a memory file and remembering pertinent data.

Example: "What is the name of your medication?"

Comprehension

Comprehension is the next cognitive level and the lowest level of understanding. Comprehension means that the client has advanced beyond the capacity to recall. The client has knowledge of what is being communicated and has acquired the ability to make some use of it. Emphasis is placed on grasping the meaning and intent of the material under consideration.

Example: "What is your medication for?"

Application

In addition to knowing and understanding information, the client at this level can apply that information and use the idea in a particular situation. At this level the client remembers and makes appropriate generalizations or principles. The client can and does use a general rule in a particular situation.

Example: "Why is your disease called arthritis?"

Analysis

Analysis is concerned with the breakdown of the material into its parts. The client can recognize unstated assumptions and distinguish facts from hypotheses. This level of complexity also includes the ability to distinguish cause-and-effect relationships from coincidences. The client can detect the relationships of the parts and the way they are organized.

Example: "Identify the factors that contribute to your arthritis."

Synthesis

Synthesis is the formation of a whole by putting together its elements. The client at this level of complexity can perform induction and develop a structure or pattern not clearly there before.

Example: "Explain how gout is related to your sore foot."

Evaluation

Evaluation means the formation of criteria by which to judge the value of an idea or a method. The client is able to judge the value or purpose of an idea or method.

Example: "How clear/useful has the teaching you received been in managing your gout?"

The above examples were questions that illustrated how the nurse might explore the client's level of understanding of gout. In the following list, the taxonomy of cognitive objectives is combined with Mager's three-point method of forming learning objectives. Examples refer to a client who has heart disease. In each of the examples **performance** will be in **bold** type, *Criteria* will be *italicized* and (conditions) will be surrounded by parentheses ( ).

1. Knowledge—Client **states** pulse rate *under which* to hold her Lanoxin.
2. Comprehension—Client **states** *two hazards* of taking Lanoxin (when her radial pulse is less than 60 bpm).
3. Application—Client **reports holding Lanoxin** *2 days* (since last visit).
4. Analysis—Client **differentiates** the significance of a *slow pulse upon awakening and a slow pulse after mopping the kitchen floor.*
5. Synthesis—Client **explains** the action of Lanoxin on the *circulatory and nervous systems* and their *relation to its side effects.*
6. Evaluation—Client **appraises** the success of her *ability to regulate her pulse* (since her last visit).

Figure 9-1 illustrates the levels of complexity in the cognitive domain. Note how each higher level of cognition builds on the cognitive processes at the lower levels.

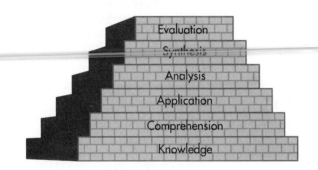

Figure 9-1 Cognitive domain: The increasingly complex levels of knowledge and the associated increase in ability to use that knowledge.

Affective Domain

The next classification of objectives addressed are those in the affective domain. The cognitive domain was listed in increasing order of complexity, but the second group, the affective domain, is listed in increasing order of depth, incorporation into the client's personality and/or value system. These affective objectives are more difficult to express accurately. One reason is that the affective-learning concept is not directly transferrable from the educational field to client teaching.

Another reason for difficulty in measurement is that affective changes are difficult to isolate. Changing your attitude is such a complex phenomenon (King, 1984). It is important to keep in mind the above cautionary remarks regarding specificity.

The following taxonomy, which has five successive parts, is presented with examples appropriate for communication with a parent whose child is mentally or physically handicapped.

Receiving

In the receiving phase of affective learning the client shows awareness, consciousness of a situation, fact, or event. The client shows movement beyond denial by selective attention to the desired field of focus, and a willingness to receive data.

> *Example:* A client cries when told about his or her child's disability.

Responding

At the next level of affective learning the client, although not initiating a particular event, shows a willingness to respond, and might find satisfaction in responding. At this level of acceptance the client may be able to entertain an opposing view.

> *Example:* The client is able to enjoy holding the child as evidenced by the client's smiling.

Valuing

When the client has reached the *valuing* level, it means that the client regards a thing or event as having value. The client shows acceptance of this value and a willingness to be identified with it. A further progression of valuing is a preference for things that have value and an exhibited commitment to those things. This becomes evident when the individual demonstrates behavior that is consistent with this value.

> *Example:* The client verbalizes a realistic picture of the child and states plans for enrolling the child in a special preschool.

Organization

The *organization* level involves the conceptualization and classification of a value system. The client considers how the new value fits into his or her current system of functioning and believing. At this level reorganization begins. The client attempts to incorporate the value with efforts to resolve conflicts with previously held values.

> *Example:* The client gets a babysitter and goes off to dinner with his or her partner.

Characterization

When the client has reached the characterization level, you see consistency in the response to related situations. The individual has adopted a basic philosophic position and orientation to the world with regard to the value under consideration. A client often arrives at the characterization level of incorporation through painful intellectual and affective work (Krathwohl & others, 1964). Characterization is not easy, and it takes time. You are not likely to see this step unless your client has been grappling with the problem for a long time. Evidence of characterization might be seen in psychotherapy and in relationships that develop in a family practice setting.

> *Example:* The client integrates care of the child into the needs of the rest of the family. When asked, "How are things going?" the client mentions concerns and activities with each member of the family.

The following examples demonstrate the use of the affective domain in describing behavioral objectives for which one might strive while relinquishing an addiction to smoking. **Bold** type will be used for **performance,** *italics* will be used for *criteria* and parentheses ( ) will be used for possible (conditions).

1. Receiving—(When asked about smoking while pregnant) the client **agrees** that, according to the Surgeon General's report, *smoking is a hazard to one's health.*
2. Responding—The client **agrees** with admonition to *try* to stop smoking.
3. Valuing—The client **cuts** *down to one bedtime cigarette.*
4. Organization—Client **adheres** to *no smoking decision.* The client finds other things to do with hands and mouth and takes up walking.
5. Characterization—The client **volunteers** the opinion that smoke is *irritating and unpleasant* and requests that meetings be smoke free. The client reduces other hazardous behaviors and increases healthy behaviors.

Figure 9-2 illustrates the affective levels in terms of the degree of integration and the depth to which the client has made a particular attitude or value a part of him or herself. Because this is an internal process, it is not easy to measure. The client may or may not choose to share his or her values with you about particular issues. To complicate matters fur-

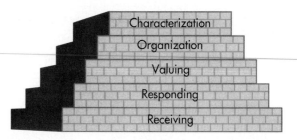

Figure 9-2 Affective domain: Increasing the depth of incorporation of a new attitude.

ther, we human beings are not always congruent. What we say we believe and what we actually believe, do not always match. We are often ambivalent and hold conflicting values.

Psychomotor Domain

In contrast to affective learning, psychomotor skills are much easier to identify and to measure because they are readily observable. Psychomotor learning refers to the third group of objectives that we consider. Learning a physical skill, such as walking with crutches, manipulating a new dialysis machine, or doing a procedure, usually involves substantial psychomotor learning. More than one level of learning exists in the psychomotor domain. For example, applying a diaper is a much less complex task than using a portable heart-lung machine. In such psychomotor activities as these the level of skill that has been achieved by the client is also readily observable.

A number of systems for defining psychomotor learning are available in the literature. We have chosen to adapt and abbreviate the system developed by Simpson (1972) because it appears to have the most relevance for client teaching. The clinical example we outline in the next six paragraphs is crutch walking.

Perception

Perception means that the client has attained sensory awareness of cues that are associated with the task to be performed. The client has the ability to attend to relevant cues.

> *Example:* The client watches the nurse demonstrate crutch walking.

Set

The client exhibits readiness to undertake a particular action and may display this readiness by verbal expressions of willingness to attempt a particular action. The client may also indicate readiness through body language.

> *Example:* The client gets ready to try crutch walking.

Guided Response

During guided response the client exerts efforts to imitate the behavior observed earlier. The client also attempts to comply with directions and coaching.

> *Example:* The client tries to walk with crutches and attempts to modify behavior in response to coaching.

Mechanism

At the *mechanism* level, the client has achieved the ability to perform the desired skill with a degree of confidence. Reaching this level also implies that the client has mastered each of the steps in the complex task to the point where the individual steps are blending into a meaningful whole. The skill is becoming a habit that is available to the client when it is desired or required.

> *Example:* The client can walk up and down the hall with a measure of confidence.

Complex Overt Response

When the *complex-overt-response* level has been achieved, it means that the client can perform the desired skill easily and independently. The entire sequence of the complex pattern can be performed

without the need for full attention to the details.

> *Example:* The client can scoot up and down the hallway with no hesitation. The client visits with other clients and talks while moving.

Adaptation

Adaptation means that the client has achieved such mastery that she or he has the ability to alter the skill to suit various conditions. The client no longer concentrates on varying responses but performs them automatically as the need arises.

> *Example:* The client can get in and out of cars or up and down stairs without difficulty.

The following examples illustrate the development of possible behavioral objectives in the psychomotor domain regarding self care of a colostomy. As in previous sections **performance** will be in **bold** type, *Criteria* will be *italicized*, and (conditions) will be surrounded by parentheses ( ).

1. Perception—Client **watches** *nurse do colostomy care.*
2. Set—Client **expresses** *willingness* to try doing part of procedure.
3. Guided Response—(Given a syringe and a basin), client **can irrigate** *while nurse gives verbal assistance.*
4. Mechanism—Client **can irrigate** colostomy *without assistance.*
5. Complex Overt Response—(Given the equipment), the client **can do complete colostomy care** *without nurse assistance and without leaks in colostomy bag seal.*
6. Adaptation—Client **can do colostomy care** *while on a camping trip.*

Figure 9-3 depicts an individual enjoying a psychomotor skill. Figure 9-4 depicts the increasing levels of complexity that are illustrated in Figure 9-3. The skier spent considerable time watching, getting set to try, and falling down during guided responses before he mastered the skill.

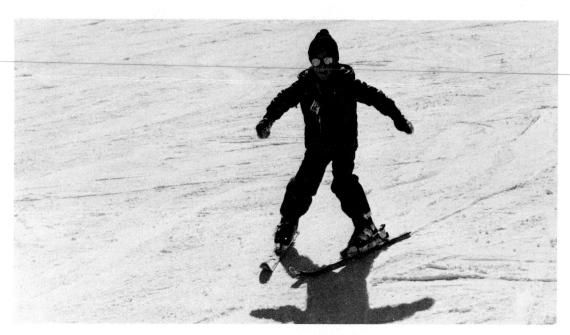

Figure 9-3 The skier demonstrates psychomotor skills.

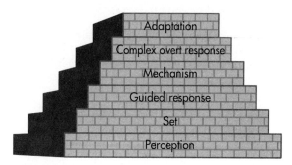

Figure 9-4 Psychomotor domain: The increasing levels of competency involved in performing a physical skill.

Verbs for Cognitive, Affective, and Psychomotor Objectives

We have included a list of suggested verbs in Figures 9-5 to 9-7 that you might find helpful if you are just learning to write objectives. Do not view these lists as fixed or as the only correct words. Such use can stifle your ability to think critically and to be creative. Use these lists as inspirations or stimuli

for your own productivity. Another point to keep in mind is the context in which you use a specific verb. Although we have placed a verb at a particular level of complexity, you might decide that the verb actually fits at another level of complexity for your client. We expect you to use this type of critical thinking.

Selection of Content

Now that you know how to write behavioral objectives, you will examine your assessment data and determine appropriate content for your client to learn. Your client and involved family will be included in this process. To walk you through the development of a lesson plan, we will present a vignette and expand on it in the next several chapters.

Case Example: Lincoln Perez

Our client is Lincoln Perez. Mr. Perez, a 45-year-old black male with Hispanic heritage, was recently diagnosed with hypertension. He is a very busy merchant who owns a construction business that waxes

EVALUATION	appraise assess audit calibrate choose compare compute	conclude contrast convert corroborate criticize debate deduct	defend discriminate distinguish estimate evaluate gauge interpret	judge justify measure rank rate revise score	select stipulate support value
SYNTHESIS	arrange assemble blend combine categorize classify collect compare compile compose	condense confirm construct contract contrast correlate create defend define design	devise estimate formulate fuse generate integrate manage mix modify order	organize paraphrase plan prepare propose rearrange reconstruct relate reorganize revise	rewrite simplify summarize teach transpose write
ANALYSIS	appraise analyze arrange assign break	calculate categorize classify compare contrast	criticize debate delineate detect diagram	differentiate discriminate dissect outline question	select separate sort subdivide test
APPLICATION	apply calculate change compute construct demonstrate design develop draft	dramatize draw edit eliminate employ formulate give illustrate implement	infer interpret investigate measure modify negotiate operate order predict	prepare produce propose revise relate search schedule select shop	show solve transpose use utilize
COMPREHENSION	describe discuss draw estimate	explain express generalize give example	identify increase locate outline	paraphrase reiterate restate review	rewrite summarize translate
KNOWLEDGE	circle color define identify indicate	label list mark match name	note number point recall record	repeat report select show state	tell underline

Figure 9-5 Verbs for cognitive objectives. *Adapted from Gronlund, N.E. (1978) Stating behavioral objectives for classroom instruction (2nd ed.). New York: Macmillan.*

and wanes depending on the local economy. Lately, the economy has not been too good. He is aware of the risks of hypertension because it runs in his family, but he is reluctant to take medication. Following a thorough assessment of his biologic, psy-chologic, sociologic, and cultural characteristics, we have decided that he has needs in the three domains of learning: cognitive, affective, and psycho-motor. Although we recognize that he has many learning needs—such as the concept of hyperten-

RECEIVING	accept accommodate admit allow attend	heed focus follow listen look	note observe pay attention regard stay
RESPONDING	agree answer assist attempt choose comply conform describe	discuss explain express label participate perform practice react	relate reply report select show state willingness try verbalize
VALUING	ask assert assist attempt choose complete describe	defend disagree explain give help initiate join	justify propose state volunteer work
ORGANIZATION	adhere alter arrange choose combine commit compare	complete contrast defend generalize explain express integrate	modify persist relate resolve synthesize
CHARACTERIZATION	adhere assert assist commit	continue defend describe discriminate	display endure explain

Figure 9-6 Verbs for affective objectives. *Adapted from Gronlund, N.E. (1978) Stating behavioral objectives for classroom instruction (2nd ed.). New York: Macmillan.*

sion as an invisible disease, multiple factors in the etiology and treatment of hypertension, nutrition, and weight management—at this point we are only focusing on stress reduction. In Table 9-1, you will find sample objectives in these domains. This is how you begin the construction of a lesson plan. Our lesson plan will have three columns. The first will contain the learning objectives, the second will identify the content in outline form, and the third column will identify the teaching strategies and ma-

terials that we plan to use. Evaluation, an important part of this lesson plan, is not included on the lesson plan itself but will immediately follow. We have included only three columns because we expect you to teach from the lesson plan. Three columns is all we believe is practical to include on one page.

With this lesson plan as begun in Table 9-1, you can look at your learning objectives, then look immediately to the right to remind yourself of the content you will teach the client. It is important that

ADAPTATION	adapt	compose	invert	reverse	swap
	alter	modify	modify	revise	switch
	change	convert	rearrange	rotate	vary
	convert	design	remodel	shift	
	correct	divert	reorganize	reformulate	
	create	exchange	replace	substitute	
COMPLEX OVERT RESPONSE	align	construct	lean	push	squeeze
	apply	cool	lift	raise	stand
	arise	coordinate	locate	read	start
	arrange	count	lower	reassemble	stick
	assemble	connect	make	recline	stimulate
	attach	cover	manipulate	remove	stop
	attempt	crawl	mend	repair	synchronize
	auscultate	cut	mold	replace	stoop
MECHANISM **GUIDED RESPONSE**	avoid	demonstrate	navigate	restore	tear
	balance	disconnect	open	rub	test
	bathe	discriminate	operate	run	tie
	boil	dissect	palpate	scrub	turn
	breathe	examine	part	secure	transfer
	brush	find	place	separate	type
	build	fold	pickup	sew	ventilate
	catheterize	freeze	pinch	shake	walk
	change	grasp	pivot	sharpen	wash
	choose	guide	plunge	shorten	weigh
	clean	heat	pour	simulate	wipe
	cleanse	hop	practice	slide	
	close	hold	press	solve	
	comb	insert	produce	splint	
	compile	join	pull	spread	
SET	aim	begin	get ready	react	start
	align	copy	position	respond	try
	attempt	display	prepare	stand up	volunteer
	ask	express	proceed	show	
PERCEPTION	attend	contrast	distinguish	look	select
	choose	describe	focus on	observe	separate
	compare	detect	identity	perceive	
	concentrate	differentiate	isolate	relate	

Figure 9-7 Verbs for psychomotor objectives. *Adapted from Gronlund, N.E. (1978) Stating behavioral objectives for classroom instruction (2nd ed.). New York: Macmillan.*

the information (objectives and content) correspond. By doing so, you will know exactly what you plan to teach and will not wander off into another area.

Summary

In this chapter we focused on analyzing the data, as in Figure 9-8, you have collected about your client. We addressed the issue of choosing objectives that are realistic given your own philosophy and that of the clients, the physicians, and the hospital on client education and client self-direction. Other variables we considered were time constraints and the effects of the situation on how you and the client relate. We discussed the selection of learning objectives in the three domains—cognitive, affective, and psychomotor. We concluded the chapter with a sample lesson plan that demonstrates how to organize your material and relate content to learning objectives.

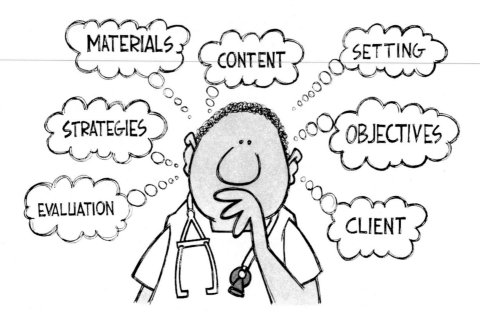

Figure 9-8   Your lesson plan includes client, objectives, content, setting, strategies, materials, and the means of evaluation.

T A B L E   9 - 1
Sample Lesson Plan for Lincoln Perez

Learning Objectives	Content Outline	Strategies and Materials

By the end of this lesson, the client will be able to:
   Select from a list three benefits of relaxation.
	Introductions
	Relaxation
	   Definitions
	   Balance with exercise
	   Benefits
	      Reduce blood pressure
	      Reduce tension
	      Increase efficiency
		(This column will be completed in subsequent chapters.)

Agree to experiment with walking and various relaxation techniques.	Medications
	   Fears
	   Side effects
	Life-style change
	   Costs
	   Benefits	

Count his pulse within three beats of what the nurse counts.	Techniques for pulse taking
	   Location of artery
	   Finger placement
	   Counting
	   Multiplying
	   Recording method
	Techniques for relaxation
	   Deep breathing
	   Yoga
	   Meditation
	   Imagery
	   Prayer
	Wrap-up	

SELECTING VERBS

Purposes:

- Think critically about clarifying objectives
- Differentiate cognitive, affective, and psychomotor domains
- Integrate nursing diagnoses with appropriate learning outcomes
- Choose clear, complete, and concise statements to describe client learning outcomes

Directions:

1. In the following statements you will find a list of incorrectly written behavioral objectives.
2. Notice the domain(s) inferred by each incorrect objective. Notice also the implied level of complexity.
3. Correct the statements so that each objective contains no more than one verb and one set of criteria.
4. Feel free to rewrite more than one correct objective for each incorrect objective.
5. You may use the verbs listed on the preceding pages.

Incorrectly Written Objectives

- Client will be integrating the master and competency of passive exercises to support attitudes of adequacy and self-esteem.
- Client will be able to perform at some level a return demonstration of the presented passive exercises despite his physical limitations.
- To teach the client to cough and deep breathe preoperatively.
- To demonstrate to the client the use of the circle bed traction and abduction splint preoperatively.

WRITING BEHAVIORAL OBJECTIVES

Purposes:

- Apply theory to clinical situations
- Practice using the concepts contained in this chapter through several learning channels
- Gain proficiency in writing objectives before using them in the teaching module
- Relate nursing diagnoses to learning objectives

Directions:

1. Develop the teaching module you plan to use.
2. Think about possible learning deficits/potentials among your anticipated clients.
3. Write nursing diagnoses (Kim, McFarland, & McLane, 1989) that are germane to the needs you assessed while you were visiting the potential clients at your anticipated teaching site. If you have not yet selected a site, pick a real situation from your recent client teaching opportunities. If you do not

have client contact at this time, think about children, neighbors, or friends who might benefit from your teaching.

4. Write one nursing diagnosis for each of the three domains. Each diagnosis should address a different domain: cognitive, affective, and psychomotor.

5. Work on the objectives until they are:
   a. Stated as outcomes.
   b. Measurable.
   c. Specific.
   d. Composed of **one performance** and *criteria*. (Conditions may or may not be applicable).
   e. If the performance is a complicated procedure, then the criteria should be listed step by step. See examples in Chapter 14: Sample checklist for correct pulse taking and the box on p. 279.

6. After you are satisfied that each objective contains a **performance** and *criteria*, refer back to the information in this chapter. Determine the level of depth or complexity at which you have written the objective. If you decide the level as you wrote it is too high or too low, rework your objective until you are satisfied.

7. After you are satisfied that the objective is at the level you believe is appropriate, write the appropriate level beside that objective.

8. Work in small groups and consult with each other.

References

Andersen, J. & Briggs, L. (1988). Nursing diagnosis: A study of quality and supportive evidence. IMAGE: Journal of Nursing Scholarship. 20(3), 141-4.

Bandman, E. & Bandman, M. (1988). *Critical thinking in nursing.* Norwalk, CT: Appleton & Lange.

Bloom, B.S, Englehart, M.S., Furst, E.J., Hill, W.H. & Krathwohl, D.R. (1956). *Taxonomy of educational objectives: The classification of educational goals. Handbook I: Cognitive domain.* New York: Longman.

Gronlund, N.E. (1985). *Stating behavioral objectives for classroom instruction* (3rd ed.). New York: Macmillan.

Hamilton, E.M., Whitney, E.N. & Sizer, F.S. (1991). *Nutrition concepts and controversies.* St. Paul, MN: West.

Harrow, A.J. (1972). *A taxonomy of the psychomotor domain: A guide for developing behavioral objectives.* New York: David McKay.

Kim, M.J., McFarland, G.C. & McLane, A.M. (1989). *Pocket guide to nursing diagnoses.* (3rd ed.). St. Louis MO: Mosby.

King, E.C. (1984). *Affective education in teaching.* Rockville MD: Aspen Systems Corporation.

Kleoppel, J.W. & Henry, D.W. (1987). Teaching patients, families and communities about their medications. In C.E. Smith (Ed.), *Patient education: Nurses in partnership with other health professionals* (pp. 271-296). Orlando, FL: Grune & Stratton.

Krathwohl, D.R., Bloom, B.S. & Masia, B.B. (1964). *Taxonomy of educational objectives: The classification of educational goals. Handbook II: The affective domain.* New York: David McKay.

Litwack, L., Linc, L. & Bower, D. (1985). *Evaluation in nursing: Principles and practice.* New York: National League for Nursing.

Mager, R.F. (1984). *Preparing instructional objectives* (3rd ed.). Belmont CA: Pitman Learning, Inc.

McFarland, G.K. & McFarlane, E.A. (1989). *Nursing diagnosis & intervention: Planning for patient care.* St. Louis: Mosby.

Neufeldt, V. (1991). *Webster's new world dictionary* (3rd ed.). Cleveland: Webster's New World.

Simpson, E.J. (1972). The classification of educational objectives in the psychomotor domain. In *Contributions of behavioral science to instructional technology: The psychomotor domain.* Mt. Rainier MD: The Gryphon Press. (3rd ed.). Englewood Cliffs, NJ: Prentice Hall.

Teaching Strategies

. . . for we learn a craft by
producing the same product that
we must produce when we have
learned it, becoming builders,
e.g. by building and harpists by
playing the harp. . . .

Aristotle (Irwin, 1985, p. 34).

10

Objectives

Upon completion of this chapter you will be able to:

- Contrast informal and formal teaching.
- Compare and contrast nine teaching strategies according to the following: technique, advantages, and disadvantages.
- State at least two examples of strategies for achieving objectives in each of the following domains: cognitive, affective, and psychomotor.
- Identify five principles that serve as guides in selecting a teaching strategy.
- Demonstrate selected teaching strategies when presenting a teaching module.

Key Words

preparation	lecture	programmed
organization	discussion	instruction
deliver	demonstration	simulated
formal	return	environment
informal	demonstration	role playing
strategy	modeling	team teaching

Introduction

In this chapter we focus on *how* clients are to learn. We will discuss the strategies listed on the summary chart at the end of this chapter. We also will think about how each strategy might best facilitate clients' learning. In other words we will present the process of selecting and designing teaching strategies to most effectively lead to the outcomes that are selected.

You have assessed yourself and the situation and analyzed the client's learning needs in terms of their learning-domain potentials and/or deficiencies. You have given thought to what clients will know, feel, or do in order to move to higher levels of wellness. You have also thought about what material clients should learn. In addition to promoting the outcomes you anticipate, you will want to choose strategies that suit the clients, your teaching style, and the content to be mastered.

Types of Teaching

A teaching strategy may be defined as a method of presenting content that is designed to bring about specific changes in learners. A teaching strategy includes activities that will be done by the learners as well as the teacher. An effective teaching strategy also includes a design of the environment that is most conducive to the desired learning. There are a number of teaching strategies available. Fundamental in the discussion of these strategies is the distinction between formal and informal teaching. Nurses engage in teaching/learning interactions much of the time, both formally and informally.

Informal Teaching

Informal teaching is the casual unstructured teaching that takes place in nearly every nurse/client interaction. Whenever you encounter clients, you usually talk to them. The conversation may sound friendly and casual to the uninitiated, but you will be engaged in purposeful communication and have a definite goal in mind: reducing anxiety, conveying information, and testing clients' sensorium.

Asking and answering questions is another important part of your role when you encounter clients. You will be expected to continuously assess and be cognizant of clients' learning needs and to make some educated guesses about the purposes behind clients' questions. During encounters with clients, you will find yourself frequently drawing sketches on facial tissue boxes and giving impromptu demonstrations. You do this for good reasons; you intuitively or rationally comprehend that you have encountered clients at the teachable moment. The other main teaching strategy you will use is reflection, which will promote affective learning in the informal setting.

You will also teach informally by the example you set. Clients notice what kind of care you take of yourself in your appearance (trim, glowing), behavior (energetic, smiling), and conversation (language that is self-enhancing and respectful of others). They also notice the odors emanating from you, and they make judgments about how you care for yourself (clean, smoke-free). This phenomenon was brought home to one nursing student by some nonnursing students. They asked why the nursing students were selling candy and coffee as money-raising projects if these products are bad for the health. There was no answer, except to blush and say, "You are right!"

Formal Teaching

Formal teaching is different from informal teaching in that it is planned in advance and occurs at a specific time and place. When teaching formally, you have objectives in mind, and you have a plan developed that includes the content you want to address. You might teach formally to an individual, family, or a group. The main difference between these formal and informal methods therefore is planning.

In this chapter we will describe the use of several teaching strategies: lecture, discussion, demonstration, modeling, programmed instruction, simulated environment, games and activities, role playing, and team teaching. While exploring the first method of teaching, lecture, we will discuss several principles that are applicable to most of the other strategies as well. We will also integrate principles that are treated elsewhere in the text in more depth.

Lecture

The *lecture* is defined as an exposition of a given subject delivered before an audience or class for the purpose of instruction; discourse (Neufeldt, 1991) as illustrated in Figure 10-1. An effective cognitive structure for planning the lecture and every other strategy consists of a design that takes into consideration its preparation, organization, and delivery. In other words, the guidelines we provide for preparing a lecture are equally applicable to all of the other methods that follow.

Preparation

It is important to clarify the objectives of your lecture. By the time the lecture is completed, what do you hope the listeners will have gained? Another important preparatory activity is analyzing your au-

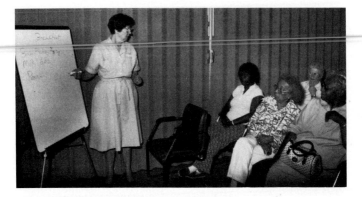

Figure 10-1   The well-prepared and well-developed lecture conveys more information more efficiently. *From M. Stanhope and J. Lancaster,* Community Health Nursing: Process and Practice for Promoting Health, *3rd ed, Mosby, 1992.*

dience. What generalizations can you make about the biologic development, health, handicaps, and other physical characteristics that would impinge on the lecture/learning process? When approaching teenagers you would need to use a much different approach than when you approach retirees. What is the educational level of most of the audience? What reading and media preferences do audience members have? Is the audience relatively homogeneous in composition, or is the group composed of diverse individuals?

The socioeconomic characteristics of your audience will also give you clues to the level of sophistication that is most appropriate. For example, if you were preparing a lecture on nutrition for welfare recipients, then you would focus on the value and preparation of foods known as excess commodities. Excess commodities are foods supplied by the government for free. You would need to know what these foods are and how they could be used in recipes. If members of the audience are from another culture, you may need to consult literature on portions of that culture's belief system that are relevant to the topic you will cover. The topic you choose, and the way you present the material should be determined by the culture's views. This was aptly illustrated when a nursing student was teaching in a home in response to an Asian woman who asked her to talk about "no babies," or birth control. It was important for the nursing student to under-

stand that if any men came into the home, the class would end immediately. Samples of birth control equipment had to be such that they would be easy to hide in an instant. This meant the nursing student could not bring a poster and other bulky teaching materials with her. She could only bring items that were small and could be hidden easily if men were to enter the room.

You must also note the expectations of the audience. What do they want to learn or hear? What have they heard before? What is the occasion? Are clients expecting to be entertained? Informed? Inspired? It has been our experience that effective teachers include both entertainment and inspirational factors in their lectures. People learn better in an aroused state. They are more likely to remember information that brings them amusement when they recall it. Most health teaching involves persuading people to change their behavior. They often need inspiration and persuasion to go to the trouble of changing. Changing behavior is work; it's easier to stay the same. Inspiration can help you find the motivation to start that process and to continue it.

Content selection is based on conclusions reached from thinking about the above-mentioned phenomena. If you are very well-informed on the subject, your main preparatory task may be translating that knowledge into a frame of reference that suits this particular audience. What analogies and real life examples will be meaningful to them? For example, while preparing a talk on public speaking for a large gathering of operating room nurses, a nurse consulted with colleagues who practiced in that arena (Babcock & Zak-Dance, 1981).

If the content is less well-known to you, you may need to research the subject itself. Some nursing students, who wanted to teach nutrition to a group of girls who were earning scout badges, assumed that they knew enough to do so without further research. They failed to check their information against recent data. When they presented the pyramid they included butter in the milk, yogurt, and cheese group. The illustrations of cooked vegetables that they chose to illustrate the fruit and vegetable group also featured melting butter as a "condiment." Although butter is indeed a dairy product, it is classified in the fats, oils, and sweets group because it is pure fat. The category of milk, yogurt, and cheese should contain only those milk products that are rich sources of calcium. Searching for appropriate audiovisuals and trying them out is a time-consuming process that should be started as early in the preparatory phase as possible.

Organization

The organization of the lecture should be appropriate to the topic. One way to sequence ideas is to use a logical progression, such as cause and effect. Chronologic order is very useful for describing events that have historical relationships to one another. Geographic positions may be useful when you discuss populations, ecologic systems, or the map of the fitness stations around a building. Moving gradually from the simple to the complex is another effective method. Describing the problem and then possible solutions is another useful way to organize the learning.

Babcock and Zak-Dance (1981) pointed out that the best mix for communicating new ideas is to use material that is 70% familiar and 30% unfamiliar. How can information that is totally new to the audience be presented with such a mix? One solution to this dilemma is to develop a familiar context in which to present the new content. You can translate the new information into analogies that are familiar to the audience. You can also use personal stories that include the new information.

The presentation of audiovisuals throughout the speech should be timed to accomplish several objectives. A picture often conveys an idea much more clearly than words. A graph can help to clarify the meaning of statistics. The graph, cartoon, or other display can stay on the screen for the audience to absorb. Spoken words are much more short-lived. An audiovisual also provides variety. Very few speakers are so spellbinding that voice and body language are sufficient to keep the audience's attention and interest.

Group the ideas to make them easier to grasp and remember. Poon and colleagues (1980) found that generally people are unable to hold more than seven thoughts in their minds at once. These thoughts include both those that you intend to convey and the associations that are evoked in each listener's mind by your presentation. In applying this information, remember that three groups of three are easier to remember and less formidable to the listener than nine separate ideas. You can also make use of memory principles by organizing the ideas into comprehensible and associated groups, which will make the information easier for the audience to grasp and remember. An illustration of this technique has been used in organizing this part of the chapter. Although several ideas have been addressed, they have been organized into three basic categories: preparation, organization, and delivery.

An outline of your speech is another useful organizational activity. The outline should begin by specifying the purpose of the speech so that you stay mindful of the main objective. Communication experts often recommend that you spell out the opening line, the closing line, directions, and questions (Babcock & Zak-Dance, 1981). The opening line should be catchy, arresting and designed to focus the group on the topic at hand. If you have not had much experience speaking publicly, we recommend that you pay special attention to the axiom: Know thyself. A joke is a fine way to begin a speech if you are a good joke teller. If you are not, the attempt can unnerve you as well as your audience. One caution: Do not make other individuals or groups the butt of your joke. It is insensitive and can backfire on you. Telling a story about yourself is often fun because you are then sharing a human experience and give the audience a sense of who you are. The story, however, is most meaningful when it relates to the topic. Don't make another cultural group the source of humor in your story, unless you are a member of that culture. We discourage you from putting yourself down, ever. It is simply not respectful of yourself.

Speech specialists disagree on the value of sharing your feelings of nervousness with the audience (Carnegie, 1980). If the audience is a very warm, nurturing group, their general feelings of compassion may reach and comfort you. If the audience is cold or critical, such a tactic may backfire. If you convey nervousness to the audience, then they too may begin to feel uncomfortable. This phenomenon can interfere with learning because the listeners might be focusing on their own discomfort instead of the importance of the topic under consideration.

Another way to capture the audience's attention is to start with statistics that are particularly meaningful to the group. Statistics also help convey that you are well read and current on the topic at hand. It establishes your authority as a speaker if you are knowledgeable about the topic. You will want to be adequately prepared to support the impression you are making.

Delivery

Your language should be appropriate to the audience. A professional audience will expect you to use technical language during a lecture. An audience of citizens might find such an approach incomprehensible. They also may feel put down by your choice of words. An audience of college-educated people would enjoy a different vocabulary level than a group of day laborers.

The pace of your speech must be geared to the clients. If the clients are older, as mentioned previously, your voice should be low, slow, and loud. If this is difficult to accomplish with your natural voice, use a microphone, even for a relatively small group. Clients from large, urban areas, particularly on the northeast coast, would probably enjoy a pace that is more brisk than individuals from a rural community or from the South.

Individuals who are familiar with the topic would be able to comprehend the point of the lecture much more quickly than people to whom the information is very new. Think of yourself when you read an article on new medical discoveries. You can not only comprehend it better than your clients but also make some educated guesses about the accuracy of the reports.

Because the human attention span is limited, we recommend that you deliver no more than 15 minutes of straight talk before introducing a change of pace (Babcock & Zak-Dance, 1981). The change may be in the form of a transparency, a slide, an exercise, or a question that requires a show of hands from the clients. The rare orator who can capture an audience's attention for an extended period usually does so by creating visual imagery, painting pictures with words.

Talk *from* your notes; do not read your paper. There are several reasons for this advice. One is the effect that reading a paper has on the audience. Think of your own reaction to a teacher who stands in the front of the room and reads. Many students express a feeling of outrage because such teachers make it clear by their behavior that the topic is more important than the learners. The audience members might say to themselves, "Why doesn't she just photocopy the information and pass it out? Then, I could read it when it suits my schedule!" The speaker who reads a prepared lecture is engaged with the topic and not the audience, but a good speaker is able to do both.

Another reason for avoiding the temptation to read the lesson is the effect it has on you as the teacher. If you read, you are looking at a piece of paper rather than the audience. It is easy to lose touch with clients and not notice their nonverbal feedback. If you lose touch with your clients you may fail to notice when they are interested, puzzled, or getting restless. If you are nervous, you tend to speed up. When you have complete sentences in front of you, you are further tempted to talk faster. Because notes are incomplete clues rather than sentences, they help you pace your lecture. As you look at the next line and reconstruct what to say, you will pause. During your pause, clients have the time to absorb what you just finished saying. It thus allows time for the clients to reflect on the idea and to associate it with experiences they already know. Notes that stimulate recall also allow for more spontaneity in you, the teacher. A fresh example may occur to you during the reconstruction process. This helps keep your presentation more lively and avoids the feeling that it is a "canned" speech.

Your voice should be clear, loud enough to be heard, and conversational in tone. A monotone is usually a sign of anxiety. If you concentrate on how important the topic is and how much clients will benefit from the information, your natural enthusiasm will modulate your voice. If you have a high, soft voice, become familiar enough with a microphone that it becomes a friend and communication enhancer.

If possible, relinquish speech patterns that are distracting. One nursing instructor used the phrase "in terms of" so much that its use irritated her students. One of the students started making cross-hatches each time the teacher used the phrase. Classmates soon realized what the student was doing because they too were annoyed by her overuse of this phrase. All of them thought it was funny at the time. The subject has long since been forgotten, and only the memory of the class's annoyance and the student's amusing solution remain. Looking back, the student says, "It did not occur to me then to take her aside and give her feedback on her irritating mannerism. No one knows whether or not she would be receptive to a helpful suggestion. To my chagrin, I'll never be able to find out."

In the past, some speech teachers emphasized formalized gestures borrowed from the repertoire of professional actors. There are indeed gestures that convey certain meanings. For example, a raised fist is a well-recognized gesture for inviting the audience to participate in a battle. There are gestures that convey emotional messages, such as putting your hand in the middle of your chest. Leaning your

upper torso forward conveys sincerity and interest.

A number of studies have been reported on the definition and effects of enthusiasm (Practical Applications of Research, 1981). Frequent demonstrative gestures, dramatic body movements, and selection of varied adjectives all add to your presentation. A common approach today is to emphasize loosening up your body to allow natural enthusiasm to guide your gestures. Distracting gestures, however, can diminish the effect of your message. Remember to check your appearance closely before beginning your lecture.

Eye contact is very important for effective teaching. If you are a neophyte and insecure as a teacher, you may be tempted to avoid this, but if you are brave enough to face your audience you may find that it can actually diminish your anxiety. A helpful way to deal with trepidation is to pick out a few friendly faces and talk to them. These friendly individuals should be located on both sides and in the front of the audience so that all of the clients will feel they are important and worthy of your attention. Dancing, wide-open eyes will enhance your delivery. Members of the audience characteristically respond to this kind of attention in a warm, encouraging way. Eye contact also allows you to determine when clients have not grasped the point under discussion. At that point you can slow down and repeat information, or you can ask a volunteer what seems to be the trouble.

Your appearance establishes a set before you begin to speak. As a health teacher your appearance should be that of a well-educated and well-prepared individual who is worthy of the audience's undivided attention. Within those parameters your appearance should be suitable to the topic and your audience. If the lesson of the day covers physical exercises, then a becoming sweat suit would be appropriate. If the audience is composed of little children and you are a female, we recommend that you wear a pant suit or slacks so that you can sit comfortably on low chairs or participate in the activities that are mandatory for young, restless children. A dark suit would be suitable for a business audience. If your audience is older, you will also be more easily received when you present a more conservative appearance. A woman with a wild hairdo or a man who wears a ponytail when talking to an elderly audience may create barriers that are insurmountable. On the other hand, if the audience is a group of individuals with low socioeconomic status, a very sophisticated and expensive outfit can feel like a putdown. The point is: If you want to be heard, be sensitive to your audience.

When speaking to a very large audience that is far away from the podium, when speaking to an audience of older citizens, and when appearing on television, you will need to make some modifications in your usual appearance. Put bright, attractive colors close to your face and if you wear makeup, make it more exaggerated than usual. If you are a woman and makeup is not against your religious convictions, you should wear bright lipstick. If you are a man who is not used to professional television appearances, you may not realize how important makeup can be to the effectiveness of your delivery. A mustache, which hides your lips, can interfere with your intelligibility. This will be particularly true for members of your audience who have hearing deficits and are used to lipreading. If you have a mustache, trim it to expose your lips and use lip gloss to make it easier to read your lips. This will facilitate communication. If you find it intolerable to wear any other kind of makeup, at least add gloss to your eyelashes and eyebrows. This will increase the visibility of your facial expressions.

Whether or not you choose to wear a new outfit when you teach depends on your personality and your taste in clothes. Some speakers find that a new outfit gives them a psychologic lift and enhances the liveliness of their presentation. Others feel more secure in an outfit that is familiar and comfortable. One speaker routinely checks with her adult daughters. They have good taste and will tell her honestly if the outfit is too outdated or unbecoming. A last-minute check on your appearance and smile in a full-length mirror is an excellent feedback device. It is also a fine opportunity to give yourself a final "pep talk." More hints for dealing with anxiety follow.

Practice cannot be overemphasized. It is a very effective device for easing anxiety. Practice is important for the neophyte as well as the experienced teacher. Practice should be done with feedback and can be done in front of a mirror. One experienced teacher would not dream of going before any audience without two complete dress rehearsals. These rehearsals help reduce her anxiety and are an indication of her respect for the audience.

If you have a soft voice, we urge you to rehearse with an audio cassette tape recorder. Many individuals with soft speaking voices have acoustic feedback inside their skulls regarding their own voices, which is not helpful in gauging their volume. These people experience themselves as shouting before the volume of their voice is even up to "normal." They have described sounds that reverberate very loudly inside their heads. If this description fits you, place a cassette tape recorder across a sizable room and record your voice. The tape recorder will give you more accurate feedback than your internal feedback system.

The next step when practicing is to do so with trusted friends or relatives who will give you honest and helpful feedback. If the lesson will be delivered to an unfamiliar group, then we advise you to talk to a small group of similar individuals. Several nursing students who planned to talk to a class of youngsters enlisted their own children and young neighbors to critique them. Children enjoy being consumer groups and are able to give forthright, concrete advice on what is likely to be successful. Before giving a presentation on public speaking to an audience of 200 operating room nurses, one speaker arranged to give a talk to the operating room nurses at a nearby hospital. This smaller group, when invited, gave excellent feedback and wonderful examples that were meaningful to their own area of specialty. The speaker was able to illustrate various aspects of the talk with those examples when presenting to the larger audience.

Dealing with Speech Anxiety

Sprague and Stuart (1992) report that one out of five people experience enough fear when speaking in front of groups that it interferes with their performance. One out of 20 people find public speaking so upsetting that they cannot get through a public speech. In one survey, people ranked fear of public speaking higher than the fear of death. It is normal to feel tension before speaking to any group, although larger groups of strangers are more likely to be anxiety provoking than smaller groups of trusted friends. Many public speakers and other personalities report that they still experience some feelings of anxiety before they begin each performance (Sprague & Stuart, 1992).

One way of coping with anxiety is to reframe the experience. Note the "butterflies" and have them fly in formation. Redefine your raised epinephrine level as excitement. Recall that an epinephrine rush makes your eyes shiny and gives you an alert posture. Both of these visible characteristics will make you more attractive and interesting to watch. An exuberant overall energy level increases the amount of time the audience pays attention to you (Practical Applications of Research, 1981).

There are several ways to use up the excess energy that is released with the adrenaline surge. One of these ways is physical exercise. One speaker, who likes to run, runs in the morning before she gives a presentation. Another speaker arrives at the speaking site very early and rearranges the furniture in the room and runs back and forth arranging and gathering equipment. Yet another arranges the day in such a way that everything remains calm and under control until after the presentation. Things that are anxiety provoking are simply delayed until after her talk.

Ways to calm yourself include breathing deeply, chewing gum, eating clear candy, praying, and employing comforting magic. For instance, famous artists have described ritualistic behaviors such as special meals before performances and the use of charms, such as a rabbit's foot. Covert rehearsal, or fantasy, is also helpful and can significantly improve performance. Imagine yourself very poised while delivering an excellent presentation, then imagine smiling while the audience applauds vigorously.

Self-talk is an essential mechanism for calming yourself (Fishel, 1988). Self-affirmations are very useful to many individuals in many situations. The way you talk to yourself greatly influences your self-esteem, your posture, and your many bodily processes. The following phrases are affirmations that may help you assume a positive attitude.

Example: "I have a right to speak. I know this subject well. I have practiced thoroughly. They need to learn this for their own future well-being. What I want to share with them is important."

Most of the guidelines we have offered in connection with the lecture strategy are also pertinent to the other strategies. The rest of the chapter will highlight special considerations.

Discussion

Discussion is a two-way verbal interaction that involves talking, listening, asking questions, and answering questions. Discussion implies an egalitarian approach to teaching. An assumption underlying the use of discussion is that your clients have some knowledge and experience in the area under scrutiny and that their thinking, knowledge, opinions, and conclusions provide valuable input. You are more likely to succeed when your clients are actively involved in addressing the objectives of the session. Discussion is particularly useful when the aim of the learning includes intellectual skills beyond comprehension. These levels of cognition include application, analysis, synthesis, and evaluation, which we explained in Chapter 9.

Figure 10-2 illustrates discussion as a common strategy in health education. One of the major components of a productive discussion is the skillful use of questions. Questions can serve many purposes in the teaching/learning process. Questions can help you find out what clients already know, stimulate interest in a new topic, discern whether or not clients grasped the main points of your lesson, explore ideas with your clients, and promote higher levels of thinking (Browne & Keeley, 1986).

Listening can provide you with substantial information for guiding the rest of the lesson. The way you listen and to whom you listen shapes the discussion. If you regularly call on the first person who

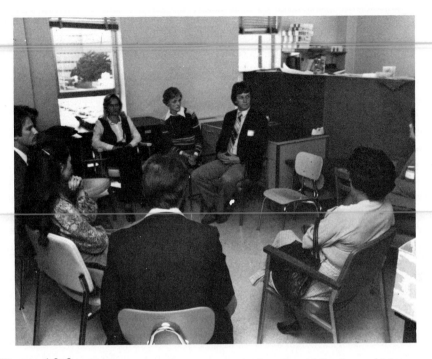

Figure 10-2 Discussion is two-way communication. *From M. Stanhope and J. Lancaster, Community Health Nursing: Process and Practice for Promoting Health, 3rd ed, Mosby, 1992.*

responds, then others who conceptualize or translate their thoughts into words more slowly may not make the effort. You also shape the discussion by the manner in which you treat contributions. Ready, animated acceptance of ideas and feelings boosts participation as well as learning (Practical Applications of Research, 1981). If clients feel that their contributions will be valued and used, they experience more freedom to express themselves. If they see another client ridiculed, or if they perceive that only certain kinds of contributions are welcome, they tend to produce those contributions or produce fewer of them. One of the most important points to keep in mind while planning a discussion is to *PLAN CAREFULLY and BE READY TO FLEX.* We thought presenting this message this way will help you keep it in mind.

One of your first tasks is to get the discussion started. It is often helpful to review the objectives of the session with the group. Sometimes a summary of past information helps when it is followed by asking audience members' opinions. Other skilled

teachers stimulate the group by making a controversial statement calculated to arouse the participants. A warm, friendly attitude, a smile, and an expectant look also help the group to get started. If no one answers immediately, we recommend that you take a deep breath and concentrate on twinkling your eyes. This will help you tolerate the group's hesitation and be more patient until some brave soul "takes the plunge."

Once the discussion is in progress, there are several ways to keep it on track. deTornyay and Thompson (1982) discussed the following substrategies: focusing, refocusing, changing the focus, and recapping what has been said. In the following section of this chapter we have used their concepts as our organizational themes.

Getting the Discussion Underway

Because people often process phenomenon through associative thinking, they branch from one idea to another. It is your responsibility to help keep the discussion on a path that is related to the objectives. One way to center the discussion is to ask questions that specifically direct the group's attention to the point(s) you wish to make. Centering-type questions may be open-ended or questions that evoke single answers. For example, if the class was covering parenting techniques, an open-ended or divergent question would be: "What do you find to be the most fun part of being a parent?" The following is a single-answer, or convergent, question: "How many people in this room have children between the ages of 0 and 2?"

Keeping the Group on Target

Getting the group back on target is necessary when the group has strayed from the original topic and you wish to lead the group back to it. This can be done directly with the following statement.

> *Example:* "Let's get back to the topic at hand."

You can also accomplish the same thing by repeating what the client has said, and then asking a question that is related to the last client's remarks but prompts the group back to the subject. For example, if a discussion group on toddlers was underway and a participant drifted into describing how stubborn a teenage daughter was, you might begin with the following:

> *Example:* "Yes, a stubborn teenager can at times remind you of a two-year-old. How many of you are trying to cope with the challenge of a stubborn *toddler* right now?"

When to Move On

When a group has discussed a topic sufficiently and no new information or ideas are forthcoming, then it may be time to change the direction of the discussion. Using the above example of children, you might say,

> *Example:* "Now that we've discussed the darling and impish behaviors of toddlers, let

us examine ways to respond to them, to increase their cute ways and to decrease their impish behaviors, at least the ones that drive us crazy."

Ending the Discussion

You will decide when to summarize what a group has said so far. Its purpose is to lift out ideas that have been offered to make the ideas more understandable to the group. This summary helps clients see relationships and draw conclusions. The following is an example of such a summary.

> *Example:* "We have talked about toddlers and how they can be so cute at some times, while at other times they can get on our nerves. We have noted that our own moods affect how we react to specific behaviors at any one time. We have also noted that when we stay calm, we can get more of the behavior we want by paying attention to it. We also talked about ways to ignore or distract children away from the behaviors we don't want."

Problems with the Discussion Strategy

Whenever you use the discussion strategy, you give up some control because you are allowing clients to share some of the leadership. At times, this may mean that clients diverge to a topic that is very different from what you had in mind. At that point, you must make a decision about whether or not to attempt to refocus the group or to go with the energy of the group. When making the decision observe how many of the group members seem more interested in the new topic. When you get a response to this question, you must determine if the new topic is in some way relevant to the content that needs to be learned or if it will simply lead the group astray and will not facilitate achieving the learning objectives. This is a judgment call because the new topic may be important for the group to discuss. Another aspect you may need to consider is the purpose of the divergence. Is the topic you raised too uncomfortable for the group to handle? Did you collect insufficient preliminary data on the needs and interests of the group? Does the group need to deal with a community crisis that just arose?

There are times when audience members' need to discuss the topic of their choosing is so strong that an attempt to refocus would be futile. Attempts to go on might be perceived as insensitive, and might deteriorate the learning environment. The group may need to deal with the new issue before they can focus on anything else. Your attempt to refocus under such circumstances might be an attempt to avoid an issue that you find uncomfortable to consider. To explore some of the above considerations, you can ask the group members a question to focus their concerns.

> *Example:* "It seems that your concerns about the health care crisis are more pressing right now than the behavior of your toddlers. How many of you have worries about paying for your family's health care? How many feel the need to cope with that worry right now before we discuss your toddlers?"

Another way to respond to a shift in energy is to just let it flow. An interesting axiom to follow is: "Want to be a leader? Find a parade and get in front!"

There are times during a group discussion when the participants lose interest. Clues to diminished interest include slackening contributions, side conversations, yawning, restlessness, and glassy-eyes. At this point, it may be profitable to change your strategy. For instance, you could conduct a group activity. It may help enliven the group and regenerate interest if you have the participants do a few deep-breathing exercises or encourage them to move their chairs into a new arrangement that is more appropriate to the group activity. Another possibility is to change the topic.

Nonparticipants are a challenge, especially if you believe that everyone should participate. If you and the group are relatively new to one another, the general rule is to leave the nonparticipant in peace. Part of this decision may be based on the contract you have with the group. A group of parents who have been ordered by the court to attend your classes would have a different contract than a group in which you are a guest. If you are running an assertiveness training course, participants cannot meet the objectives if they remain silent. There are strategies that you can use to engage the nonparticipant. Dividing the large class into smaller, less formidable groups may make the atmosphere less threatening and might promote interaction. Another possibility is to give a reluctant person time. Many people will participate after they decide they are safe doing so. These people very carefully note your response to less-than-brilliant contributions of other individuals. If you welcome every contribution and manage to use it to enrich, the discussion is much more likely to get a response from the client who is slow to risk.

Another challenge that you will face is the overparticipant. One response to this individual is a direct message.

> *Example:* "Thanks, now let someone else work."
> "Do you all agree with . . . ?"
> "Does . . . speak for all of you?"

Standing by the overparticipant, even touching that person on the shoulder, while asking others for answers sometimes helps. In planning how to deal with an overparticipant, you might wish to make an educated guess into the dynamics of this client as a learner. A client who is very kinesthetically oriented may need to be physically active to grasp the information being imparted. The overparticipant may be "stroke-hungry" and in need of attention. The client may be inappropriate and insensitive to the restlessness she or he generates in the rest of the group, or the individual may be a very enthusiastic and/or articulate person who, by coincidence, is in a group of people who are unable or unwilling to fully participate. If often helps to put such willing participants to work by having them write group contributions on the chalkboard, be secretary for the group, control the lighting, control the slide projector, put the equipment away, or help with displays.

If the group is ongoing and the above suggestions do not seem to help, you might offer to meet with the overparticipant outside of class. At that time, you can give extra attention and provide individual counseling. You can gently confront and negotiate a contract.

> *Example:* "Are you aware that when you speak at length or contribute for the third or fourth time that everyone else in the group gets restless?"

Wait for response and use it to tailor further confrontation.

> *Example:* "I do not want you to do that because you might end up alienating yourself from the others. Will you agree to speak only once in group? After that, write down anything else you want to say, and we will meet to discuss every point you wish to make."

The rude participant can be unnerving, especially if you are a neophyte. One way to deal with rude people is to ignore them and pay enthusiastic attention to the listeners. This method works particularly well with young children. A strategy that sometimes works is to stop speaking and look at those having a private conversation. This usually evokes some pressure from the talkers' immediate neighbors to rejoin the group. Asking the talkers to share their burning thoughts with the rest of the group sometimes helps. The assumption that their thoughts are related to the topic at hand is often correct. If you have an easy wit, you might be able to confront them with humor. Sometimes a direct polite plea works.

> *Example:* "The rest of us are having a hard time concentrating. Would you wait on your private discussion till after group?"

Demonstration

Demonstration may be defined as an activity that describes or illustrates by experiment or practical application; during *demonstration* one displays, operates, and explains (Neufeldt, 1991). You will frequently use demonstration when parents need to learn skills to care for their ill child, as illustrated in Figure 10-3. Heidgerken (1965) offered nine characteristics that are essential for a good demonstration.

Guidelines of a Good Demonstration

1. Understand the entire procedure before attempting to perform for others. After being able to perform the demonstration with ease, you become free to pay attention to your clients and to the parts of the demonstration that are more difficult and need further discussion or clarification.

2. Assemble and pretest before you demonstrate. It is distracting to clients to watch you gather equipment or fumble with equipment that is not working. Fumbling around uses up energy that should be available for focusing on the essential steps in the desired skill. Clients do better when they have confidence in you. Fumbling and false starts detract from this mystique.

3. Advance knowledge of the general procedure to be followed helps clients develop a mind set that will facilitate their learning. They then know how long they need to pay attention and how complicated the procedure is likely to be.

4. Use a positive approach. Emphasize what to *do* rather than emphasizing what not to do. Messages, such as "Do not do this, and do not do that," emphasize the likelihood of errors and interfere with your clients' confidence in whatever procedure you are teaching them. If such warnings are necessary, follow them with the "do's" that are likely to avoid the hazard.

5. Ensure a good view for everyone watching the demonstration. You can accomplish this by having everyone gather around you. If you are speaking to a large group, use a video camera to show the demonstration on a television screen for those seated farther away. Be sure to focus the television camera on your hands. If this procedure is used, any size audience can watch, as long as each client is close enough to a television screen to have a good view.

6. Offer running comments that focus the attention of your clients on the relevant components of your demonstration. Nonessential elements need not be mentioned.

7. Use a true-to-life setting for the demonstration,

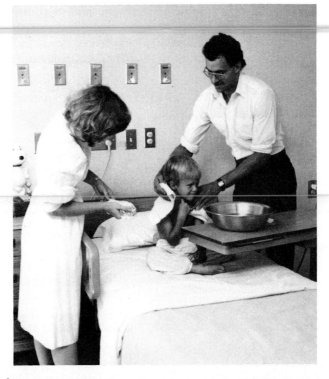

Figure 10-3   Psychomotor skills are learned more easily with demonstration and return demonstration. *From L.F. Whaley and D.L. Wong,* Essentials of Pediatric Nursing, *3rd ed, Mosby, 1989.*

if possible. A demonstration in the actual place where clients will carry out the procedure is ideal. In community health nursing, when you demonstrate a procedure to clients in their homes, you will get the most realistic picture of their resources. Professionals who have had experience in community health nursing are more apt to be sensitive to the limitations under which clients must operate. In the acute care setting, if you provide a situation that simulates the client's home environment, you will promote the transfer of learning.

8. Hold a discussion period following the demonstration. This provides an opportunity for reemphasis, questioning, recall, evaluation, and summary while the procedure is still fresh in the clients' minds. Discussion also allows clients to request the rationale for any part of the procedure they find puzzling. Those who fear the actual performance, however, may stall by prolonging the discussion.

Clients vary in how much discussion they find useful; you will learn to judge how long to continue the discussion before it reaches a point of diminishing value.

9. Have clients practice as soon as possible after the demonstration. The sooner they can practice the skill, the more effective their learning will be.

It has been our experience that information that seemed quite clear can be less so if the client actually tries to do the procedure. Psychomotor learners may catch on very quickly, while other clients who thought they understood, can become overwhelmed during the actual practice. "Would you like me to talk you through it?" may be very reassuring words to such a client. Coaching and using positive reinforcement principles are very effective means of supporting clients through the learning process. By following a demonstration with actual practice, clients can become aware of gaps in comprehension that they had not noticed during their observation period. Another discussion period after the return demonstration, therefore, helps solidify the learning.

Modeling

You teach a great deal by your personal example alone. You are teaching whether or not you are aware of your effect as a good (or poor) role model. If you smell of smoke or appear to practice other life-diminishing habits, clients are aware of this. Many of our nurse colleagues laugh when they talk about the obese individual who taught them nutrition. It is obvious that this teacher's appearance decreased the effect of the information she attempted to convey. Action speaks louder than words. The way in which you perform a procedure influences how clients will perform it. Those with compulsive needs and good memories may mimic you with much more precision than you expect (see Figure 10-4).

Enthusiasm is contagious. If you are excited about what you are doing, clients find it easier to learn from you. Your enthusiasm also helps tense clients convert their anxiety into more useful energy.

Programmed Instruction

Programmed instruction is prepackaged in the form of a book, booklet, or computer software. All of the steps necessary to systematically learn the information are anticipated and presented to the client in a logical fashion in one of these three forms. Programmed instruction provides for client reaction at the completion of each step before the client proceeds to the next step. Programmed instruction has three basic steps.

1. The material is broken into small steps called frames.
2. The client is required to make frequent responses.

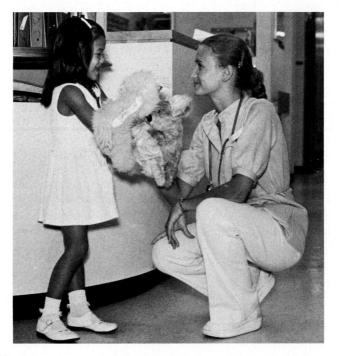

Figure 10-4   Role modeling often occurs at unconscious levels of learning. *From L.F. Whaley and D.L. Wong,* Essentials of Pediatric Nursing, *3rd ed, Mosby, 1989.*

3. The client receives immediate feedback as to the correctness or accuracy of his or her responses.

Programmed instruction is particularly useful for clients who learn better when they have no time constraints, and when they can repeat steps as many times as they choose in order to feel comfortable. Increases in technology have made more and more interactive strategies available for the client who may benefit from programmed instruction. The program must be written by experts who are fully aware of the learning that is desirable. Teachers with very logical minds and very meticulous personalities seem to be best for writing such programs.

You will find programmed instruction is more useful for training clients in cognitive skills involving certain kinds of judgment. Programmed instruction is also useful in teaching certain psychomotor skills, such as listening to breathing sounds, correctly taking blood pressure readings, or identifying the appearance of an infected wound. It is less useful for helping clients master affective and experiential learning, which are dependent on intuition, process, and gestalt-type operations. Inter-active video productions are proving useful in experiential learning.

Simulated Environment

The simulated environment is an artificial situation designed to evoke in the client the same coping responses that are likely to occur in the real situation. The simulated environment provides the client with an opportunity to practice, under low-risk conditions, the coping skills that are needed for an activity that *must* be done correctly, such as starting intravenous fluids. Your instructors probably made use of this strategy to teach you how to give injections to oranges and each other. A simulated environment, as shown in Figure 10-5, is often helpful in teaching children.

Youngsters in primary education classes are sometimes assigned to raise a plant and carry it with them all of the time or to babysit a raw egg. Such experiences give children some experience in the amount of care and attention parents must provide a real baby. Teachers who wish to promote anticipatory learning in adolescents sometimes take students through the life cycle of a marriage: engage-

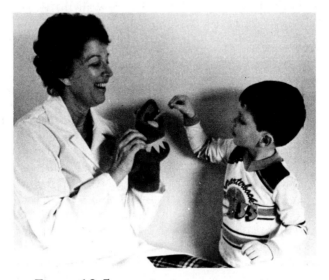

Figure 10-5 Simulated environment evokes coping responses similar to the real event. *From L.F. Whaley and D.L. Wong,* Essentials of Pediatric Nursing, *3rd ed, Mosby, 1989.*

ment, planning a wedding, shopping for furniture on varying budgets, planning meals, encountering crises over which they have no control, and getting a divorce or dealing with the death of a spouse by the end of the semester.

Group Activities

A group activity is any activity directed by the teacher and designed to enhance learning in a group. In addition to providing variety, an activity arouses group interest and enhances learning because more channels of input and output are involved in the process.

Be sure to spell out the objective(s) the activity is designed to promote. This will allow your clients to get their minds in the framework of your content. Explain to the group in a general way what they will be expected to do. For example, if you want them to do aerobics, they need to put down their pencils and get up. If you want them to divide into smaller groups, they need to take their chairs and writing implements with them.

Spelling out directions is an important task, but it is not an easy one. We urge you to first try the directions out first on friends or colleagues. We guarantee you will learn a lot by doing this. It is like a pilot study to a research project: You iron out the kinks so that when you use the directions with clients, everything will run more smoothly.

Pay attention to timing and give participants a chance to develop trust in you and each other so that they are willing to participate. Take into account the environment and the setting when assigning activities. Many group participants are willing to do more emotionally risky activities when they are insulated from individuals toward whom they feel vulnerable. For example, if you are running a group at a work place, and the boss is next door or in the same room with the group, you cannot expect low-level employees in the organization to take many risks.

Allow the group time to discuss what they learned from their participation in the activity. At the conclusion of every activity, participants need time to process the learning experience. After having them engage in an important learning activity, it is time to reflect on what they learned. The primary learning objective should be discussed along with any learning related to it. However, the additional insights clients gain might surprise you. Group activities are holistic learning opportunities and might stimulate many areas of learning besides your target objectives. Expect that the learning will include more than just your learning objective.

Role Playing

Role playing may be defined as assuming the characteristic and expected behaviors of an assigned individual as illustrated in Figure 10-6. The individual may be oneself in an anticipated position, or the player may take the position of another in order to better understand that other individual or role. This strategy is quite useful in learning new social behaviors. It is helpful in skills such as assertiveness training. Clients who experience conflict when there is no easy answer can learn how to cope more successfully with their own feelings. They can also practice various behavioral options.

Role playing has become an integral part of developing successful refusal skills for individuals of any age, including youngsters (Bauer, 1981). The ability to "Just say 'no' " is enhanced when youngsters have practice in real-life situations and have tried out the principles they have learned (Bingham & Bargar, 1985). Children in general seem to role play more easily than adults. If the teacher tells young children, "Be a carrot," "Be a police officer," or "Be a fence," they will know just what to do. Adults, however, are more inhibited and worried about how they look and whether or not they will play the role correctly.

When you plan to use role playing, look for good role models in the group. The other clients can then imitate the model until they come up with their own personal style of more effective coping. Because this is a specialized group activity, the guidelines we provided for group activities also fit here.

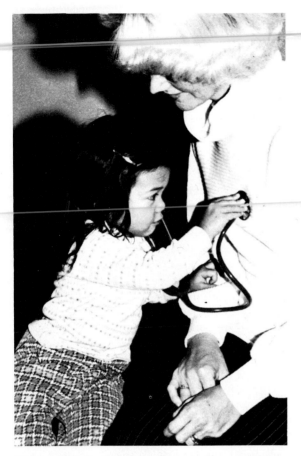

Figure 10-6 Role-play allows each person to "try on" the behavior of the other. *From L.F. Whaley and D.L. Wong, Nursing Care of Infants and Children, 4th ed, Mosby, 1991.*

Special Considerations

Rapport among you, the clients, and each other is especially important in role playing when the clients are older and more self-conscious. You must allow time for the group to reach a certain level of trust, because role playing so frequently elicits emotions from the participants. Because role playing can evoke strong emotions, you should build in some safety rules before proceeding.

> *Example:* "Remember, you should go no further than you choose when dealing with this situation."

You will also check periodically with the clients in the spotlight.

> *Example:* "Is that enough for now? Do you want to go further?"

Be sure to allow time for clients to practice responding to the situation under discussion, until they are satisfied. Resolution occurs when an individual expresses better understanding of the situation and describes new or more options for responding to it. If the role play does evoke emotions in the players, be sure to reintegrate these individuals with the rest of the group. You can do this by having the others share their own emotional reactions to the scenes.

Team Teaching

Team teaching exists when two or more teachers with different preparation, abilities, and skills cooperate and share with one another the responsibilities for planning, teaching, and evaluating the learning of clients. You will find guidelines for effective team teaching in the box on the next page.

In team teaching, different types of teachers combine their strengths to make the workshop more positive for all. For example, a teacher who is quiet prefers to avoid discussion because she is afraid that she will not know what to do with spontaneous discussion. However, her partner is very spontaneous and laughs very often. The quiet partner, using the microphone, gave a very well-prepared lecture. Her partner was easily able to evoke a lively discussion.

In another situation, two experienced teachers, who planned a workshop for a large convention of nurses, combined their strengths. During the preparation phase of the presentation one teacher—who had a doctoral degree in public speaking, the specific topic of the workshop—researched the literature. The other teacher, who had a master's degree, was an expert in group process, so she researched typical work situations in which this specific group of nurses practiced. She went to local units and observed the transactions of these nurses. She arranged to give these nurses a shortened version of the material and asked them all for real-life examples of the theory being studied. The teacher with the research background in the subject presented the lecture portion of the workshop in a very logical and clear manner. The process-oriented teacher provided examples to which the audience could relate. The latter teacher also led the exercises, using experiences that were appropriate to the work situations of the audience. Both teachers critiqued the group's practice speeches.

Selecting the Right Strategy

Select the strategy that best suits the objectives, the content, the clients, you, and the reality of the learning situation. Think about the situation in which the new learning will be used. An example of this involved an experience with family counseling. A family asked a nursing student in community health nursing for help in dealing with the family's problems. During the assessment phase the family members reported that they had been to many classes and workshops on family communications and related experiences, but they said that although what they learned sounded good, attempts to apply the theories to their own family situation were un-

successful. The student chose to engage them in learning new behaviors in their own home. This strategy pushed the student to try interventions tailored for the family's situation. The problem also gave the student the opportunity to see what the family was doing with what they had learned. In their home, the actual patterns of communication became apparent and on-the-spot coaching was provided. The family reported that this type of approach was much more meaningful, practical, and successful.

The strategy should also suit the domain in which the learning is to take place. If the objective is to gain new information, lecture is one of the most efficient methods for imparting knowledge. Programmed instruction is another excellent tool to promote the learning of new facts. This can be done at your client's pace. Provide clients with the opportunity to gain new information in context. Hearing about a resource and actually visiting it are not the same, particularly for an experiential learner. A good example of this is having youngsters visit the hospital before surgery. A lecture given by a person who has participated in a particular program, such as Reach for Recovery or Healing the Child Within, can provide new knowledge as well as hope for individuals who also want to change attitudes or values. Such speakers are able to model options while talking about them.

Attitude adjustments are facilitated by modeling, discussion, and participatory activities, such as games, role playing, and simulated environments. These methods of unconscious influence and personal confrontation are also helpful for helping clients change their values. One such approach is to have clients enact simulations or role play situations that confront the attitudes they hold. To be most effective, you will want to provide a positive consequence for clients who risk trying on the new desired value.

Skill building is facilitated through modeling and through demonstration. Interpersonal skill building is facilitated through both these methods and role playing. Team teaching is particularly useful when clients' needs exceed the expertise of any one individual teacher.

The strategy should suit the client's learning style and abilities. If the client cannot read, a strategy that involves the client's reading or writing would be ineffective. If the individual is a kinesthetic learner, then at least one of the strategies should provide an opportunity for hands-on experience.

The strategy should also suit you, the teacher. We recommend that you strike a balance between practicing strategies that play to your own strengths—logical, calm, or flamboyant—and challenge you to stretch and grow a bit. During practice you can discern whether or not you find a particular strategy so uncomfortable that it would negatively affect the learning experience of the audience. This type of rehearsal is very worthwhile for a number of reasons. When you try something that is new and uncomfortable, you grow and expand your experience. You have the opportunity to know on firsthand what you are asking of clients. Nurses frequently expect clients to try some behavior that is totally foreign to them although it is quite familiar and common to the nurse. Whenever you stretch yourself and remind yourself of what it is like to change, this, in turn, increases your sensitivity to others and broadens your repertoire of adaptational strategies. Even a strategy that is not the most comfortable allows you more flexibility. In case a change of plan becomes necessary, you have that other option at your disposal.

A small space or a large auditorium with fixed seats will eliminate certain activity options. If the learning situation is not conducive to privacy and uninterrupted time, you would not choose a psychodrama. If in the real situations the clients are homeless as well as diabetic, you are going to be challenged to choose realistic strategies to teach them proper nutrition, relaxation, exercise, and insulin preparation (Witt, 1991).

Expanding the Lesson Plan for Lincoln Perez

In Chapter 9 we started a lesson plan for Mr. Perez. We are now expanding on this lesson plan to include teaching strategies. Refer to Table 10-1 to see how we included teaching strategies in the lesson plan. One of our objectives is increased knowledge, and because our situation is one-to-one, we will use the strategy of discussion to increase his knowledge about the relationship between stress management and blood pressure management. Discussion is also a useful strategy for altering attitudes. We have spelled out specific questions you should ask him during this discussion. During discussion we can also have him select soothing prayers or engage in deep relaxation, a psychomotor skill. We will use the strategy of reading him directions for deep breathing, meditation, and imagery. We will demonstrate some simple yoga positions, have him copy our movements, and tell us how he feels as he does them. Because one of our longterm objectives is to reduce his blood pressure and heart rate through a combination of better eating, exercising, and effective stress management, we wish to give him skills he can use to monitor his own progress. Pulse rate is easier for Mr. Perez to access than his blood pressure. If he succeeds in relaxing deeply, he can lower his pulse rate on the spot, and he can easily tell if he has succeeded. To accomplish this objective, he needs the psychomotor skill of measuring his pulse accurately. We have, therefore, included in our strategies the demonstration of pulse taking.

Summary

In this chapter we have reviewed nine of the most common teaching strategies used in health care settings. No one teaching strategy is better than the others. Each strategy has advantages and disadvantages, and each is more suitable than others for various types of learning. You will find that you are more skillful and comfortable using some strategies than others. We urge you to try new strategies and become flexible in applying them to various learning situations for clients. You will find what all good teachers have discovered—a variety of strategies greatly enhances the amount of learning that is retained (Claxton & Murrell, 1987). Table 10-2 summarizes the advantages and disadvantages of the previously mentioned strategies.

TABLE 10-1

Sample Lesson Plan for Lincoln Perez

Learning Objectives	Content Outline	Strategies and Materials

By the end of this lesson, the client will be able to:
  Select from a list three benefits of relaxation.
	Introductions
	Relaxation
	  Definitions
	  Balance with exercise
	  Benefits
	    Reduce blood pressure
	    Reduce tension
	    Increase efficiency
		Discussion Question: "What does relaxation mean to you?"
		Discuss the relationship of stress to blood pressure.

Agree to experiment with walking and various relaxation techniques.	Medications
	  Fears
	  Side effects
	Life-style changes
	  Costs
	  Benefits
		Discuss fears and mixed feelings.
		Question: "Who else in your family has been diagnosed with hypertension? What did it do to them? What have they done to control it, and what were the results?"

Count his pulse within three beats of what the nurse counts.	Techniques for pulse taking
	  Location of artery
	  Finger placement
	  Counting
	  Multiplying
	  Recording method
	Techniques for relaxation
	  Deep breathing
	  Yoga
	  Meditation
	  Imagery
	  Prayer
	Wrap-up
		Demonstrate pulse taking.
		Have the client demonstrate pulse taking.
		Develop a record-keeping system for monitoring his pulse rate.
		Read directions for deep breathing, yoga, meditation, and imagery.
		Have the client select soothing prayers.

T A B L E   1 0 - 2

Teaching Strategies

Strategy	Advantage	Disadvantage
Lecture	Makes it easier to organize and transfer a large amount of information. Is predictable, efficient, good for a large group, and quicker. Allows teacher control over the material she or he presents. Makes focusing the easiest.	Lacks client feedback. Allows for information overload. Makes sustaining interest difficult. Makes it difficult to tailor material for the group.
Discussion	Allows for continual feedback, attitude development, and modification. Flexes according to motivation of the audience. Picks up confusion and helps resolve difficulties. Serves as a vehicle for networking.	Increases the chances of getting off focus. Makes it easy for discussion to become pointless. Allows some participants to be dominant and others passive. Takes a lot of time.
Demonstration	Activates many senses. Clarifies the ''why's'' of a principle. Commands interest. Correlates theory with practice. Allows teacher to see learning and diagnose the problem. Helps learner get well-directed practice.	Takes a lot of time. Does not cover all aspects of cognitive learning.
Modeling	Facilitates affective learning. Bypasses defenses. Proves effective with children.	Proves ineffective without rapport. Does not always make what is learned visible. Allows for learner ambivalence.
Programmed Instruction	Allows students to go at their own pace and repeat a section at will. Breaks material down into manageable increments. Saves the teacher time.	Depends on motivation of learner. Does not account for unplanned feedback, which can distance clients.
Simulated Environment, Games, Activities, Role Playing	Promotes the greatest transfer of learning. Helps client learn what she or he needs to cope with specific problem or environment. Allows for practice that is most transferrable.	Facilitates unpredictable occurrences. Appears threatening for clients. Takes lots of time. Makes achievement of outcomes difficult.
Team Teaching	Enhances teaching by using competencies of more than one teacher. Allows teachers to learn from each other. Accentuates divergent points of view.	Lacks continuity and internal consistency. Requires more planning time. Makes group processing slower. Forces teachers to give up autonomy.

OBJECTIVES AND STRATEGIES

Purposes:

- Apply theory to practice
- Think critically about the relationship between strategy selection and objectives

Directions:

- Divide into small groups and read the following vignette.
- Your job is to hold a coordinators' meeting. Come up with a menu of objectives (one from each learning domain) and strategies for teaching these clients so that they can achieve the objectives you have outlined.

Lan Chu, RN, works at Community Health Clinic with four other nurses. She discovered that they were all worried about their hypertensive clients. She asked the coordinator to put these concerns on the agenda for the next conference to see what could be done. During the conference the five nurses shared with each other their concerns about patients who did not take their medications and were not controlling their blood pressure. The nurses agreed that a series of classes with the clients might be a way to intervene. Lan agreed to do the classes and set them up using what she had learned in her Client Education class at the local college. She noted that a change of attitude and behavior was as important as increased knowledge.

During the first class, Lan learned that some clients were fearful that their children and grandchildren would begin popping pills if they saw Mom or Grandpa doing it regularly. Other clients had heard that if you eat right you do not have to take pills. Lan told them that she would not promise freedom from pills, but they could discuss that with their physicians. She offered to arrange for a meeting with a dietitian for those who needed more intensive nutritional evaluation and consultation. She started thinking about where in the neighborhood there might be a free or coin-operated blood pressure machine.

SELECTING STRATEGIES

Purpose:

- Review advantages and disadvantages of each strategy

Directions:

- Divide into small groups so that all strategies are assigned.

- Each group is to write a brief vignette about a client that would be suitable for the strategy to which you were assigned. Explain how the advantages and disadvantages of that particular strategy are evident in the client situation you design.
- Share your report with your peers.

References

Babcock, D. & Zak-Dance, C. (1981). Developing skills as a public speaker. *AORN Journal, 33*(5), 994-1000.

Bauer, K.G. (1981). *Improving the chances for health: Lifestyle change and health evaluation.* San Francisco CA: National Center for Health Education.

Bingham, A. & Bargar, J. (1985). Children of alcoholic families. *Journal of Psychosocial Nursing, 23*(12), 13-15.

Carnegie, D. (1980). *The quick and easy way to effective speaking,* 2nd ed. New York: Dale Carnegie & Associates.

Claxton, C.S. & Murrell, P.H. (1987). *Learning styles: Implications for improving education practices.* ASHE-ERIC Higher Education Report No. 4. Washington DC: Association for the Study of Higher Education.

deTornyay, R. & Thompson, M.A. (1982). *Strategies for teaching nursing.* New York: John Wiley & Sons.

Fishel, R. (1988). *Time for joy: Daily affirmations.* Deerfield Beach FL: Health Communications.

Heidgerken, L. (1965). *Teaching and learning in schools of nursing: Principles and methods.* Philadelphia: J.B. Lippincott.

Irwin, T. (1985). *Nicomachean Ethics.* Indianapolis: Hackett.

Neufeldt, V. (ed.). (1991). *Webster's New World Dictionary* (3rd ed.), Cleveland: Webster's New World.

Poon, L.W., Fozard, J.L. Cermak, L.S. Arenberg, D. & Thompson, L.W. (eds.). (1980). In *New directions in memory and aging: Proceedings of the George A. Talland memorial conference.* Hillsdale NJ: Lawrence Erlbaum Associates.

Practical applications of research. (1981). *Newsletter of Phi Delta Kappa's Center on Evaluation, Development and Research.* Bloomington IN: 3(4), 1-4.

Sprague, J. & Stuart, D. *The speaker's handbook* (3rd ed.). (1992). Orlando FL: Harcourt Brace Jovanovich.

Witt, B.S. (1991). The homeless shelter: An ideal clinical setting for RN/BSN students. *Nursing and Health Care, 12*(6), 304-307.

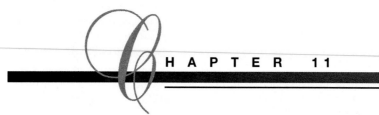

Selecting Teaching Materials

All education is self education.
Teachers may help define
procedure, collect equipment,
indicate the most propitious
route, but the climber must use
his own head and legs if he
would reach the mountaintop

Russell, 1938, p. 385.

Objectives

Upon completion of this chapter you will be able to:

- State three purposes of teaching materials.
- Critique the advantages and disadvantages of 15 types of teaching materials.
- List 10 questions to consider when selecting appropriate teaching materials.
- Develop a list of resources for obtaining teaching materials.
- Evaluate the readability level of selected health education materials.
- Design and alter teaching materials so that they are more appropriate for a particular client or group with regard to readability.

Key Words

videorecording	overhead projector	bulletin boards
motion pictures	opaque projector	computer-assisted
objects	chalkboard	instruction (CAI)
models	pamphlets	flip charts
slides	posters	public address
filmstrips	photographs	system
audiocassette tapes	cartoons	readability

Introduction

In the previous chapter we focused on the strategies and methods that will facilitate client learning. In this chapter we examine a number of teaching materials that will help you achieve your objectives. Teaching materials are the actual matter or substances that will be physically manipulated with the aim of promoting the client's learning. These materials may be manipulated by you as well as the client. Teaching materials provide the visual component that is essential for learning. In addition, some materials allow for the physical contact that kinesthetic learners need. Other materials invite emotional involvement, which is crucial for changing attitudes.

Teaching materials serve several purposes (Pohl, 1981). These purposes include extending the client's sensory experience, introducing variety into the teaching process, giving meaning to abstractions, and making otherwise complicated explanations understandable. Pohl outlines a number of factors that must be considered when you are determining teaching materials to use. These factors include assessment of the topic being

—Continued next page

presented, the client(s) being addressed, and the materials available. Pohl emphasizes that materials are *not* a substitute for the teacher.

There are a variety of teaching materials available to you, and each has its own advantages and disadvantages for any specific teaching/learning situation. This chapter discusses advantages and disadvantages of certain materials along with purposes and helpful hints.

Videorecordings

A videorecording is the substitute closest to the actual experience because it stimulates both hearing and sight. A videorecording can evoke imagery and intense emotion as it invites the client to experience with the actors the scene that is being enacted. The television usually evokes very positive associations, such as relaxation and entertainment. These associations help clients start out with a positive attitude toward the learning.

Videorecordings allow clients to view the action very closely or to move back for a panoramic view. Such recordings are excellent to use for a close-up demonstration of a procedure regardless of the group's size. This medium is also excellent for generating an affective response in the audience and for promoting discussion. A videorecording can be stopped to discuss a particular action or to elicit predictions and problem-solving options from the audience. A video can also help clients anticipate possibilities for which they must prepare.

Technology has made it possible to project a videorecording onto a giant screen, which means better visibility when showing the video to a larger group. Videotapes are able to tolerate pauses for frame-by-frame viewing, with less risk of overheating, than motion picture films. Once the initial investment in a videocamera is made, the followup cost of buying, recording, and showing videotapes is relatively low. In just 1 year the number of students in our classes who owned video cassette recorders (VCRs) tripled. Now, most nursing students own them. Even though a VCR is bulky, it is readily available in many settings. However, it is important

to explore in detail whether or not compatible equipment is accessible. A VCR and monitor would be very cumbersome to transport especially if inappropriate equipment renders them unusable.

Videotapes themselves are easy to store and transport. Those that are "homemade" are available for showing immediately after they are recorded, which means you can avoid the delay of processing. If you are dissatisfied with the results, you can recycle the tape immediately. Video cameras and players are excellent tools for giving immediate and accurate feedback to clients who are attempting to learn a particular process. A videotape is also helpful for rehearsing and critiquing emergency procedures. Videotapes are widely used in helping athletes, such as skiers and swimmers, study their motions. They are also excellent training devices for clients who are learning to be more assertive.

The videotape can also be recycled if its message becomes outdated. Commercially prepared videotapes are comparable in price to motion pictures for both rental and purchase. Whenever you intend to use a videotape, you must plan well in advance. If a popular videotape is to be borrowed or rented, it must be reserved weeks or months ahead to ensure that it is available on the desired date. We strongly recommend that you preview the videotape and test the equipment on which you will use it.

Because modern VCRs are relatively easy to operate, the machines may engender a false sense of security in you: "I know how they work; I have one at home." The trick is making sure the desired tape will play on the available player. You must take as much care in checking compatibility as you do when preparing to administer a blood product. The most common videotape formats are the ½ inch (for VHS) and 8 mm (for camcorders). At this time, VHS is the most common format for professional use in the United States. Another compatibility factor that must be assessed is the speed at which both parts of the system run. Most VCRs in the home have automatic speed adapters. Equipment borrowed from a library (and of an earlier vintage) may not have this feature. Therefore when you borrow equipment, you need to practice using the actual tape on the actual machine on which you will show it. Because a VCR depends on electrical power, you should have a backup plan ready in case the power fails.

As with any learning experience, the tape will be most valuable if prefaced by advance organizers. An introduction to the tape includes its title, its length, a synopsis of the message or story, and what you expect the clients to gain from viewing the tape. It may also be helpful to tell the clients specifically what they should notice and what they will be expected to do with the experience afterward: take a test, discuss the plot, or perform the procedures. If unfamiliar words are used in the tape, we suggest that you introduce them beforehand. Put the words on a transparency or on the chalkboard before the videotape is shown.

Motion Picture

Motion pictures have many of the same advantages as videorecordings, and they can be shown to any size audience, limited only by the size of the available screen. However, the film used to make motions pictures is very fragile,. and it cannot be recycled. Because this type of film breaks easily, it must be protected from moisture changes as well as extreme temperatures. Because science and technology change so rapidly, films relevant to health and illness become outdated rather quickly (Kemp & Dayton, 1985). In the past 8 years the cardiopulmonary resuscitation (CPR) procedure has been changed five times, making each previous film outdated. Because films are very expensive, the individual responsible for choosing should exercise caution during the selection process. Each motion picture projector threads a bit differently than others. Therefore we urge you to practice the threading procedure. While doing this you can wind the film to the desired spot in an atmosphere conducive to calm and concentration. Sometimes these films are wound incorrectly. Rewinding the films is not only time consuming but also challenging—especially if the film is backwards, inside out, or both.

The use of motion pictures can be problematic for a number of reasons. Because the lights must be dimmed during the film, some clients may fall asleep. In addition, films of any length are cumbersome and bulky to store. The projector necessary for showing the film is even more unwieldy than the film. Most projectors are noisy while they are running, which can be annoying in a small room.

Before you plan to show a film, you should get some technologic training regarding the principles and procedures of running a film projector, in addition to hands-on experience with the particular projector you will be using. We recommend that you refrain from mending a film that breaks in the middle of the showing. This means that you should have an alternative plan ready in case the intended film presentation goes awry.

Objects and Models

Actual objects should be used for demonstration whenever possible. For example, use a real syringe when you teach self-injections, and use a real dressing when you teach self-application of a dressing. Models are used when the real object, such as a heart, is not available or not feasible to use. Three types of models are a replica, an analogue, and a symbol.

Replica

A replica is a model that resembles the real object. A replica is a scaled construction that magnifies the features of the original object. The increased size of the features makes demonstration easier. This type of model can be picked up and manipulated and helps convey the concept of dimensions. A replica is useful for the kinesthetic client who learns better with hands-on opportunities. Such a client can take the model of a kidney apart and put it back together again, thus getting a better idea of how the parts fit together. Because the client will learn by handling the replica, the client is able to control the pace of his or her learning.

A replica may be constructed larger than life. For example, the enormous plastic sculptures of the heart that have been placed in museums and institutes allow clients to walk through various chambers, envisioning themselves as blood cells wandering through the heart. In addition to being fun, these sculptures contribute to learning by exposing clients kinesthetically, auditorily, and visually to the concept of circulation. Models through which people can stroll have proved fascinating to the young as well as the young at heart. Such gigantic sculptures of the circulation allow people to get a better understanding of the structure of that system as well as the process of the blood flowing from one part of the body to another. Although as an individual teacher you will probably not be able to afford such a production, you might arrange a field trip to an appropriate display.

A replica can be used to help clients develop a skill. Learning to clean a central line and to examine breasts for lumps are each challenging procedures best learned on something other than a human being. Although replicas exist for practicing these particular skills, they are expensive and fragile. Such replicas require bulky storage space and protection from atmospheric extremes. They are also unwieldy to transport.

Replicas, unless they are enormous, usually serve only a few clients at a time. You can compensate for this by using team teaching and by arranging different replicas at different "stations." Such an arrangement divides the larger group into several smaller ones and allows each station to become an area of concentrated focus with fewer competing stimuli.

Analogue

An analogue is a model that acts like the real object because it features properties of a system that are essential to the learning under consideration. The analogue model can be used effectively to describe, explain, and/or represent certain crucial features of a dynamic system. Mechanical circulation devices, heart-lung machines, and dialysis equipment are examples of analogues. They do not resemble the real anatomy of a person, but they perform similar physiologic functions; dialysis equipment is frequently called an artificial kidney for this very reason.

A popular example being used currently to explain intellectual processes compares the human brain to a computer. Your mind is like a computer. It will work for you as long as you input good information into it. Some people have million-dollar computers and some people have five thousand dollar computers in their head, but if they are well cared for, get good input, and are allowed to go at their own pace, they both work just fine. An analogue demands conceptual sophistication and a measure of similar understandings. Because not everyone perceives the same way, you should practice using the analogue on others to find out how many understand the point. It also helps to explain to the test group how the analogue fits the message you intend to convey. Table 11-1 contains a little memory crutch for helping you differentiate analogue, replica, and symbol.

Symbol

A symbol stands for something else that it represents by association, resemblance, or convention. The treble clef sign and notes on lines are examples of musical symbols. Often a printed or written sign is used to represent an operation, element, quan-

---

TABLE 11-1
Differentiating Models

	Analogue	Replica	Symbol
Mnemonic device	Acts like	Resembles	Stands for
Example	Artificial kidney	Red heart model	Stop sign

tity, quality, or relation, or something invisible (Neufeldt, 1991). Examples of symbols are words, which are combinations of circles and lines arranged in special patterns to convey a certain meaning. The meaning varies according to the language familiar to the speaker, writer, listener, and reader.

Words are symbolic models that you will use to convey a concept or idea to the client. Words are such familiar symbols that you no longer perceive the circles and lines with which words are drawn unless you are dyslexic. In fact, unless you have a photographic mind, you could not even report the exact words on this page. You would probably report the ideas, general concepts, and meanings you attached to what you read.

You may draw diagrams, signs, or cartoons, all of which are attempts to convey meaning through the use of symbols. The international traffic signs are examples of such symbols. The picture conveys the meaning. Circles have many meanings. Arranged on top of each other and colored red, yellow, and green, they would probably be perceived in this country as parts of a traffic light. "Smiley" faces are recognized by most people in this culture as conveying happiness or approval.

The practice of representing something by association, resemblance, or convention is so widespread in this culture that it is difficult to describe by example. The symbol "+" means *plus,* and the symbol "=" means *equal to.* Stick figures can be used by any teacher to symbolize people regardless of artistic talent. Such a figure can really help you focus a client's attention on the desired point. A basic stick figure is symbolic of a person. If that same stick figure is next to a stick figure with a triangle

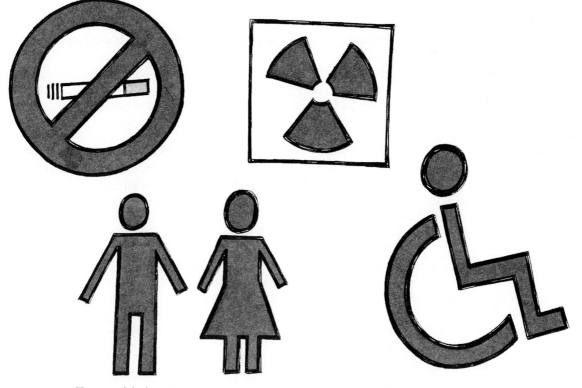

Figure 11-1 Symbols are arbitrary signs that represent widely recognized concepts.

over the lower portion of the figure, then the first figure is thought to represent a man and the second a woman. A good example of the power of symbols can be illustrated by noting the difference between your understanding of our message described in this paragraph and your familiarity with stick figures.

Symbols are gaining widespread application in areas that cater to multilingual groups. These areas include airports, research hospitals, and businesses in ethnically diverse neighborhoods. You should avoid using abbreviations that are common among medical personnel but are not common among consumers. These abbreviations include NPO, PO, GNP, GTTS, and PRN. Although these abbreviations convey meaning to certain groups they might add to the confusion of other groups. Figure 11-1 illustrates some common symbols.

Slides and Filmstrips

Slides are relatively easy to create if you own or have access to a camera. They are also relatively inexpensive to have developed. However, slides take longer to process than prints. Children can make their own slide shows, which could help you understand how they see the world. Although there are varying degrees of expertise and artistic skill necessary for composing pictures, you could arrange slides in interesting and colorful ways to convey the points you wish to make. Slides allow you to capture real people doing real activities that are relevant to the lesson. Pictures of real people are easier to relate to for people with limited literacy skills (Doak, Doak, & Root, 1985). A slide presentation is excellent for the visual client and helps clarify the lecture. You may find that an extensive slide show may contain all of the clues you need to jog your memory. You may need no other cue cards or notes.

If a few slides are unsatisfactory or become outdated, they are easy to replace without disturbing the others. If you decide that a different sequence of slides would be more conducive to learning, you can easily rearrange them. Homemade slides can be tailored to the specific needs of your audience. There may be times when you wish to make a slide of a poster or a picture. If so, the camera should have a short focal length. To obtain the best possible result you must find a way to flatten the material you intend to copy. Keep in mind that black and white pictures look better if they are surrounded by color.

If you wish to have slides transferred into a film chain for video, we advise you to consult with the video transformer before buying the slide film or having it processed because this method requires a degree of technical assistance not discussed in this text.

A commercially prepared slide show can be used with its accompanying audiocassette, or you can select pertinent slides and construct your own script. Slides are very useful when you wish to spend time on a particular scene while conveying knowledge related to that scene. It can serve as a focal point to keep the audience on track. Many families own their own slide projector. The equipment, therefore, is relatively easy to obtain. Slide-audiocassette combinations are more complicated and expensive. They may be available at the school or local library. They also take practice if you are going to use them effectively.

Slides are easy to store and to transport. However, because slides are made of film, they need the same kind of protection as any film. They should be protected from moisture and temperature extremes. Once you have your slides organized be sure to mark each of them in a consistent spot. We recommend marking the slides on the upper, right-hand corner because this spot is readily visible. If you should need to remove the slides and replace them at a later date, the numbers will help you replace the slides much more rapidly. Once your slides are arranged in the tray, remember to fasten the collar on the tray to prevent the slides from falling out if the tray falls.

If there is no slide carousel at the teaching site, you can bring your own carousel, but it will be bulky to transport. If those in charge of the teaching site are willing to provide a slide projector, then the materials you will have to bring will be significantly reduced. Compatibility and operability are two important considerations. We urge you to try out the equipment with the tray of slides at least one day before the teaching session. This will allow you time to find an alternative slide projector or to purchase a spare bulb that is compatible with the machine you intend to use. We also urge you to avoid slide trays that hold 140 slides because trays that hold 80 slides work more predictably and become stuck less often.

Filmstrips are materials that have some properties in common with slides. One of the advantages of commercially prepared filmstrips over motion pictures and videotapes is the cost. Filmstrips are much less expensive, and they are less bulky to store. When accompanied by music and taped narration, filmstrips can be quite entertaining. However, filmstrips are less flexible than slides because their sequence is preset. Because you have no control over the sequence, you have fewer options in displaying this type of teaching material. Many filmstrips are accompanied by matching audiocassettes.

Audiocassettes for filmstrips typically have two sides: an automatic side and a manual side. With the right projector, the automatic side advances frames automatically. The other side makes a subtle signal that indicates the frame should be advanced manually. If you wish to use the filmstrip and replace the dialogue, you can do so. There are levers on the filmstrip projector that allow this option.

Filmstrips are delicate and can begin to burn if you focus on one frame for too long. Both slides and filmstrips are best viewed in a darkened room, but this makes note taking relatively difficult. The darkened room can also be hypnotic for bored or weary clients. Both filmstrips and slides are frequently shown while you stand in the back of the room behind the audience. This positioning may interfere with your ability to track the audience's response.

Audiocassette Tapes

Audiocassette tapes are easily obtainable today, as are cassette players. This teaching material is particularly useful when the skill the client must learn is auditory. For example, if you are trying to teach the parents of an asthmatic child to recognize various breath sounds, an audiocassette might be particularly helpful. By listening to different types of breathing on an audiocassette, parents can learn which types of breathing require an emergency response and which types can be improved by cupping. Tapes are also useful for hearing directions when the client cannot look at the speaker. An example is a client who is lying prone while following directions for exercise or relaxation. Many people find it easier to concentrate when their eyes are closed or when they listen to soothing music or directions for creating healing images.

Audiocassette tapes are excellent devices for learning while traveling. For example, it is possible to study a foreign language and practice pronunciation while driving. Memorization and other repetitive tasks can be accomplished while you wait in traffic. Instead of being aggravated by traffic jams, you can end up with mastery of a vocabulary list.

In these days of early discharge, clients often leave the hospital before they or their families are confident of the procedures they must do at home. By recording your voice, during the client's final teaching or coaching session you can talk the client through the procedure with a minimum of extra effort or time. First you quiz your client on the equipment she or he needs to proceed. The list of equipment will then be at the beginning of the tape. During the procedure itself you will automatically pause and allow the client enough time, because you will actually be watching the client's behavior. You will also offer words of reinforcement and encouragement during this transaction. When the client and family go home, they will hear your reassuring words, which can be very comforting to those who must now handle the procedure on their own. In addition to being a reassuring experience that lowers tension, the familiarity of your voice recreates a mind set that more closely approximates the last teaching session. Both of these variables promote more accurate recall.

The only equipment you will need is an audiocassette tape and a cassette recorder and player. If the family owns a tape recorder, this should be used to ensure compatibility between materials. If no tape recorder is available among family or friends, see if the hospital could lend the family a tape player.

Make sure the family understands that the instrument will be returned during the third home visit or the first office visit.

Audiocassette tapes can also be used to promote bonding between sick and hospitalized infants and their parents from whom the babies are separated. The mother can hold the microphone near her abdominal cavity and her heart, to record the sounds the infant heard during gestation. The mother can record lullabies and other messages of endearment that she would say if she could hold her baby. These messages can then be played within the baby's hearing range. Listening to a heartbeat has a favorable effect on an infant's sleep and weight gain (Anderson, 1989).

When you are in community health settings and clients live far away, such as in rural settings, you might depend on the telephone between home visits. A tape recorder could be left with the family containing reminders, complicated instructions, or both. The audiocassette could also be used for blind clients or those with reading disabilities. In addition to being mailable, audiocassette tapes are easy to make and small enough to transport readily. A tape recording can capture nuances of speech that are impossible to convey in written communication.

Although audio tapes have many advantages, they also have some drawbacks. The listener may find it difficult to listen for more than 15 minutes without other stimuli because he or she gets bored. Remember that audiocassette tapes are somewhat fragile and need protection from moisture and temperature extremes.

Overhead Projector

The overhead projector is a very popular audiovisual aid that can display transparencies or silhouettes of items to any size audience. The only limitations are the size of the screen and the distance from the projector to the screen. We recommend that you stand to one side of the projector and look at the audience when giving a presentation. The projector is arranged so that, while you face the audience, you can look at the projector table and see the same scene that is being displayed in larger proportions on the screen behind you. This means you and the clients can view the same scene while still facing each other.

A transparency can be seen with lights on unless there is unusual glare, such as direct sunlight. A transparency is an excellent medium, therefore, to aid clients who wish to take notes. You can use transparencies to highlight verbal presentations. The highlights can be in the form of brief, well-spaced outlines, pictures, simple drawings, or cartoons. You can prepare transparencies in advance or on the spot in response to dialogue with the clients. Transparencies are relatively inexpensive to purchase and can be stored flat in a pocket envelope that fits a standard note binder. Some teachers prefer to bind their transparencies. This method keeps transparencies looking very nice and gives them more protection, but they must be stored in a large, separate folder.

You can prepare transparencies in many ways. One way is to construct an attractive line drawing on paper, copy the drawing on a copy machine that makes quality copies, and then run the copy together with a blank transparency through a thermofax machine. You can use a Kroy machine to get a variety of large type for labeling. Arrange the letters into brief statements and then copy the product on a copier. This then would also be suitable for running through a thermofax with a blank transparency. You can also design a poster on a computer, copy it on a copy machine and then make a transparency of the copy by running it through a thermofax.

In the above paragraph we emphasized using a copy of your design when you plan to use a thermofax. This is necessary because it is the carbon on the copy that interacts to make the transparency in the presence of heat. Inks that are used in printers will not work in a thermofax or other heat transfer device. Pages designed with Kroy letters also contain the transparent tape on which the letters were printed. If this tape were run through a thermofax, it could ruin both the document and perhaps the roller that transported the paper through the machine.

Some photocopying machines can now make

transparencies, but these transparencies are produced by a different process than the one described above. Instead of burning a figure into the film in the presence of carbon, the copy machine deposits layers of carbon on the film, just as it would if the film were a piece of paper. Because the machine deposits layers of carbon on the transparency, the transparent tape that holds Kroy letters is not a problem; the figures, however, may be more fragile and therefore more temporary. The carbon deposit has a tendency to flake off the film.

You can use colored felt pens to enhance cartoons or to create variety in transparencies that contain standard printed words. You could put a colored box around a key word or underline it. Pens are available in washable and permanent inks. We recommend that you use pens with washable ink for several reasons. If the information is likely to change, or if you occasionally misspell or make other mistakes, you can easily wipe the film clean and begin again. The ink used in permanent ink pens contains strong chemicals, which add another bit of environmental pollution.

Guidelines for Use of an Overhead Projector

Do not block the audience's view. Sitting may be better than standing. Not only is it easier to stay out of the audience's view of the screen, but also you can rest your hand more easily on the edge of the projector for pointing.

Use the on/off switch. Arrange the transparency on the glass stage and take care of any problems before turning on the switch. Turn the switch off as soon as the transparency has served its purpose. As long as the transparency is up, it will draw the audience's attention away from you and the other points you wish to make. In a small room, the whir of the fan can also be distracting.

Keep it simple. The message on transparencies should be simple and easily grasped. A good transparency has no more words on it than a poster. If the idea and words are complex, then clients should have a handout that matches your transparency. In that case you merely use the transparency to help orient clients to the particular graph or sentence under consideration.

Mask any distractions. You may wish to mask the edge of the glass stage itself or enclose each transparency in a cardboard mount. If you have listed several ideas on one transparency, mask the other ideas while you talk about the first one. This focuses the audience on your point and lowers anxiety for avid note-takers. Clients who are note-takers have learned that some speakers may not leave the transparency up long enough to copy, so they copy everything they can see. If you display only one point at a time, note-takers can get it and still have time to hear what you are saying. Each transparency film comes with a thin piece of paper, which you can use to mask the other thoughts. The draft from the projector motor keeps the thin paper in place. Regular-weight paper reacts differently to the draft.

Use a screen large enough for your audience. The larger your audience, the larger your screen should be. If the only screen available is too small, look for a blank wall of a light color. It may suit your needs better.

Keep transparencies free from hand oil. When you draw on a transparency, it is best to protect the film, by keeping a piece of paper under the surface of your hand that rests on the film. If there is oil on the film, the ink will "bead up" and not make a clear drawing.

Try before you buy. All films do not react alike to washable pens, and all washable pens do not wash off freely, so we recommend that you try out the pens and the film before purchase. You may be able to recycle discarded x-ray films, and use them as transparencies. If you are using a new film, buy a small amount until you see how it works for you.

Look for ways to introduce color. Colored films can be used as background for the figure or words.

The tinted film helps provide variety and reduce the glare of the strong light used to illuminate the field. The figures themselves can also be colored. This can be done ahead of time or it can be done when you are referring to a particular item on the transparency. Another way to use color is to print three main ideas in three different colors. Use each main idea as a heading for three subsequent transparencies on which the headings are further outlined. Make the subheadings the same color as the main idea to which they relate.

Color may help clarify an issue as you lecture. For example, to inform a group about the circulation of the heart, first display a black outline of a heart showing the chambers and valves as well as the main veins and arteries. While discussing the circulation of the right side of the heart, add blue color to the right side of the heart on the transparency. Begin by giving or eliciting the names of the superior and inferior venae cavae. Then add blue color to the right atrium and then to the right ventricle. After identifying the pulmonary arteries and tracing blood out to the lungs, use a purple pen to begin discussing carbon dioxide and oxygen exchange. When the blood leaves the lungs to return to the heart, switch to a red pen. If the clients are younger, have them color a handout of the heart that matches one on your transparency.

If you decide to present a complex idea to a group, you may wish to consider using an overlay. The above example of the heart could also be done with overlays. There is a limit to the number of overlays that can be added before the picture becomes fuzzy. Try it on the overhead projector and see how may layers you can see clearly. You can use overlays to demonstrate various options. For example, overlays will help you to illustrate the effect of a coronary artery obstruction on the heart of a sedentary person, and the effect of a similar obstruction in a person whose heart has increased vascularity from aerobic exercise. Exercise I at the end of this chapter will give you experience in working with overlays.

Although overhead projectors are very useful, they have some disadvantages. The machine itself is bulky and awkward to transport, although portable models do exist. As with other projectors, the light bulb can burn out. Most machines have a convenient space for a spare bulb built into the body of the projector, but always be sure you have a replacement bulb at hand.

Opaque Projector

An opaque projector is a piece of audiovisual equipment that usually has a very short focal length and a limited range of flexibility. Such a projector works best in a darkened room. It is the one machine that can show a picture out of a book to a group of clients all at once. The projector is also an ethical way to use the picture without infringing on the author or publisher's copyright. It is also excellent for showing tables, figures, and graphic models. If you choose well, you have an excellent, high-quality picture that will make your point. Using this equipment to illustrate your point may be easier, more accurate, and quicker than converting the same illustration to transparency film. The other main use of the opaque projector is to trace a picture and enlarge it into a poster. To do this:

1. Fasten a piece of large poster board to a wall.
2. Put the picture to be traced in the opaque projector.
3. Focus the picture, and trace it right onto the poster board.

One of the disadvantages of using an opaque projector is its bulkiness, which means it must be transported on a cart. Many graphics departments now have alternative machines, such as the Art-O-Graph, that are more stationary but more versatile. The Art-O-Graph has an updated ventilation system that helps prevent overheating. Old opaque projectors would sometimes get so hot that they would burn the paper being displayed.

Chalkboard

The chalkboard is available in most classroom settings. It is very valuable for making a spontaneous drawing, diagram, or illustration right at the time of concern for your clients. You can add to, or take away from the drawing while using it to explain the meaning or purpose of the topic under discussion. You may remember the chalkboard as being called the blackboard, but it is now called the chalkboard because black is no longer the universal color. In fact, most chalkboards today are colored green. In the near future, they may be replaced by whiteboards.

The chalkboard or whiteboard is an excellent device for involving your clients. To promote contributions, ask a question and then start writing down the responses from the audience. Most individuals find it very reinforcing to see their words written on the chalkboard. The chalkboard is also an organizational device. You can link ideas in a circle, or you can list problems on one side and solutions on the other. A chalkboard also allows you to compare and contrast various points of view or to organize contributions from the audience into whatever schema you choose.

Whenever possible, we recommend that you transfer complicated ideas to a handout that clients can use during your presentation. However, there are times when electric failure, human error, or budgetary restrictions make the chalkboard the more practical way to convey information. The following section contains guidelines for effective use of the chalkboard.

Guidelines for Use of Chalkboards

Print or write in large clear lettering.   Test legibility by deciding whether or not your cursive writing is more legible than your printing.

Put a brief notation on the board and then step aside and face the audience.   This will allow you to maintain contact with your clients and to receive feedback on the clarity of your point. By stepping aside, you also allow clients to copy the message, which means they will be able to integrate both visual and auditory stimuli. Stepping aside will also keep you from becoming so involved with your creation on the board, that you start talking to the board instead of your clients.

Start as high as possible on the board.   If you are very short, bring an easy-to-handle step stool with you. You should consider such a stool part of your audiovisual equipment. Avoid writing below the clients' line of vision.

If the board is wide, draw a vertical line down the middle and use each side to outline several related ideas.   You can also use one side of the board to list causes, but reserve the other side for a list of effects. You might also consider writing signs on one side and symptoms on the other. You may also choose to make three or four columns to elicit related ideas from the audience. For example, you might discuss the effects of certain conditions on the mind, body, and spirit. This also works when you present an extended outline. If you are right-handed, start on the right half of the board, against the drawn line. If you are left-handed, start on the left half of the board, against the left edge.

Fill up one side of the chalkboard before moving to the other.   As you begin to fill up the second half of the chalkboard, note-takers in the audience will have a clear view of the first column. Whenever possible, write down complicated ideas in the form of a handout for clients.

Ask a good note-taker to save a new design before you erase it.   Frequently, spontaneous designs will be very cogent and a result of creative interplay between you and the clients. When this occurs, remember to capture it. This is particularly important if you are forgetful because you may not be able to recall it later.

Be sure that the chalkboard is located in an area that is suitable for the learning purpose.   If it is permanently affixed to the wall in a place that does not work for you, you might want to bring your own board as well as chalk and an eraser.

Use the chalkboard or whiteboard to elicit audience participation.   It is a very effective device for eliciting responses from your clients. The best questions to ask first are those to which everyone can respond, such as questions about personal experience.

> *Example:* "How can you tell when you are stressed out? What do you do or what have you seen others do when they are stressed out?"

You can then write audience contributions on the chalkboard. If you are team teaching, the questioner can keep attuned to the audience while the writer concentrates on writing legibly.

Avoid wearing dark and textured clothing, such as black or navy velvet. Chalk shows up on dark surfaces, and it may be embarrassing if you have it all over yourself.

Pamphlets and Posters

Pamphlets are portable, attractive, readily available, and often free. You can use them before, during, or after a presentation. Clients can hold pamphlets and use them to study and learn at their own pace thus exercising more control over the learning experience. It is important that you give careful consideration to the timing of pamphlet distribution. If the pamphlets contain the actual information you wish to discuss, they may be used as advance organizers and substitute for note-taking. If you decide they would be distracting, you may wish to keep them out of sight until the presentation is completed.

Pamphlets may be purchased at minimal cost or obtained free from many organizations. We have included information about where you can obtain pamphlets in Appendix G. Learning where and how to obtain relevant pamphlets can be an interesting adventure. As you develop your interest and skills in teaching, you will start to notice good pamphlets wherever you go. Commercially prepared pamphlets are frequently designed by marketing experts who incorporate experience and readability principles into the production of their pamphlets. Study particularly attractive pamphlets and identify their appeal. If you cannot find an appropriate pamphlet, you may decide to design one. It is helpful if you are

artistically inclined. If not, you may be able to persuade an artistic friend or relative to help out. It is your responsibility, however, to decide on the message and the basic information. In addition to readability principles, the following guidelines may be useful to you when you design pamphlets of your own.

Guidelines for the Use of Pamphlets and Posters

Illustrations in a pamphlet should have space on all four sides. The space keeps the page from looking too cluttered.

Words should be large, pleasing to the eye, and arranged in short easy-to-read paragraphs. Lines of text should be short enough to scan, and each paragraph should be separated from the next by an illustration or drawing. Illustrations are particularly important for lower-level readers, who would include individuals with poor comprehension of English as well as people with little education. The vocabulary level should be carefully chosen to suit the intended audience. The sentence length should also be within the client's reading level. We have found that it helps to try out the pamphlet on assertive individuals whose reading and vocabulary levels are similar to the target audience. You can then ask these trial readers if they believe the pamphlet is written in plain English. These trial readers also serve as consultants for improving the pamphlet.

Artists' renditions can be very beautiful and pleasing, but they are not necessary to make your point. An understandable illustration is more important than an artistic or entertaining one. The more important the subject matter is to the client, the more she or he would prefer clarity over artistic qualities. You can even use stick drawings, which are usually very easy to understand.

Organizers, such as headings, should be clearly marked and easy to differentiate from the body

of the text.   Color is an excellent organizer. It can be used to differentiate headings, ideas, and sections. Key words are highlighted with color, boldfacing, or underlining.

Posters make excellent advance organizers. A poster can be used to market an upcoming teaching module. It may be color coded or have a particular design that is suggestive of the theme of the lesson. Posters that will be on bulletin boards open to close scrutiny can contain more information than those used during a teaching module.

Posters can also be used to provide you with clues. An excellent speaker frequently impresses her audience by her recitation of statistics from memory. When quizzed about how she manages that feat, she shared this secret: "Put the statistics on the back of the page. As you flip it, you can look at the figures you wish to quote." The following paragraphs contain guidelines for using posters.

The poster should contain a sizable portion of empty space.   The message should contain only key words—not sentences—in large, bold letters. A picture or figure should be clear and large enough to be understood immediately.

Keep the poster simple.   If words are displayed they should be key concepts or brief cues to your progression. If a quote is more than a few words long, you should be silent long enough for your clients to read the message. We recommend that you do not read the message word for word because it is deadly to audience interest. You may want to consider another medium that is more appropriate, such as a handout.

Use color to enhance contrast.   It may help to outline each letter with black.

Be sure that any posters or cartoons you develop or use are appealing to the age, sex, socioeconomic, and ethnic characteristics of your audience.   Sensitivity and delicacy are important, especially when you inject humor.

If your clients are older, use larger, bolder, and plainer letters.   The larger the audience, the larger, fatter, and plainer the letters should be. The 6 W formula means that the last row of the audience should be no farther from the poster than six times the width of the poster. For example, if the poster is 2 feet wide, the last row of viewers should be no farther than 12 feet from the poster. For a larger audience transform the poster into a transparency or slide.

Plan and practice when using the poster.   Provide a place and/or an easel for propping up the poster. During team teaching, you and your colleagues may serve as poster holders for each other. You may also decide to request help from members of the audience. In any event, you should delegate the holding chore to another. This will allow you to pay attention to the audience and to look at them while pointing to the key idea on the poster.

Use a pointer to focus your clients' eyes on a key word or place on the poster.   If you are a dynamic speaker, you may tend to wave your hands while speaking. Do not do this while holding a pointer and referring to a poster. It is distracting and confusing to the audience.

Analyze the effectiveness of the poster from a distance.   One suggestion is to have a near-sighted friend remove his or her glasses and read the poster from across a room that is similar in size to the teaching site. This will give you an approximate idea of the effect your poster will have.

Use soft, removable, gummy, stickum-type products or brown masking tape if you plan to hang the poster on a wall temporarily.   Clear tape has a tendency to lift wall paint and tear the poster or wallpaper.

Photographs and Cartoons

Unless photographs and cartoons can be converted to slides or transparencies, they are best used on an individual basis, or in a small group. When they are passed around, they are distracting to the audience.

Each member of the audience is not paying attention to you while viewing the photograph or cartoon.

Photographs and cartoons are easily personalized, and they are excellent media for clients to hold and study at their own pace. Photographs stimulate emotions and conversation. Humorous cartoons can provide comic relief and/or make a point much more clearly than many words. Before you decide to use humor, test it out on people similar to your intended audience. Drawings that are intended to be humorous can also evoke unexpected reactions among clients who may perceive the material differently than you do. If clients are expected to develop a psychomotor skill, the visual you prepare should portray the situation as they are most likely to encounter it. Doak, Doak, and Root (1985) give some helpful information about what is and what is not clear in cartoon drawings. For example, a photograph with all details showing may be confusing. A line drawing of the same picture with the extraneous variables removed will make the point of the picture clearer. Cartoons are not necessarily cross cultural, so you should show prospective cartoons to someone from the target culture and have them critique it for you. In general, a few, simple words are best.

Photographs tend to change color as they age. Cartoons can be protected with clear plastic wall covering, which will slow the aging process and protect them from destruction during handling.

Bulletin Boards

Bulletins boards can be used to display posters, pamphlets, cartoons, and photographs as well as more wordy information. Place bulletin boards in conspicuous spots that are suitable for browsing. Keep in mind that pausing and glancing are the usual activities of browsers. Information that is deep or wordy will languish unread or it may disappear if someone wishes to really delve into it. To be useful, learning materials placed on bulletin boards must be updated and spaced. We recommend that you use attractive colors and uncluttered designs in the background to attract the eyes of passersby.

Computer Assisted Instruction

Computer Assisted Instruction (CAI) is becoming increasingly conspicuous on the self-paced learning market (Brunt & Scott, 1986). An electronic device does not become impatient; its pace can be controlled by the client; it gives immediate, objective, and consistent feedback. Furthermore, a computer will not embarrass the client by making comments on the client's stupidity or slowness. Also, a computer does not get irritated when the client wishes to repeat all or part of the lesson. For the younger client, CAI may evoke the fun and excitement of an arcade game. The client can acquire information in private, and no one else has to know what the client thinks or how long the client takes to obtain the expected knowledge. User-friendly electronic devices can arouse the curiosity of clients of any age, especially if the clients can control the pace at which they approach use of the machine.

Self-paced learning takes initiative on the client's part. CAI may tempt you to expect too much independent learning, or you may not be available to receive a client's questions. We have seen this neglect occur with the use of earlier devices, such as the learning packages recorded on little videotapes that nurses have parked at the bedside.

If the client is uneasy with any machine that resembles a computer, the lesson may be more stressful than expected. As electronic devices become more user friendly, and as society becomes more accustomed to CAI, some of the current problems will diminish. Many software manufacturers are aware of these problems, and encase the message in a program that has "toy value" (Minnesota Educational Computing Corporation, 1990).

Because computers have become more "intelligent" and programmers more sophisticated, computers are now being used to interact with the client directly. Because of its flexibility and capacity to handle branching options, the computer provides a wide variety of learning experiences and opportunities (Bainbridge & Quintanilla, 1989). The client can explore cause and effect in safety and without embarrassment.

Public Address System

The skilled use of a microphone takes some time and practice, but it is a must if you have a soft voice or are speaking in a large room. The microphone will allow you to continue to speak in little more than a whisper, in case you come down with an inconvenient sore throat. In such a circumstance, whispering will preserve your voice, and the microphone will make the whisper intelligible to your audience. The following section outlines some guidelines on the effective use of the public address system.

Guidelines for Use of Public Address Systems

Adjust the microphone to your height. Take the time to turn the microphone off, adjust it to a convenient height, and then turn the microphone on again. This will give the audience members an impression of poise, and will set them at ease. It is very distracting to see a speaker get up on tiptoe, trying to speak into the microphone. It is equally disturbing to see a speaker hunch over in an attempt to get within range of the device. If you are going to talk at any length, your natural body position will prevail, which will take you out of range of the microphone.

Be sure you can be heard. Take the time to make sure those sitting in the last row can hear before continuing your presentation. Many speakers ask if everyone can hear, but then they go on speaking without paying attention to the audience's response. Recently Pat Schroeder, a U.S. Representative from Colorado, attended a fund-raising event to benefit a local college. A very effective speaker, she realized that the sound system that confronted her was ineffective. To compensate, she shortened and shouted her speech, and she turned out to be the only speaker the audience could hear.

Position the microphone in front of your mouth and keep it in line between your lips and the audience. As you turn to face each side of the audience to maintain good eye contact, be sure to move the microphone with you. If you do not, you will cause a distracting fading effect. If the microphone is stationary, you will need to practice turning your head around the microphone.

Use a lavaliere-type microphone to speak freely if you are a hand-waver. Empty hands are very important if you are this type of speaker. The gestures may be interesting to your audience and add charm to your presentation. However, if you have papers in your hands, the motions can be very distracting and diminish an audience's enjoyment.

Repeat questions from the audience before you answer them. This is particularly important if the question comes from a client in the front of the room.

Flip Charts

The flip chart is versatile because it is portable and you can use it like a chalkboard. Other creative uses of flip charts include composing instantaneous posters, gathering and preserving audience contributions, and having clients write out their thoughts. The flip chart combines the advantages of posters and chalkboards. You can plan ahead and prepare your charts or you can have the blank pages available for spontaneous use as you teach.

If you prepare the flip chart ahead of time, you can take the time you need to prepare exactly what you want—written messages, pictures, cartoons, or a combination thereof. A flip chart can be used as an advance organizer because it will allow you to write your outline and have the clients follow along as you move through the presentation. Everything you can put on a transparency can be put on a flip chart.

If you plan to use the flip chart spontaneously as you teach, you will want to have a good supply of colorful pens. Spontaneous use is appropriate when you want to elicit responses from the audience or when you want your clients to work in small groups and write their contributions down, so they can be shared later with the larger group. If you use this method, you can hang the finished charts around the room. When you do this, clients feel like valued parts of the teaching/learning process. Your flip charts also can be saved for future use. The material you have collected can be transcribed and sent to all the participants.

The major disadvantage to using a flip chart is that you must have at least some artistic talent to be effective. Also, your audience must be small enough so that everyone can see the flip chart. In the box above we have summarized some questions to ask yourself when selecting appropriate media.

Readability of Materials

Clients vary greatly in their ability to read and translate the symbols on a piece of paper into ideas that are meaningful to them. You may find yourself tempted to depend on reading materials to convey information to clients. This becomes more important when you feel pressed for time and depend on reading materials to expand the client's knowledge regarding the topic at hand. As a rule, we support giving reading materials to clients. However, it is imperative that these important materials be within the literacy level of the client for whom they are intended. Streiff (1986) found that more than 50% of the clients in her survey could not read any of the educational materials at the health care site she studied. In addition, 25% of the materials were beyond the literacy level of any of the participants. This part of the chapter is intended to raise your consciousness about the level of reading materials you give to clients. A secondary hope is that you will design better ones in the future. Materials can be evaluated using qualitative criteria as well as quantitative criteria (Zakaluk & Samuels, 1988). A brief list of thoughts and questions addressing qualitative criteria follows.

Qualitative Criteria

Note the cohesion of the text. Is it redundant? How are ideas linked? Ask someone who is not already familiar with the author's style to read the material and react to it. Determine what knowledge or background is necessary for comprehension. What is the writer assuming that the reader already knows?

Evaluate the number and complexity of required inferences. Must the reader combine what she or he already knows (experiential information) with what is in the text to form a conclusion, construct a new meaning, or both?

Examine the number and clarity of pronouns. When and how often are the pronouns *he, she, it, we, they,* and *you* used? Understanding of pronouns requires a certain amount of sophistication with the language, especially when the pronoun is implied. For example, in the statement "Go to bed," "you" is understood.

Judge how much and what kind of figurative language is used. Is the meaning commonly understood by the target population? For example, if the figure of speech you use refers to a coal stove, or a "bureau," or a Shakespearian character, will the target population understand the connection? How literally will the reader take the command, "Wash off your face"? Will the reader keep washing in an attempt to obliterate features? Pimples? Makeup?

Assess the reader's background. What is the client's educational level? What reading materials do you see in his or her room? What level of vocabulary does the client use? Ask the client what his or her favorite reading materials are. How does the client earn a living? How much reading is required on the job?

Evaluate the purpose of the reading materials. Are the materials to be used for explanation? Is the material a set of instructions on how to do a procedure? Should the material encourage or inspire? Is the material intended for exploration of a topic of concern?

Measure the distance between the subject and predicate. If the subject and predicate are far apart, the client faces a greater challenge when trying to understand your message. For example, "Write a sentence" is easier to comprehend than "When you are feeling the urge to express yourself, it may be advantageous to you to formulate those thoughts and transfer them to paper." The latter message is more difficult because the reader has to keep both subject and predicate in mind throughout the entire sentence before comprehending the meaning. If the concept you wish to convey is new to the client, it will be an even greater challenge and more confusing. In general, it is easier to handle complex concepts in an area with which you are familiar. It is more difficult when the area is foreign. We encourage you to use the above information as a starting point for thinking more critically about the level of the material you give to clients.

Quantitative Criteria

Quantitative criteria are those standards that can be counted. Quantitative criteria are used to determine readability. The criteria include examination of the number of syllables in each word and the number of words in each sentence. In general, words of many syllables are thought to require a higher level of reading skill than words of few syllables. Short sentences are generally considered easier to read than long sentences.

Fry's graph (Fry, 1968) for estimating readability allows you to use quantitative criteria to determine the grade level associated with a piece of reading material. This determination is made by counting the number of syllables and the number of sentences in each 100-word passage. The general assumption is that the more syllables a passage has, the harder it is to read, and the fewer the sentences it has (more words per sentence), the more difficult the passage is to read. Computer programs that can calculate readability automatically are available. The user enters paragraphs into an appropriate software package, and the program evaluates the passages according to the formulae chosen by the manufacturer. For those who do not have access to such software, we have included Fry's graph for estimating readability and directions for using the graph. See Figure 11-2.

One factor that influences a client's reading level is his or her level of formal education. However, grade level is an inexact measure, because comprehension is often lower than the number of school years completed (Streiff, 1986). Many people read at a level lower than the highest grade they completed in school. Clients' learning styles greatly influence the use they make of the material they read. To verify this statement you are invited to think about how you follow directions for knitting, sewing, or assembling a bicycle. Many readers look solely at the illustrations, turning to the printed directions only if they cannot understand the pictures. Many individuals approach assembling a bicycle or other appliance as they would a puzzle. They do not even look at the words or illustrations unless they have a great deal of trouble with the puzzle. When all else fails, they read the instructions.

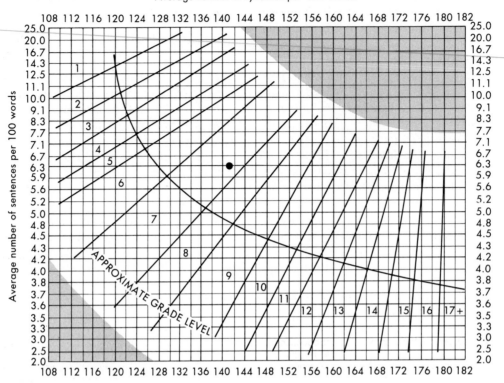

Average number of syllables per 100 words

Figure 11-2 Fry's graph for estimating readability gives a good estimate of reading level by counting number of syllables and number of words per 100-word passage.

DIRECTIONS: Randomly select three 100-word passages from a book or an article. Plot average number of syllables and average number of sentences per 100 words on graph to determine grade level of material. Choose more passages per book if great variability is observed, and conclude that book has uneven readability. Few books will fall in gray area, but when they do, grade level scores are invalid.

Count proper nouns, numerals and initializations as words. Count a syllable for each symbol. For example, "1945" is one word and four syllables, and "IRA" is one word and three syllables.

EXAMPLE:

	SYLLABLES	SENTENCES
1st Hundred Words	124	6.6
2nd Hundred Words	141	5.5
3rd Hundred Words	158	6.8
AVERAGE	141	6.3

READABILITY 7th GRADE (see dot plotted on graph)

In the acute care setting, many of the clients receiving instruction are intoxicated by drugs they are receiving for a disease or surgery. It is not at all unusual for certain drug-induced states and other postsurgical or disease conditions to blur vision and slow intellectual processing. Age is another factor that takes a toll on vision. Visual acuity may be affected by mundane problems, such as the unavailability of a client's eye glasses. The client may be too proud to ask or too sick or sedated to figure out that eye glasses would make the page easier to see. Fear and anxiety can lessen reading ability or even make it impossible for the client to grasp the meaning of any printed words.

When the reading material is beyond the skill of the reader, comprehension is decreased and recall is sketchy and inaccurate. In addition, motivation to seek further instruction from printed sources is reduced. It may be that all handout materials should be prepared for the sixth grade level, unless the material is intended for people with less than a sixth grade education.

Whatever the reason, it is quite possible that the client may not be able to read materials that should be within that client's ability level, so you might want to assess the individual client's reading ability. One way to assess a client's ability to make use of a pamphlet is to ask.

Example: "I want to give you a paper that explains things clearly. Will you look at this and tell me if it suits you?"

Another way is to ask the client to read a pamphlet and report its comprehensibility.

Example: "Tell me what this pamphlet says to you. Is it boring? Confusing?"

Look carefully at the client while he or she is attempting to read it. Does the client show signs of tension such as hair twisting or scratching? Watch the client's eyes. Do they move across and down the

---

TABLE 11-2
Sample Lesson Plan for Lincoln Perez

Learning Objectives	Content Outline	Strategies and Materials
By the end of this lesson, the client will be able to: Select three benefits of relaxation from a list.	Introductions Relaxation Definitions Balance with exercise Benefits Reduce blood pressure Reduce tension Increase efficiency	Discussion question: "What does relaxation mean to you?" Discuss the relationship between stress and blood pressure. Give the patient the pamphlet: Balancing Relaxation and Exercise.
Agree to experiment with walking and various relaxation techniques.	Medications Fears Side effects Life-style change Costs Benefits	Discuss fears and mixed feelings. Question: "Who else in your family has been diagnosed with hypertension? What did it do to them? What have they done to control it, and what were the results?"
Count his pulse within three beats of what the nurse counts.	Techniques for pulse taking Location of artery Finger placement Counting Multiplying Recording method Techniques for relaxation Deep breathing Yoga Meditation Imagery Prayer Wrap-up	Demonstrate pulse taking. Have the client return demonstration of pulse taking. Develop a record-keeping system for monitoring pulse rate. Read directions for deep breathing, yoga, meditation, and imagery. **Obtain a clock with a second hand. Develop a chart for record-keeping at home. Obtain an audiocassette for recording directions for deep breathing, yoga, meditation, and imagery.** Have the client select soothing prayers.

T A B L E 1 1 - 3

Features of Teaching Materials

Type	Advantages	Disadvantages	Helpful Hints
Video recordings	Best possible substitute for actual experience. Easily obtainable. Easy to remake and update. Can be stopped and rerun. Familiar to many.	Size of monitor limits audience distance. Technical skill with film making helpful. Expensive initial investment.	Must be compatible with the VCR. Can take three times longer than you expect to make a tape.
Motion pictures	Usable for any audience size. Generate positive mind set. Facilitate emotional involvement. Allows for "over the shoulder" close-ups.	Expensive and fragile. Require technical competence. Break easily. Require a darkened room. Become outdated quickly. Require the use of bulky equipment.	Must be ordered in advance. Require a back-up plan. Require pretest of equipment. Must be rewound correctly afterwards. Require teacher to learn how to center the film in the frame.
Objects and models	Depict the real thing as closely as possible. Can be handled and studied at the client's pace. Replicas—static. Analogues—dynamic. Appeal to kinesthetic learners.	Can be bulky and heavy. Inconvenient to transport. Time consuming. Expensive. Analogues—Demand conceptual sophistication.	Require advance planning if borrowed. Work well with several stations around a teaching area. Require the use of a teacher at each station.
Slides and filmstrips	Slides—Easy to make, update, store, and rearrange. Filmstrips—Relatively inexpensive, easy to store, good for individuals and groups. Allow learners to go at their own pace. Colorful and realistic. Can be used with taped narration or music.	Contain no movement. Can burn. Filmstrips—Must be remade to be updated.	Require learning how to synchronize narration with pictures. Require learning how to center the film in the frame. Require attention to detail, such as fastening of the collar on the slide tray before turning it over. Slides—Should be marked in the upper-right-hand corner after they are properly inserted in the slide tray.
Audiocassette tapes	Can be used with individuals or groups. Good for developing listening skills. Accessible. Cheap. Can be tailor-made, erased, or remade. Good for enhancing stress management skills.	Can be dull if used by itself. Can be damaged easily.	Must be protected from temperature and moisture extremes. Should be of high quality. Must be long enough.
Overhead projectors with transparencies	Versatile, cheap, and reusable. Enable you to face learners. Eliminate verbal repetition. Can be used with the lights on. Allow for use of overlays.	Bulky. Use bulbs that often burn out. Boring when used exclusively. Noisy. Transparencies—Time consuming to prepare.	Transparencies—Must be protected from hand oils and fingerprints. Require the use of washable pens, which should be tested before you buy too many.
Opaque projectors	Allow for projection of book or picture to a large group. Allow for projection of a picture on the wall so that it can be enlarged and traced.	Bulky. Require a darkened room and technical competence. Can burn the book if left on too long.	Require understanding of how the machine flips the image. Require the teacher to practice focusing and determining the correct distance from the screen or wall.

Features of Teaching Materials—*cont'd*

Type	Advantages	Disadvantages	Helpful Hints
Chalkboards and whiteboards	Widely available. Useful for spontaneous illustration at the time of client's concern. Offer reinforcement to respondents. Erasable. Allow the teacher to add to and take away from illustrations. Good back-ups.	Two dimensional. Messy. Require chalk or pen and an eraser. Require good lighting. Can be time consuming to use. Require a teacher with good writing skills.	Require teacher to supply chalk and eraser. Can be messy and get on dark clothing. Require the teacher to start high on the board and to refrain from writing below the viewers' line of vision. Should be divided in half to accommodate lengthy lists.
Pamphlets and posters	Portable, attractive, and attracting. Can be used before, during, and after a presentation. Can be studied at client's pace. Readily available. Often free.	Time consuming to make. Provide limited viewing. Need a prop. Bulky to carry and store. Useful only to readers. Pamphlets—May overwhelm client if too many. Do not have auditory accompaniment.	Pamphlets—Must be checked for currency and must be passed out at the most propitious time. Should contain few words and lots of space.
Photographs and cartoons	Easily personalized. Can elicit emotions. Can portray many more thoughts than words alone. Allow the client to control the pace.	Inappropriate for large groups. Can be distracting if passed during talk. Yellow with age. Cartoons—Can inadvertently offend or confuse.	Should be tried out on people of similar ages and backgrounds as your clients. Look more lively if in color. May require explanations.
Bulletin boards	Attract browsers.	Can get cluttered and outdated. Unsuitable for long or complex messages.	Should be changed often and kept attractive and lively. Should contain a minimal number of messages.
Computer Assisted Instruction (CAI) programs	Allow the client to control the pace. Reinforce correct responses immediately. Good for sequential thought processes. Allow the client to repeat the lesson if necessary.	Depend on client initiative. Time consuming to monitor and do. Are of a limited value if the teacher is not available. Require clients who are visual learners and computer literate. Can be boring.	Allow the teacher to select the most user-friendly software available. Work best if the teacher spends enough time with the client to ensure that he or she is comfortable with the program.
Public address systems	Augment your voice to any size audience.	Can be ineffective if faulty equipment is used.	Microphones—Should be tested before clients arrive. Should be adjusted to the correct height. Should be held in front of your mouth. Step back and aside if squeals are produced. Be sure the audience can hear you.
Flip Charts	Versatile, portable, used like a chalkboard. May be prepared before the presentation or spontaneously during presentation.	Require artistic talent and good handwriting. Provide clients with a limited view.	Teacher should have a good supply of black and colored pens and should use masking tape or soft, gummy adhesive to affix flip charts to the wall.

page in a systematic manner? You could also compose a test in which the reader fills in the blanks. You could use this as a diagnostic test before choosing materials. Your test could also be used as an evaluation tool to assess comprehension after the client reads the materials.

Ways to adjust reading materials include shortening the words, shortening the sentences, rephrasing the paragraphs, adding pictures, interspersing stick figures, and inserting diagrams. In the exercises at the end of this chapter, you will find several tools for evaluating and correcting the reading level of materials. These tools should also be useful for designing materials that are appropriate for clients of varying ability.

Expansion of Lesson Plan for Lincoln Perez

We will now expand on our sample lesson plan for Mr. Perez by adding suitable materials. See Table 11-2 for these additions. To assist Mr. Perez in learning to count his pulse, we will need a clock, a paper, and a pencil. To help him learn the relaxation methods, we will need written directions for deep breathing, yoga, meditation, and imagery. We might have these same techniques recorded on an audiocassette tape. Mr. Perez could bring in a blank audiocassette tape on which we will record verbal instruction. We might give him the assignment to go to a local store for commercially prepared cassettes that will suit his needs. We should also seek his consultation to see if there are prayers he finds most soothing. One of his options is to bring the prayers in, and we will record them onto the audiocassette tape.

Summary

In this chapter we examined the following teaching materials: video recordings, motion pictures, slides and filmstrips, audiocassette tapes, overhead projectors, opaque projectors, chalkboards and whiteboards, pamphlets and posters, photographs and cartoons, CAI, bulletin boards, and flip charts. These materials are designed to help you achieve your teaching objectives. The materials you select

should be based on what you want clients to learn and the strategies you have selected to facilitate learning. Materials should be appropriate to you as the teacher and to the clients as learners. Each medium has advantages and disadvantages that you must consider when you make your selection. You will find these features summarized in Table 11-3. In the box that follows, you will find a list of recommendations for preventing and solving common problems with equipment.

Preventing and Solving Media Equipment Problems

1. Be sure the equipment is plugged in.
2. Check all cord connections.
3. Turn the power switch on.
4. Find the focus knob and know how to use it.
5. Test all equipment before your presentation.
6. When all else fails, read the instructions.
7. Get someone who is familiar with the equipment to teach you how to use it and to supervise your first experience with it.
8. Prepare a back-up plan that does not require power.
9. Bring a three-prong, long extension cord and a two-prong adapter.
10. Return the equipment properly packaged.
11. If something breaks, report it so that it can be repaired.
12. Locate the light switch in case you need to make the room darker.
13. Arrive early to test and set up your equipment.
14. Arrive early to test the equipment set up by someone else.
15. If a technician is involved, find out his or her phone number in case you run into problems.
16. When you put in a request for equipment, specify what you want. For example, specify what kind of projector you want. Slide? 35 mm? Overhead? Opaque? Do you want extra reels?
17. Be specific about the location, date, and time you need the equipment.
18. If your presentation will take place outside of regular hours, clarify the entrance you will use, how you should manage security, and how you conduct the correct lock-up procedure.

EXERCISE I
USING OVERLAYS

Purposes:

- Integrate kinesthetic learning with cognitive learning
- Practice using multiple overlays

Directions:

- Start with an outline of the surface of a sedentary heart.
- Add an overlay portraying a clot and the resulting damage from oxygen deprivation.
- Remove the clot overlay and add an outline of an exercised heart (with increased vascularity as a result of aerobic exercise).
- Add a final overlay of a smaller clot in the same location depicting a decreased area of damage, due to improved flow of blood to the area.

EXERCISE II
NOTICING DIFFICULT WORDS

Purpose:

- Increase awareness of consumer perceptions of medical jargon

Directions:

- Look at the words in the left-hand column.
- In the middle column, write what a client might think the words mean. If you cannot think of a possible client meaning for the word, ask friends who do not have medical backgrounds, or clients who could use some entertainment.
- In the third column put the medical meaning.
- In the last column put an alternative word or phrase that would convey the desired meaning.

Medical Terms and Client Understanding

Word	Client Meaning	Medical Meaning	Easier Synonym
Ambulate			
Cancer			
Concussion			
Culture			
Decubitus			
Discharge			
Force fluids			
Fracture			
Heart attack			
Hematocrit			
Hemorrhage			
A negative test			
NPO			
BID			
Reflux			
Stool			
Void			

ASSESSING READABILITY OF CLIENT TEACHING MATERIALS

Purposes:

- Practice assessing readability of materials
- Use the Fry readability formula
- Analyze the readability of selected reading material, such as a pamphlet, intended for client education

Directions:

- Follow the instructions for assessing readability that accompany the Fry Graph for Estimating Readability. See Figure 11-2. Use a list of common words to adjust the reading material if necessary.

GIVING A SPEECH

Purposes:

- Practice public speaking
- Increase awareness of the health educator's role
- Become more familiar with teaching resources

Directions:

- Give a talk on a resource you have investigated. The resource should be some place where you and your peers can obtain teaching materials, such as pamphlets from the local branch of the American Heart Association, materials from a teacher's store, or a teaching package from the American Dairy Council.

- Your speech does not have to be comprehensive. Select the features that your audience will find most interesting. Be sure to dress in a way that enhances your image, gets your audience's attention, or highlights a feature of your presentation.
- The instructor will set the amount of time you can take for your speech. Be sure to introduce yourself and make a concluding remark so your peers will know when you are finished.
- Be sure to provide the group with the name, address, phone number, and summary of materials available at your resource so you can share them with your peers.

References

Anderson, G.C. (1989). Skin to skin: Kangaroo care in western Europe. *American Journal of Nursing, 89*(5), 662-666.

Bainbridge, L. & Quintanilla (Eds.). (1989). *Developing skills with information technology.* New York: Wiley.

Brunt, B. & Scott, N. (1986). Factors to consider in the development of self instructional materials. *Journal of Continuing Education in Nursing, 17*(3), 87-93.

Doak, C.C., Doak, L.G., & Root, J.H. (1985). *Teaching patients with low literacy skills.* Philadelphia: J.B. Lippincott.

Fry, E. (1968). A readability formula that saves time. *Journal of Reading, 11,* 513-516, 575-577.

Kemp, J.E. & Dayton, D.K. (1985). *Planning and producing instructional media* (5th ed.). New York: Harper & Row.

Minnesota Educational Computing Corporation. (1990). *Writing and publishing in multimedia computer file version 1.0.* St. Paul: Author.

Neufeldt, V. (Ed.) (1991). *Webster' New World Dictionary* (3rd ed.). Cleveland: Webster's New World.

Pohl, M.L. (1981). *The teaching function of the nurse practitioner.* Dubuque IA: Wm. C. Brown.

Russell, J.E. (1938). Insights about adult learning. *Journal of Adult Education, 10*(4), 385-386.

Streiff, L.D. (1986). Can clients understand our instructions? *IMAGE Journal of Nursing Scholarship, 18*(20), 48-52.

Zakaluk, B.L. & Samuels, S.J. (Eds.). (1988). *Readability; its past present and future.* Newark DL: International Reading Association.

Implementation

All genuine education comes
about through experience.

John Dewey, 1938.

Objectives

Upon completion of this chapter you will be able to:

- Analyze 18 principles of teaching.
- Apply selected principles of teaching to a given clinical situation.
- Use positive reinforcement in a teaching situation.
- Select various types of teaching models and use them appropriately.
- Discuss how to use descriptive, clarifying, and higher-order questions in teaching.
- Create positive mind set in selected teaching situations.
- Achieve closure in selected teaching situations.
- Demonstrate the use of eight different types of media equipment.
- Formulate your criteria for good teaching to critically evaluate a teacher's performance.

Key Words

principles of teaching	clarifying questions	humor
openness	higher-order	mutual respect
psychologic safety	questions	enthusiasm
organization	critical thinking	patience
advance organizer	implementation	reinforcement
factual questions		

Introduction

Using the nursing process model, we have devoted the last several chapters to planning: objectives, strategies, and materials and their readability. It is now time to implement the teaching module and to actually do the teaching. In this chapter we will focus on a number of issues that are cogent in any teaching situation. The principles we state will also help you select the best strategies and materials for accomplishing your objectives.

We assume that you have lifelong experience speaking (oral communication) and in-class experience with public speaking (giving a report to the class). You have also been recipients of different kinds of teaching, so the teaching principles in this chapter will not be new to you. As you read, we encourage you to think of role models who used the particular teaching principles and practical examples that follow. We also invite you to think about the various pieces of teaching equipment to which you have been exposed over the years. In this chapter we will examine principles of teaching, and we will provide guidelines for using some of the equipment with which you

—Continued next page

should be familiar. Later in this chapter, you will find considerable attention devoted to teaching technologies. Each piece of equipment you use should come with instructions. If your institution is connected with a well-equipped audiovisual department, you may be able to obtain training from the staff. In our experience, many pieces of equipment do not come with directions, nor do beginning teachers get much training on how to use various pieces of equipment. For these reasons, we have devoted considerable attention to the use of common pieces of equipment. No two film projectors or overhead projectors are alike, but the general principles and guidelines we have included should help you pay attention to the important points.

Teaching Principles

Many think of the teacher as one who tells and gives information. Telling in a clear, organized, and interesting manner is indeed an important communication tool for effective teaching. Nurses who mumble, fail to maintain eye contact, and speak too rapidly greatly reduce the effectiveness of their communication. If you are willing to agree that the main role of teacher is to facilitate learning, other phenomena besides clear speech become important. We asked more than 800 adult learners to describe teacher behaviors that facilitated and impeded their learning. These data were collected over a period of 11 years from learners whose ages ranged from 18 to 65. We have used the data to create the following teaching principles.

Attitude

Project an attitude of ease and self-confidence. People—whether they are college students, school children, colleagues, or clients—learn easier and better from an individual who has self-confidence and self-respect. When you feel confident, you radiate ease with yourself, and you help put the audience at ease. This, in turn, makes you more believable, and a better role model for whatever health teaching you do. Confidence is contagious

and so is its counterpart. If you act nervous and insecure, clients are likely to feel uncomfortable. Some clients react as nurturing parents and others react with more negative responses. In any event their energy and attention may be diverted from the task at hand by the attitude of the teacher who lacks self-confidence and self-respect.

Maintain a friendly, warm, and open attitude. Simple courtesies such as starting the teaching/learning session with a smile and greeting your clients are examples of such an attitude. Your response to questions is also very closely observed. No matter what you say about your openness to questions, your actual responses to questions are more significant. Intimidation and ridicule block learning in clients and frequently affect others who fear they may be scapegoats for ridicule in the future.

Responsiveness to the group's tenor is as important as sensitivity to individuals in the group. A number of glassy-eyed stares may indicate the need for a distinct change of pace, perhaps a break or a strategy shift. An example would be an exercise that requires the formation of small groups. Individual clients appreciate the teacher who is alert to facial expressions and invites them to put words to their puzzled expressions.

Another characteristic of an open teacher is adaptability. When you are open, you can take most client contributions and weave them into useful items for consideration. For example, a nursing student was discussing constructive ways of handling anger with high school students. After announcing that there was a paradigm for "fighting right," the nursing student turned her back to write the model on the chalkboard. One of the students whispered something to a neighbor, and the nursing student (who had good ears and was alert to the class) asked him to repeat his comment out loud. The student sheepishly grinned, "No hitting below the belt." After laughing with the rest of the class, the nursing student said, "You're absolutely right. In this case the rule is no hitting below the psychological belt. It's not fair to accuse your partner of having certain traits or quirks that you do not like, especially those that your partner cannot change. It's not fair to say words for which you will be sorry later. You can apologize, but once those words are out, they sting. The pain and hurt can permanently alter your relationship. Another way to hit below the belt is to blame your partner's relatives and ancestors: '. . . and furthermore your mother and your brother. . . .' "

Learning Environment

Practice sensitivity to the psychologic safety of that particular learning environment. This principle is of crucial importance when affective learning is the goal. When your strategies include the promotion of self-disclosure, it is important that you establish a commitment to confidentiality and other related issues. It helps to plan for steps of increasing risk, so that each individual has an opportunity to see how others respond to that risk. A client's tolerance of public exposure should also guide you in how far to push that person to reveal faulty thinking patterns or the inadequacy of his or her sources.

Clients need to know when they are in error. There are times when the error is due to faulty logic. You may be able to help the client immediately by reviewing the steps that led to the error. This is an information processing approach. At other times, you may find that the problem is the client's inability to distinguish between sound and questionable sources of information. It may be helpful to the client and others to ask questions that will promote critical thinking (see Chapter 2).

We find that nursing students welcome correction and criticism when it is presented constructively and in a form they can use, such as coaching.

> *Example:* "Your voice is too soft. You cannot be heard in the back of the room and what you have to say is worthwhile. Please stand up and turn around so your peers can hear you."
> "You should use a microphone because your voice does not carry. You should plan to use a microphone even when you are talking to a modest-size group."

A clear explanation of why something is wrong followed by an explanation of the right answer can be very straightforward and helpful.

Organization

Organize the material to suit the clients and the purpose of the learning. Your organization can be logical, linear, historical, simple to complex, free association, or circular. Clients appreciate it when you are well-prepared and can get right to their learning goals. A well-planned teaching module takes time and thought. One of your tasks, as you organize your teaching module, is to think about what kind of mind set you wish to invoke, and how you will elicit the mind set most conducive to your objectives. *Set* has many meanings; Neufeldt (1992) devotes well over a column of space to defining the word. As we use it, *set* is the learning climate and refers to the response system that predisposes clients to view and approach a situation in a predetermined manner. *Set* can also be defined as an attitude of mind and an organizer of information, which includes the atmosphere you create and the beginning activities you conduct. The preconceived attitudes clients bring with them to the learning environment, and the learning environment itself are all part of the set.

Set induction refers to your actions that evoke the attitudes and expectations in clients that will be most conducive to effective learning. To promote the proper set you will want to clarify the goals of instruction, to motivate clients to learn and to help them see the relevance of your presentation to their improved health. A set assists in organizing information by providing a common frame of reference and evokes an attitude of mind that helps clients accept or reject the learning experience. A set can also be used to help your clients see the relationship between what they already know and what you hope to impart.

Set predisposes clients to view and approach a situation in a certain way. For example, if you are told that a given speaker is an expert in the subject, you tend to regard the speaker's comments with more credibility. If you are led to believe that a given task is difficult, then you will find it so.

Our own internal predisposition (internal set) to learning influences us to use skills and solutions we already know when learning anything new. We automatically make associations, good or bad, to previous situations that are similar somehow to the present learning situation. Your job is to capitalize on that human process and/or to change it. In order to do that, you must assess your clients' set as you encounter one another. For instance, when we teach a class entitled Clinical Teaching Methods, we ask nursing students to fill out a diagnostic tool that has them describe their previous teaching experiences. You can find a sample of that tool in Appendix A. If many of the students report few or negative experiences with client teaching, we shape the course differently than we would if most of the students reported that they had had quite a bit of positive teaching experience.

Set induction is particularly appropriate at the beginning of a class and at the beginning of any change in activity, such as moving from the lecture strategy to a discussion or a group exercise. A preinstructional set can vary in length and elaborateness. You as the teacher always have some control over the learning environment, and you should take responsibility for influencing it as much as possible. This may mean rearranging the furniture, providing light refreshments, or bringing long extension cords to rearrange the placement of equipment. If the auditorium has fixed seats, you can still influence the set by arriving early and greeting clients just like a host or hostess would. Such actions give you some information—intuitive as well as observational—about the audience and help you establish rapport.

Try using an advance organizer. Slavin (1991) defines an advance organizer as "an initial statement about a subject to be learned that provides a structure for the new information and relates it to information students already possess" (p. 167). From an information-processing perspective, you can think of it as creating a file in which you will generate and store information.

Example: The sun reflected off the water and made it look so inviting. The sun had been out all day, and she knew it had warmed the water and made it even more desirable. Where were Victor, Margaret, Barbara Jean, and Annie Lou? She knew they were somewhere having an adventure and would join her soon. The blackberries were especially abundant that year, too delicious to resist. That aside, Consumas awaited her. She looked carefully across the south bank. It was constructed of medium-sized rocks that widened the swimming hole. Once she had seen a bull snake slithering there, and she did not want to encounter it again, especially when she did not have her brother to protect her. Was the rope still in place? She looked up and sure enough, it was there, but it had been swung up over a limb. She had two choices, wait for Victor or try and climb up the tree and get it down herself. She was feeling energetic, so she climbed up and freed the rope. It was great swinging on the rope and splashing into the water.

As you read this passage you may have enjoyed the imagery, or you may have found that the imagery does not make much sense. You may have gotten frustrated or even lost interest as you plowed through it. You could deduce that the scene was set outdoors and involved several people. You might have also recognized that if you had known something about the passage, it would have made more sense. An advance organizer would have put the passage in context for you. Had we told you that this passage was shared by an 85-year-old client in a nursing home as she reflected on her youth, you would have thought back to an earlier time and tried to imagine the client as a youngster, frolicking during the summertime. It would also have helped you to know that *Consumas* is the name of a creek.

If the preceding paragraph had been used as an advance organizer, the passage would have made sense to you. The advance organizer would have prepared you to receive and incorporate the information into your concept of this 85-year-old woman for whom you have been caring. The paragraph would have helped you orient yourself to the material and would allow you to incorporate the new information into a structure you already possess.

Clarity of Purpose

Clearly define your objectives. Adult learners want to know what they can expect to gain from their efforts. Those in situations where they will be given grades appreciate clearly stated expectations. They do not welcome unexpected assignments that give them no opportunity to budget their time. Clients who are seeking health or recovery want clear ideas about the kind of commitment they will be expected to invest. They also want to know what they will get and whether or not they are likely to gain anything new.

Select audiovisual materials that clarify, organize, simplify, or amplify your message. Using a variety of teaching strategies enlivens learning. The variety is also more likely to address the different learning styles of individuals. In Chapter 10 we addressed the advantages and disadvantages of various strategies, as well as selection guidelines. In general, strategies that involve the client actively are more effective.

Questions

Sustain a pace that allows for thinking and absorption of the material being presented. This should be balanced with a flow that is lively enough to prevent boredom. You will find that the skillful use of questions helps you establish an appropriate pace. Questions help clarify, verify, or substantiate concepts, and serve many purposes in the teaching/learning process. You can use questions to assess what clients already know about the topic you intend to teach. Questions can stimulate interest in a new topic, and they can be used to elicit feedback to evaluate a client's mastery of the intended objectives. Furthermore, both you and clients can use questions to explore ideas, problems, and possible solutions.

Three types of questions have been identified: the factual or descriptive question, the clarifying question, and the higher-order question. These questions are categorized in terms of the type of answers they elicit.

Factual, or descriptive, questions elicit a recall response from the client, and they can be answered from memory. Factual questions include words such as who, what, where, or when.

> *Example:* "What is the normal blood sugar range?"
> "What is the normal range of blood pressure?"
> "Who is eligible for food supplements in Colorado?"

Descriptive questions also focus primarily on facts, but they require another level of thought. The client would be required to organize thoughts in a logical relationship and to respond with a longer answer than a factual question would require.

> *Example:* "What has your blood sugar range been during the last 2 years?"
> "What are signs and symptoms of insulin shock?"
> "Describe the path in your house from your bathroom to the kitchen."

Clarifying questions require that clients go beyond a superficial response. You can ask for more information, more meaning, or both either by direct quizzing or by stating a problem. You use this type of question when you are trying to help the client convey his or her thoughts. Such questions may help the client clarify an idea that is based on his or her own observations.

> *Example:* "I don't quite understand what you mean."
> "What do you mean by the term . . . ?"
> "You must have seen or been told something to come to that conclusion . . . ?"

Higher-order questions are those that cannot be answered simply from memory or perception. Higher-order questions prod clients to think beyond the facts, sequences, descriptions, and sets of circumstances in which they find themselves. Higher-order questions help clients establish relationships, compare and contrast concepts and principles, make inferences, see causes and effects, and discover rules and principles, rather than merely defining them, or accepting them because someone with authority said so.

Brown and Keeley (1986) have expressed concerns about the dangers of uncritical thinking. These concerns are very applicable to clinical teaching. As the complexity of medical science and technology increases clients feel pressured to become passive absorbers of unclear information by uncritically accepting what medical authorities say and recommend. In your role as advocate, you will encourage clients and their families to make active choices regarding the quality of their lives. You can, in fact, facilitate clients' judgments about what to accept and what to reject in the way of medical care and procedures, as well as life-style.

Higher-order questions help clients use ideas freely and critically. "Why" questions require clients to go beyond the factual answer by generalizing, inferring, classifying, and/or concluding. One way to stimulate higher-order thinking is to ask questions about inferences. To infer is to draw a conclusion or make a deduction based on facts or indications (Neufeldt, 1992). Browne and Keeley (1986) point out that "inferences are not facts, nor are they something we know automatically; they are beliefs, which require other facts or beliefs to prove or support them" (p. 19). Questions that elicit inference may be used when you wish clients to relate something newly learned to something they had previously learned. They may be used to derive a reason or motive from a set of circumstances, and they may help you uncover clients' assumptions by asking clients to justify their responses.

Example: "Why must a surgery consent form be signed before your operation?"
"Do you know what will happen to your father if you tell the doctor to do all she can for him?"
"After reading this pamphlet about the risk of heart attacks in people with high cholesterol, what would you infer about the foods you are accustomed to eating?"

Another way to stimulate higher-order thinking is to seek comparisons. Comparison questions help clients establish whether ideas are contradictory to one another, similar or dissimilar, and related or unrelated. This type of thinking is very important because clients so often hear contradictory opinions when they are under the care of several specialists. Clients need to recognize that they may be getting conflicting information and not just assume that they are confused or unable to comprehend what they are being told. Examples of promoting comparisons follow.

Example: "Contrast what will be done for your father if you call an ambulance and what will be done for him if you have him transferred to hospice."
"Your regular doctor and the surgeon said very different things to you. How about if you compare and contrast the benefits and risks of each option. What are the long-range results of having open-heart surgery or taking medication and changing your life-style?"
"Compare and contrast the signs and symptoms of drunkenness and the onset of diabetic coma."

Questions that seek evaluation have no right answer. They deal with matters of judgment, value, and choice. To arrive at answers, clients must set up standards and measure their observations against such standards. Your attitude when asking an evaluative question is crucial. You can very subtly inject your own viewpoint when you question clients about their values. Try to lay aside your own biases when you attempt to help clients discover theirs. You are likely to experience difficulty with this when it is obvious that clients and you differ.

Example: "What did you hear the doctors say about your baby's chances of having a normal childhood? What options did you hear? How can we support you in deciding what to do?" "What did you think of the instruction you received from the home health nurse regarding your wife's Broviak catheter?"

Questions can be used to prompt youngsters to volunteer their ideas by giving them hints or clues to the answer the teacher is seeking. They can also be used to prompt the client to engage in lateral thinking to connect ideas previously unassociated in his or her mind. Questions can also be used to broaden the participation of other clients in the group.

Example: "Can you think of an amphibian? I'll give you some hints. It starts out as a fish and ends up as a small animal. It likes water, it's usually green, and it says, 'Cricket!'" "You all have the principles of immediate response to a bee sting very clearly. Now how would you carry out those principles while you were on a camping trip?" "Do you all agree with Anne's response to that question?"

One of the difficulties you may experience is waiting for answers from your clients. Silence appears to be very threatening. Sometimes nursing students tend to jump in and unintentionally cut off clients who would answer if given enough time. An early way to promote full participation is to ask questions that can be answered by a show of hands and then to react to the audience's response enthusiastically.

The extrovert, who will answer immediately, is most welcome to you if you are feeling insecure. However, if you repeatedly call on this individual, you will miss an opportunity to enrich everyone with the contributions of quieter participants. Another unhappy consequence of calling on only the most extroverted is that the others will stop trying. They also may stop listening.

The purpose of waiting before calling on a vol-unteer is to encourage other clients besides the most extroverted members of the group. In many groups you will find many people who raise their hands before you have finished the question. These clients are either mind readers, quick processors, or superficial thinkers. It is more apt to occur in younger groups. To encourage wide participation, you should think through the question ahead of time, make it clear, and tell the group what kind of response you want—opinion, recall, or experiences. It helps to invite the group to write down their answers before entertaining any responses. You can then write audience responses on the chalkboard. You may set the stage for the question by announcing that you want everyone to think about it for a few minutes before responding. This reduces your anxiety about silence and lets the listeners know that a thoughtful rather than a quick response is appropriate.

The box below highlights some general guidelines for the use of questions.

Guidelines for the Use of Questions

1. Determine what level of thinking is desired.
2. Determine the client's present level of knowledge, insight, and critical thinking ability.
3. Determine the meaning of the client's responses.
4. Alter the level of questioning to be congruent with the client's current level of thinking.
5. Determine what level of thinking is possible given the client's current status and capacity to focus and concentrate.
6. Begin at or below the client's current level. Begin simply and build toward more complexity.
7. Ask questions *one at a time.*
8. Wait for feedback before proceeding to the next question. This feedback will help you determine what meaning the client is deriving from your questions.
9. Use each client response to help shape the direction and level of your next question.

Reinforcement of Learning

Repeat important points. Dale Carnegie's famous quote of an Irish politician says it best: "Tell them what you're going to tell them. Tell them. Tell them what you've told them (Carnegie, 1980)."

Demonstrate and provide for return demonstration. This type of behavior is a crucial part of teaching any procedural learning. Demonstration can also serve to clarify the message. Some method of hands-on learning is also vital for the kinesthetic client. When you physically demonstrate your point you also make it more interesting and vivid for your audience.

Show substantial knowledge of the subject being taught and current knowledge of how the new information can be applied in the client's world. Your ability to do this will, in part, be dependent on your sensitivity to the clients in the audience and in part on your willingness to be exposed to the client's reality. You also must be knowledgeable about learning principles and be able to apply them appropriately. Use of consistent and liberal reinforcement generally enhances client involvement.

Using Anecdotes

Use stories and examples that help to clarify the information. These anecdotes can be sad, amusing, frustrating, or anger-provoking, but they should be chosen for their illustrative value; in other words, use examples and stories if they make the point under discussion clearer. An example helps your client understand the nature of the issue being examined. The learning principle of building from the simple to the complex also applies to the use of examples. At times you may find it more effective to use a simple example to begin teaching and more complex examples to deepen the client's grasp of the concept. For example, when you teach dialysis, you might start out with, "Have you ever used a coffee filter? What does it do? Well, a

dialysis machine does basically the same thing; it filters out the junk in your blood."

Examples that are relevant to the client's experience and knowledge should be selected. In the above example, we first asked the client if she or he had used a coffee filter. If the client had not used such a filter, we would have chosen another example. This means that you must familiarize yourself with the life experiences of each group of clients. If the clients are elderly and you were raised with a grandparent, think of your own personal experiences to guide you in your selection of examples. If you cannot relate using your own experiences, you may need to seek out a trial group as consultants. You might explain the concepts to your consultants and ask them for examples. In this way, your elderly consultants learn something interesting and so do you.

Examples must be related to the concepts they are designed to clarify. The connection between the example and the concept may not be as clear to the audience as it is to you, so try it out on others and use their feedback. You may find that you need to describe the connection in a detailed and concrete way.

Asking clients for examples is an excellent way to discern whether or not the clients have indeed grasped the message. Asking for an example that illustrates the main point will help you evaluate how successfully you have achieved the objectives of the class.

Using illustrations is helpful as well. Illustrations can be word pictures, actual pictures, or cartoons. One of the advantages of using these items is their ability to capture, in a gestalt, the notion you are trying to convey. Illustrations have the advantage of stimulating the brain longer than individual words, which are entertained in the mind only briefly. Gose (1988) reported that visual memories are easier for most people to recall than auditory memories. Communication theorists tell us that we convey only about 5% of the meaning of our messages with words. The other 95% is conveyed by other means, such as illustrations, body language, and voice tones (Babcock & Zak-Dance, 1981). Illustrations are more apt to reach both the left and right sides of the brain (Springer & Deutsch, 1981).

Display a sense of humor.   Clients find it easier to retain material they acquire during an aroused state. Anger and fear are emotions that promote arousal. However, amusement can be just as arousing and much more pleasant. Some nursing students used humor to engage some junior high school students in the topic of first aid. The nursing students prepared a skit in which the first nurse began by tripping up the steps and sprawling on the stage on the way to the podium. The other nurse, after exclaiming about the accident, administered first aid. All eyes were riveted to the scene. Students in the back even stood up to get a better view. It took the youngsters a few moments to figure out that the whole thing was staged. It was arousing, it was fun, and it was similar to a practical joke. Such a beginning was very appropriate for this age group.

Maintain Focus

Keep with the learning at hand.   Clients find it disconcerting if you stray too far from the subject they are trying to grasp. They also find it annoying if you allow certain individuals to take up too much group time wandering to tangential issues. It is your responsibility as teacher to control the learning environment. Strategies for staying on course are discussed in the discussion strategy section of Chapter 10.

Promote an atmosphere of mutual respect.   You should offer courtesy and attentiveness to all members of the learning group and expect courteous conduct in return. Do not allow yourself to be unnerved by the occasionally disruptive participant. Use the suggestions we offer in the discussion strategy section of Chapter 10.

Exercise Sensitivity

Strive for sensitivity to race, ethnicity, and gender.   Sensitivity to ethnic, racial, and gender issues is essential in our country. In general, professionals and adult clients in the United States prefer a direct and businesslike style. Eye contact is very important, and clients feel counted when you look at them. However, other cultures may have quite different attitudes toward directness. Many Asians, for whom the avoidance of "shame" is a very powerful motivator, would find too much directness very disruptive to their ability to learn. Certain ethnic groups might not ask questions for fear of "losing face." Others would not ask for fear of embarrassing you. Such clients might be willing to share concerns in private if you can establish rapport with them. This situation occurs quite frequently. Clients might not speak out during our presentation, but they will come speak to us afterward in a more private and individual setting.

Exercise patience.   Clients learn quickly how psychologically safe it is to ask questions or to ask you to repeat material that they did not quite grasp or hear. If you express amazement at their failure to understand your pearls of wisdom or the "obvious," you intimidate the one who raised the question, as well as the others in the group. If you continue to put yourself in the role of learner, you keep yourself sensitive to the struggles that accompany most learning tasks. As a busy adult, you are probably aware of how outside interests and problems can interfere with the learning at hand. Something you said a few moments ago may spur a client to begin free associating, which may keep him or her from hearing what you are saying currently.

Genuineness

Be believable.   Adult clients are particularly skeptical of teachers whose claims are not believable. Authenticity can be achieved through scholarly activity, advanced training, and experiential learning. Adults vary in what they value. If you become actively engaged in high-quality research, are familiar with the research related to the field, and can quote your sources, you will be impressive to those who value scholarship. Advanced training credentials will enhance your credibility when you teach complex skills. If you report recent clinical experience, you will be more believable to workers in the field. Your believability is greatly affected by your ability to function as a role model. Clients are very aware of your apparent health, the values you espouse, and the congruence between what you say and what you do.

Show enthusiasm. When you are enthused about your subject, you are more apt to make the subject interesting and meaningful. When you are lively and energetic, you capture clients' attention more easily. Even the way you approach the podium influences the set of the clients. If your stride conveys enthusiasm and authority, these characteristics influence the audience positively. Be sure to establish your authority, or right to speak (Carnegie, 1980). Your credentials are important and should be mentioned if the introducer fails to do so. Academic credentials, certifications in the topic under consideration, special training, and life experience may all be germane to establishing your authority. A social worker who begins by saying that she has raised six children will be perceived as someone with real life experience as well as education. Parents who are struggling with that phase of life will find her easy to believe.

If you are very young or look very young and the clients are very old, then you might describe older clients from whom you have learned a great deal. Another tactic you might employ is to begin with a story that makes it clear that you understand the challenges older clients face with regard to the learning objectives. You may begin with a story that includes personal transactions between you and a favorite grandfather or beloved great aunt. You should also describe your years in the field about which you are speaking.

Provide reinforcement. We have discussed reinforcement in several chapters because we believe it is a powerful tool for helping clients learn. From a behavioral standpoint, *reinforcement* is the term that refers to any stimulus that strengthens the occurrence of a response. Reinforcement increases the probability of a selected behavior recurring. The following section outlines basic reinforcement principles.

Principles of Reinforcement

It may help at this time to review some principles of reinforcement that have been developed by behavioral researchers and therapists.

Reinforcing desired behaviors increases the likelihood that those behaviors will increase in frequency. We are more apt to repeat actions that have pleasant consequences. For instance, if you receive compliments whenever you wear a particular color, you are more apt to incorporate more of that color into your wardrobe. If you smile each time a client contributes, the client is more apt to continue contributing.

Success that is recognized by the client as success is reinforcing. Success promotes a feeling of satisfaction that is a very powerful reinforcer. When a client is attempting to reach a goal, the client experiences some measure of anxiety and tension. When that goal is reached, the client is apt to experience some feelings of satisfaction or lowering of tension.

Rewards that closely follow the desired behavior or movement toward the goal are more reinforcing than delayed rewards. Behaviors that you are promoting may actually produce immediate discomfort in the client. It may take some imagination and enthusiasm on your part to find a factor to which the client can relate with a feeling of satisfaction. An example would be the need for the postsurgical client to turn, breathe deeply, and respond to the cough reflex, when it occurs, by splinting and coughing. You may need to provide external reinforcement, "You did a good job."

Reinforcement can be combined with the simple hypnotic technique of suggestion. Therapeutic suggestion is a very powerful healing tool. The following examples show how these concepts can be melded. Listening to the above client's chest after coughing, you could say, "Oh, good. Your lungs sound much clearer/cleaner now. All the air you breathe can now get in your body and help it mend itself." You could also say, "Each time you move you make it easier to move the next time. When you move like this, you are exercising, which will stir up your circulation and speed your healing."

Rewards the learner desires are more reinforcing than general or routine rewards. Determine what the client finds reinforcing and attempt to increase the likelihood that the personally recognized reinforcer follows the desired behavior. An example of a personal reinforcer is the woman who quits smoking because she overhears an attractive man talk about his aversion to another woman's odor of smoke. The woman's desire to appeal to the man outweighs her desire to continue smoking. For this woman, the possibility of attracting the man is more powerful than the general reward of improving her health.

The clearer the cause and effect, the stronger the reinforcement. The clearer the causal connection or correlation between the desired behavior and the reward or punishment, the more effective the reward or punishment will be. The example of smoking can be used to illustrate this point, also. The punishment for smoking—increased risk of cancer—is remote in time. It is very difficult to connect the immediate action of smoking with such a distant threat. This same principle can be exemplified by a person who practices weight control. The gratification involved in eating junk food is immediate. The negative consequences—gradual deterioration of body tone and blood pressure—are much more remote.

Behaviors learned with spaced or intermittent reinforcement are more enduring than behaviors learned with consistent and regular reinforcement. An example of this is the child-parent interaction in which the child nags the parent to buy a product that the parent knows is expensive, unhealthy, or will soon be discarded. The parent says no and accompanies the answer with his or her reasons, but the child continues to nag. If the child nags long enough, the parent may give in to get relief from the negative reinforcer. What the child receives is intermittent reinforcement—the type of reinforcement that produces the most enduring and persistent behavior. The child's nagging thus becomes very difficult to eradicate.

Behaviors that receive no reinforcement decrease in frequency and eventually cease. There may be a period of increased frequency as the client attempts to recreate the former conditions. The above example may be used. If the parent can decide that she or he will no longer give in to nagging, the first thing the parent can expect is an increase in the nagging. This can be compared to the "Pop Machine Phenomenon." If we put money in a soft drink dispenser and get no soda pop, we may put in more money. We may even wait around to see if the next customer has better luck. We also may jiggle all of the buttons, push irrelevant levers, thump on the machine, even kick it in an effort to get some kind of response. Eventually, if the machine persists in not responding, we will walk away.

If the parent can hold out *permanently,* the nagging will cease. However, the parent must be ready for the child to do a test run every once in a while, to see if the reinforcement schedule has really changed, or if the parent was just employing a temporary, new program.

Punishment can decrease an undesirable behavior. Antabuse is taken with the intention of helping the alcoholic remain sober out of fear of the consequences of taking alcohol while antabuse is in her or her system. Antabuse thus helps the individual resist momentary urges. Punishment can also decrease a desirable behavior. Pain may motivate a person to avoid the behavior, such as moving in bed after surgery, that produced the pain.

Behavioral response to punishment is less predictable. The client may respond with aggression against the punishing mechanism. Many people on quick weight-loss programs report feelings of deprivation and rebellion. Another possible response to punishment is to withdraw from the learning situation. Withdrawal is frequently offered to explain large numbers of high school dropouts. Students who do poorly find school a punishing and negative experience that they eventually avoid by dropping out.

Punishment may suppress an undesirable behavior, but it does not teach the client a desirable behavior. A more effective regimen for eliminating an undesirable behavior is to find out what need that behavior is meeting, and then teach the client a more desirable behavior that will meet the same need. If the client is reinforced for increasing the competing behavior, the other less desirable behavior will tend to lose strength. The more you reinforce a competing behavior, the more it will eclipse the undesirable behavior as illustrated in Figure 12-1.

Classical conditioning involves attending to the antecedents of the behavior to be increased or decreased. Individuals suffering from addictions are taught to change the antecedents that helped trigger their addictive patterns. Overeaters learn to shop with a list and a full stomach. They may learn to take a different route home that avoids a bakery. Overeaters may also learn to keep dishes of prepared, fresh vegetables in the refrigerator in an easy-to-reach place. Junk food is eliminated from the cupboards to decrease cues for poor eating patterns.

Operant conditioning involves eliciting a desired behavior and then reinforcing it each time it occurs. When clients are learning to exercise, they may need to join a group. Many find the activity more enjoyable when they have company. The exercise leader may be an energetic person who constantly encourages and reinforces the class. Praise, recognition, and encouragement are valued by most people. The amount of reinforcement that is most effective with an individual client varies.

Shaping or refining a behavior is accomplished by reinforcing increasingly close approximations to the desired behavior. Children learn to feed themselves by this method. At first children decorate their hair, ears, and the floor—while they are trying to put food into their mouths. Once the food actually reaches their mouth, it acts as a reinforcer.

Parental response is also a factor. In the beginning, any attempt at self-feeding is reinforced. Eventually the child is reinforced only for the food that is ingested. This same method of learning is operational during the learning of one's native language. Babies of all races are born with similar language potential. From birth onward they hear sounds unique to the language of their caretakers. Babies' universal attempts to make sounds and to babble are differentially shaped, depending on the sounds that their parents reinforce by attention, delight, and response.

Chaining is a reinforcement schedule used to teach a complicated procedure. At first the client is reinforced for learning one step in the procedure. As the client masters that step, another is added. The client is then reinforced only after the completion of both tasks. As time goes on the client is reinforced after completing a chain of related behaviors. Eventually the client can complete the entire procedure. Teaching the client to do colostomy care can be an example of chaining. In this case it often works best to teach the procedure

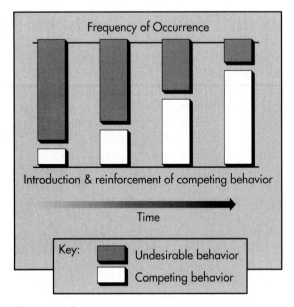

Figure 12-1 To extinguish a behavior: Elicit and then reinforce a competing behavior.

backwards. The client may first learn to apply the last piece of tape, which can be reinforcing because the client immediately experiences a feeling of satisfaction upon completion of the procedure. At the next session the client may perform the last two steps in the procedure. Eventually the client can perform all of the steps in this complicated process.

Practice is an important part of learning and retaining knowledge, skills, and attitudes. Repetition is an important component of learning skills—intellectual, psychomotor, or attitudinal. However, by itself, repetition is useful only to the point of habit fixation. When the repetition contains an improvement aspect, it moves to the level of practice. Nurses have commented on colleagues who have years of experience but who seem to have learned little. It may be that these individuals have developed a number of habit fixations but neglected to seek feedback and thus failed to integrate corrections, adaptations, and other improvements into their behaviors.

Clients with chronic diseases can fall into such habits. Conversely, some clients have advanced much further than thought possible because they were determined to keep on improving and because rehabilitation technology has advanced (Margalit, 1990).

Identification of the target or goal is an important component of reinforcement. Is the goal for the client to use the methods you choose? Is the goal for the client to think through the problem even though the solution he or she arrived at is less than ideal? Is the goal getting the client to participate in group discussion? Each of the above goals will lead to your using different applications of reinforcement principles.

Positive reinforcement is more effective than punishment in strengthening a behavior. Praise is more effective in motivating clients and increasing their performance. Praise in one subject matter may have a positive effect in another area. This may result from the increased confidence praise promotes within clients.

An interesting experiment was conducted by a school teacher who wanted to explain prejudice to children in a rural community where the children had no exposure to individuals of a different race. With the permission of the parents, the teacher designated one group of students as better than the other group based on eye color. The next week, the teacher switched the criteria. During each of the weeks, those with the preferred characteristic got special treatment and were told they were smarter. During each of the weeks, the children with the preferred trait performed better on their school work. When the children were not in the preferred group their performance suffered. This phenomenon occurred even though the children "knew" what was going on.

Knowledge of results is reinforcing. Clients want to know how well they did in any performance, whether it is intellectual or psychomotor. They benefit from accurate feedback. Knowledge of results while one is practicing a psychomotor skill helps the client improve that skill. Such feedback is equally valuable in improving an intellectual skill. Marzano and colleagues (1988) reported some interesting studies that were done by psychologists who believed they could raise the intelligence quotient (IQ) of poor students. The researchers got the students to read out loud when they were taking tests. It became clear that the students did not read the directions. Once the students began doing so, their scores immediately increased. The next step was to go over the learners' wrong answers and get them to verbalize the reasoning that led to such answers. When given feedback and very patiently taught to reason more logically, the students were indeed able to reduce their errors in logic. You are practicing an important learning principle when you provide correct answers immediately following a quiz.

Clients usually do not receive grades from nurses. Grading seems to have pronounced effects on learning but ideas vary greatly on exactly what the effects are (Slavin, 1991). If you are grade conscious you will do your best to figure out what your teachers want, and then give it to them. Students have reported to us that they learn differently when they expect a grade than when they do not. The atmosphere of the latter situation is usually more relaxed, but may also be less thorough. Students respond similarly to tests; they report studying less when they know they will not be tested on the learning.

In general, your clients will be interested in how well they are learning. Many people find quizzes and self-tests interesting. Consumers will take such tests and calculate their scores just to satisfy curiosity—consider the quizzes in monthly magazines and in newspapers. Conduct an informal survey of yourself, your peers, your relatives, and friends. Find out what kind of quizzes they take and whether or not they grade themselves.

Summarize your points.   In most circumstances, you will want to leave your clients with feelings of satisfaction. The most usual way to do this is to summarize your objectives and tell how you and the client achieved these objectives. Other ways to do this may be to have clients write a poem or a battle hymn, perform an activity, or describe what they will do with your presentation. When nursing students teach nutrition to youngsters the nurses usually provide some nutritious snacks that are illustrative of their message. Whatever your closing remarks are, they should be related to your objectives.

deTornyay (1982) identified some important components of instruction that she separated from strategies for teaching. She noted that we use these components no matter what strategies or methods we select. The components she identified are: reinforcement, examples and models, questions, set, and closure. Closure can be defined as the act of closing or bringing to a conclusion (Neufeldt, 1992). Closure is attempted when the major purposes and principles of a class, course, or program have been completed. Closure is complementary to set induction and is also used before the teacher goes on to a new topic. Some ways to accomplish closure include review and summary. Application of what has been said to similar situations is another. Closure provides the audience with a feeling of accomplishment. Closure is appropriate after explaining each concept before going on to any new concepts, ideas, or problems.

Implementation of the Lesson Plan for Lincoln Perez

Before we begin teaching Mr. Perez, we are going to arrange a room to facilitate the learning we hope to accomplish. One of the learning goals we chose is relaxation. It will be easier for Mr. Perez to learn relaxation if we provide an appropriate environment, such as one with soft lighting, controlled noise, and comfortable furniture, and if he wears comfortable clothing (you will need to instruct him ahead of time to wear this). We intend to present Mr. Perez with a menu of relaxation techniques with the understanding that he will choose the ones that suit him. We will reinforce his achievements and choices.

We will need to determine what Mr. Perez already knows about taking his pulse. If he says that he knows how, we will ask him to show us how he does it. If he uses the 6-seconds-times-10 method, we will first reinforce him for having learned this skill. We then will try to persuade him to switch to the 15-seconds-times-4 method to improve accuracy. Once his pulse-taking skill reaches the desired level, we will reinforce his accuracy with a joke, such as "You are as good a pulse counter as I am. If the construction business does not pick up, come into nursing!"

Summary

In this chapter we discussed implementation of teaching. We focused on a number of teaching principles that are cogent in any situation: openness, warmth, sensitivity, organization, questions, clarity, audiovisual use, pacing, repetition, demonstration, knowledge, stories and examples, focus, mutual respect, ethnic sensitivity, patience, authenticity, enthusiasm, reinforcement, and summarization. The chapter provides examples for using the aforementioned principles.

In closing this chapter, we wish to persuade you to consider the eclectic approach to learning. Not all clients learn best by any particular mode. Each way of learning—cognitive, auditory, visual, imaginative, associational, logical, affective, psychomotor, systematic, and process oriented—has its advantages. It is unlikely that all of your clients will have identical learning styles. Each strategy discussed has its advantages and disadvantages, and each material is more appropriate for some clients and learning objectives than others. In general, if you use several approaches you are more likely to reach more clients than if you use only one approach. Varying the strategies and materials you use is more likely to make the learning interesting and to motivate students throughout the learning process.

The way in which you learn and the ways your role models teach you will have a strong influence on the strategies and materials you choose. You are encouraged to start with ways that seem comfortable and to take the challenge of risking new adventures when they seem particularly relevant to your clients and your intended objectives. Mixed teaching strategies and materials will probably always be superior to any one method.

E X E R C I S E   I

QUALITY TEACHING

Purposes:

- Think critically about how you can integrate the principles of teaching into your own teaching style
- Raise your consciousness about the qualities of good teaching
- Search for worthwhile teaching role models

Directions:

1. Analyze the list of teaching principles in this chapter.
2. Formulate your own criteria for a good teacher.
3. Observe a colleague doing clinical teaching with a client or group of clients.
4. Prepare a report: State your overall impression of the effectiveness of the teacher using your own criteria.

E X E R C I S E   I I

TEACHING TECHNOLOGIES

Purposes:

- Prepare to implement your teaching module by practicing with equipment
- Demonstrate to a colleague how to use a piece of equipment while applying the teaching principles including positive reinforcement
- Experience the benefits of repetition through the pattern: LEARN, DO, TEACH, EVALUATE

Directions:

1. Arrange yourselves in small groups around each piece of equipment and learn what you need to know about each of them.
2. Watch as many demonstrations as necessary, before using each piece of equipment yourself.
3. After you can use the equipment satisfactorily, teach its use to the next peer in line.
4. Use principles of a good demonstration and

reinforcement as you teach.

5. Watch your peer to see how well she or he learned from your demonstration. Coach if necessary.

6. Record your performance and rotate to the next piece of equipment.

7. Continue this pattern until you have encountered all of the equipment available.

8. If you are already very familiar with a piece of equipment, please read the instructions and give the instructor pertinent suggestions for improving them. Teach use of the machine to one of your peers and then record your activity.

References

Babcock, D. & Zak-Dance, C. (1981). Developing skills as a public speaker. *American Operating Room Nurses Journal, 33*(5), 994-1000.

Browne, M.N. & Keeley, S.M. (1986). *Asking the right questions; A guide to critical thinking* (2nd ed.). Englewood Cliffs NJ: Prentice-Hall.

Carnegie, D. (1980). *How to win friends and influence people.* New York: Dale Carnegie & Associates.

deTornyay, R. & Thompson, M. (1982). *Strategies for teaching nursing.* New York: John Wiley & Sons.

Dewey, J. (1938). *Experience and education.* New York: Macmillan.

Gose, K. & Levi, G. (1988). *Dealing with memory changes as you grow older.* Toronto: Bantam Books.

Margalit, M. (1990). *Effective technology integration for disabled children: The family perspective.* New York: Springer.

Marzano, R.J., Brandt, R.S., Hughes, C.S., Jones, B.F., Presseisen, B.Z., Rankin, S.C. & Suhor, C. (1988). *Dimensions of thinking: A framework for curriculum and instruction.* Alexandria: Association for Supervision and Curriculum Development.

Neufeldt, V. (Ed.). (1992). *Webster's New World Dictionary* (3rd ed.). New York: Webster's New World.

Slavin, R.E. (1991). *Educational psychology: Theory into practice* (3rd ed.). Englewood Cliffs NJ: Prentice Hall.

Springer, S.P. & Deutsch, G. (1981). *Left brain, right brain.* New York: W.H. Freeman.

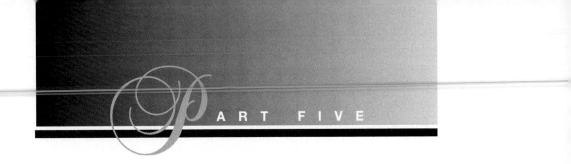

Evaluation of Learning

Client Compliance

You can lead a horse to water
but you cannot make him drink.

Rural American Proverb.

Upon completion of this chapter you will be able to:

- Discuss the changing conceptions of compliance.
- Discuss phenomena that affect and do not affect client compliance.
- Specify how compliance is affected by the client's age and cultural background.
- Apply five strategies that have helped clients adopt life-style changes.
- Discuss teaching/learning as an adaptation strategy.

Key Words

evaluation	collaboration	respect
compliance	reinforcement	choice
independence	communication	responsibility
adaptation	trust	readability

Introduction

The final step of the nursing process is evaluation. Evaluation is the process of judging how effective all of your teaching efforts have been as shown in Figure 13-1. Everything you have studied to this point has a bearing on evaluation. In the next two chapters we will consider two distinct aspects of evaluation. The first aspect is looking at whether or not the client has changed his or her behavior based on what you have taught. This is commonly referred to as client compliance. The second aspect we will address involves evaluation of the teaching module itself and the process you used as a health educator. Your findings during the evaluation step will become feedback into the teaching/learning system, so you have an opportunity to adapt what you are doing to produce more effective results. Thus adaptation to feedback brings you full circle in the teaching/learning system.

In this chapter we will focus on compliance and its meaning to the client, to the health delivery system, and to you as the health educator. We will discuss the changing conceptions of client compliance, offer some

—Continued next page

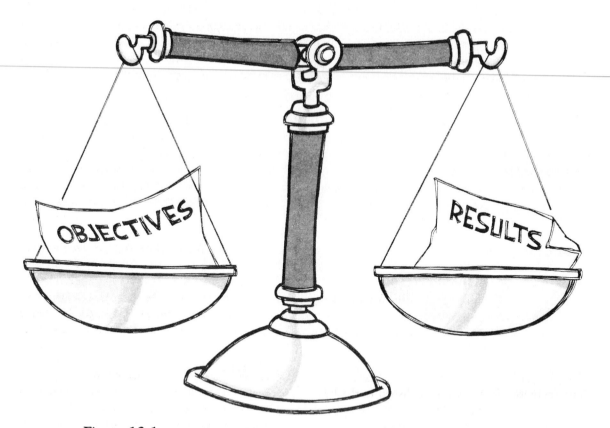

Figure 13-1   To evaluate teaching, consider its worth. Examine and judge the results (output). Do the results match the objectives?

general guidelines, and address compliance across different age groups and diverse cultures. We will also include strategies for helping people change.

Changing Conceptions of Compliance

Many nursing students and practicing clinicians have expressed concerns about getting the client to comply with the regimen the nurses are attempting to teach. It is frustrating for you when the client does not comply especially if you know from past experience that your advice, if followed, will improve the client's health. It may be equally frustrating for the client who may feel unheard or misunderstood or who may consider your recom-

mendations impractical given his or her life circumstances.

Clients choose health behaviors in which they will engage. Generally the choice is a trade-off among a variety of influences in their lives. For example, dietary modifications may be difficult to follow if there is insufficient money to buy food. It may be impractical to prepare the food as instructed. The rationale for behavioral change may not make sense to a client. It is also possible that a client's social network might not offer enough reinforcement to sustain a behavioral change such as quitting smoking.

There are many facets to the topic of compliance. The word itself means giving in to a request, wish or demand; acquiescence, a tendency to give

250   Evaluation of Learning

in readily to others (Neufeldt, 1991). Clients who do not heed your counsel and choose not to embrace the health practices you have taught them are called noncompliant. When you label a client *noncompliant*, you imply that you know what is best for the client: "If only the client will do what I tell him, he will get better and avoid another disaster." Charonko (1992) offers some insight on the concept of noncompliance. Her point is that clients are not *noncompliant* because a client's choices belong to him or her, not the health care provider. Because life is the client's choice, the client cannot be noncompliant. Health providers and health educators are the ones disappointed when the client does not follow instructions. Germain (1992) also urged health care providers to reconsider the notion of noncompliance. It may represent a failure on the part of health care providers to adequately address the client's needs.

The subject of compliance is more of an issue today because of the intense concern for clients' rights and the fact that many clients are being discharged earlier than was customary a decade ago. Many activities formerly accomplished in the hospital by the nurse are now being performed in the home with only intermittent supervision by the nurse. In other words the client and his or her family are expected to carry out the prescribed treatments. When the client was hospitalized the nurse could be sure that the client complied, but no such guarantee exists when the client is at home.

Enforcement of compliance is much less possible today than it was during the public health movements of the first half of this century (Hanlon, 1984). For example, one client who had the mumps in the 1930s in Philadelphia had a quarantine sign placed on her door, and her father was advised to live away from home until the girl was no longer contagious. In 1958, Philadelphia General Hospital had several clients in the tuberculosis unit who were in the hospital by order of the court. Since that time, attitudes toward medical authority and the effectiveness of quarantine have changed dramatically (Hanlon, 1984). Now, any kind of medical enforcement is less politically or legally sanctioned (Jane Doe, RN, 1989). It will be interesting to observe what happens to the political and legal scene now that afflictions such as tobacco-related diseases, alcoholism, abuse of other drugs, and AIDS are viewed as threats to others besides those suffering from the diseases (Froman, Owen, & Daisy, 1992).

Redman (1988) reported that age, sex, income, marital status, and educational level do not consistently correlate with compliance. This may seem confusing because education does appear to be correlated with health-promoting activities. However, we know that knowledge of health and illness is not enough to motivate lasting change and the relinquishment of addictions. For example, some health care workers smoke, abuse substances, and/or suffer from eating disorders even though they know the risks of such behaviors.

Trust and communication are integrally related issues when you are dealing with compliance. Many times clients will not tell you whether or not they will cooperate with the recommended regimen unless they know you and believe that you want to understand their point of view. We urge you to develop your skills of listening with a nonjudgmental demeanor; you have a better chance of discovering what is going on when you act truly interested (Hilbert, 1985). Although you see yourself as a caring and trustworthy person, your client's experience with the health care system may have led to disenchantment and mistrust (Thorne & Robinson, 1989). If the client is in this phase you would need to address that issue first and negotiate carefully the path along which you and the client can proceed, if at all.

General Guidelines

As the health educator, you will reinforce those clients who make the recommended health behavior modifications you see as essential for health maintenance and recovery and/or illness prevention. In this section of the chapter, we will offer some general guidelines on prevention of noncompliance and the encouragement of compliance. To begin, we recommend that you operate on the assumption that the client is interested, willing, and able to comply with your message and that the client wants to cooperate with you and learn what you have to teach, unless you have evidence to the contrary.

To begin, make sure clients can understand the written instructions. Streiff (1986) suggested that a client's compliance may be related to the comprehensibility of these written instructions, so she tested the reading level of 106 adults in a clinic and compared the results with the health education materials distributed in that same unit. Client's reading levels averaged from first grade to college freshmen, with an average grade level of seventh grade. The average pamphlet was written at a level five grades higher than the ability of the average client.

If clients are succeeding, be sure to reinforce their successes. Celebrate weight loss or improvement in a child's situation with them. In the best of situations, the changed behavior reinforces itself. The client who begins to taste food and notice odors following smoking cessation experiences this reinforcement.

In some situations, only partial client compliance with your health instruction is possible; in other situations compliance may be impossible. Avoid embarrassing, judging, or humiliating the client in these situations. Rather, take time to talk with the client about his or her circumstances and the relevance of your instruction to these circumstances. Try to determine how the client understood your instruction. Discard unrealistic goals and together establish new ones that are more workable for the client (Reynolds, 1992). In the box we have listed a number of questions that may help you evaluate the meaning of the client's improvement or lack thereof.

Special Challenges in Client Compliance

Although we may define compliance in a single way, the concept and your expectations will be applied differently to clients of different ages and cultural backgrounds. We will now look at what compliance means across various age and cultural groups.

The Child Client

For purposes of this discussion, we consider the age range of the child to be from infancy through adolescence. Obviously there is great variability in growth and development that has a major effect on clients' abilities to learn as well as to change their behavior in response to your teaching (Wong, 1990). Any teaching you do and any behavioral expectations you may have for a child must be realistically based on what the client is capable of doing. It makes little sense to expect a 2-year-old to brush her teeth with the same degree of thoroughness that you would expect from a 10-year-old. It's unreasonable to expect a very active 4-year-old to sit still for a lengthy uncomfortable procedure.

We believe that behavioral theories of learning are the most useful in the early formative years. Gestalt, humanistic, and information processing frames of reference become useful as the young

---

Evaluation Questions

The following is a list of questions to ask yourself during the evaluation phase.

1. What is the effect of the regime that you, your medical colleagues, and the client negotiated on the outcome for the client?

2. Did the client get better because she or he followed your recommendations?

3. Did the client get worse because she or he followed your recommendations?

4. Did the client get better in spite of your advice?

5. Did the client actually comply? How do you know?

6. What were the factors actually involved in the client's improved condition? According to whose perceptions?

7. How does the client perceive the effectiveness of your health interventions?

8. Is there something you missed during the assessment step that you have now discovered that affected the client's compliance?

9. Did you miss some cues that would have spared you useless effort or increased your chances of cooperation?

person matures. Reinforcement of your target behaviors is widely applicable to all clients; it is one of the most useful skills you can learn as a teacher. It is just as important, perhaps more so, when you teach children. Refrain from focusing on the negative aspect of a child's behavior. Instead, concentrate on eliciting and reinforcing the health enhancing behaviors you have targeted. Providing rewards that are recognized by the child as desirable is also helpful (Pidgeon, 1989; Smith & Nix, 1991).

A good line of investigation to follow if you are seeking to discover the causes of a child's noncompliance, is to figure out what is preventing the behavior you are attempting to elicit. An example is a toddler on the pediatric unit who was supposed to receive penicillin drops but did not. The reason the baby did not receive the drops is that the nurse had trouble getting the baby to take them. The nurse even tried mixing the drops in the baby's broth, but then the baby refused to drink the soup. Finally the nurse tasted the soup herself and agreed with the baby: The taste was too awful to eat. The nurse solved the problem by putting the medicine into peanut butter and jelly, which have strong flavors and varying textures that can overwhelm the taste of most medications, however offensive. Ever since that experience, the nurse has found peanut butter and jelly very effective in getting children to take awful-tasting medicines.

Following is an example of noncompliance involving prescription eyeglasses at two developmental levels. Each problem must be approached individually with an age appropriate intervention. A 4-year-old is supposed to wear glasses all of the time. He takes the eyeglasses off when he is actively engaged in play because they bother him, tilt, or fall off. One solution is to construct a complicated piece of head gear that will keep the glasses in place and will be difficult for the child to remove. If a teenager is resisting glasses, the motivation may be self-esteem, "Everybody calls me 'four eyes!'" A possible solution may be contact lenses. The other lesson in these two situations, is to be creative in looking for options. When people are under stress, they may get stuck and become unable to come up with options. Assist the parents or the children

themselves with the *option* mode of thinking. Even if the alternatives you suggest will not work with this family, the *idea* of options may free them to come up with a solution of their own that is workable.

Do not be put off by a 2-year-old who says, "No!" It is a favorite word, and may not be a declaration of noncompliance. We recommend that you continue with body language to elicit the behavior you have requested with words. For example, while telling the child to lie down, gently but firmly lay him or her down and tell the child that you will help him or her keep still until you have finished putting in the tiny tube, then you will let him or her move around again.

In Chapter 5 we have included helpful hints for dealing with children who resist treatment when they are afraid or in pain. When a child is outside of the hospital setting, noncompliance becomes very complicated. Not only do you need to assess the child and his or her motivation for noncompliance, but also you must examine the effect of interactions occurring among the child, the main caretakers, and peer groups (Pidgeon, 1989). Small children may be too busy with their own interests to pay attention to a set of behaviors that are at the least inconvenient and unpleasant. Adolescents with attitudes toward their own indestructibility have trouble really grasping long-term consequences of noncompliance (Hentinen & Kyngas, 1992; Schmidt, Klover, & Arfken, 1992). Connecting the behavior to consequences that are relevant to the child is an important variable. A nurse in a hospital emergency room was trying to prepare a young boy with a cervical fracture for neck traction. The boy had been in a severe accident and his life was indeed at stake. Threats that his thrashing around could cost him his life were to no avail. Finally the nurse put her face 10 inches from that of the boy's and with direct eye contact said, "I am trying to keep you from spending the rest of your life in a wheelchair." This statement apparently had meaning because the boy immediately became still and remained so throughout the rest of the procedure.

Another way to treat noncompliance is to prevent it. In general, giving children as much information and control as they can handle will raise their compliance (Hentinin & Kyngas, 1992). Todd was 7 years old when he had a tonsillectomy. He was well prepared by his mother who explained everything that would happen to him during the procedure—from the time of admission and surgery to postoperative procedures and discharge. The nurses and doctors who had assessed the parent/child system were willing to go at the child's pace and cooperate with the mother's long-standing knowledge of her child. Consequently Todd handled the entire procedure exceptionally well. Before he was anesthetized, Todd was allowed to tell the doctors when he was ready for the mask to go on. When he was ready, he applied the mask himself and went to sleep very smoothly. The point of this example is that when you allow the child as much control as he can handle, he does better complying with the procedure and the postoperative course.

The Adult Client

Adult behavior is very complex because adults can mask their feelings and motivations. Adults' noncompliance may come from a multitude of sources over which you have no control and about which you have no knowledge unless they choose to share it with you. Clients may also be reacting to forces and fears of which they are unaware.

Rosenstock (Redman, 1988) has provided a very widely used model for understanding why people take action to improve their health or to reduce health risks. Reasons for taking health action include:

1. A belief in personal susceptibility to a particular disease.
2. A belief that the disease, if contracted, would seriously affect one's health.
3. Awareness of certain actions that reduce the risk of contracting the disease or experiencing its consequences.
4. A view of the threat of change as less fearsome than the disease itself.
5. Some trigger that motivates the individual to action.

Although this model does not provide the complete answer, this model does give us some insight into why people do or do not take health actions. Levanthal (1982) discovered that clients' levels of compliance may be related to their assumptions about illness.

> *Example:* "An illness has discernible symptoms; therefore, if I have no symptoms, I am not sick. If it were a serious disease, then I would be aware of serious symptoms."

This assumption might explain the noncompliance of the hypertensive client. In this example the client has not grasped the fact that his or her blood pressure can be elevated even in the absence of perceptible symptoms.

Adults may observe with amusement the adolescent who says and/or acts as if, "It will not happen to me." Many adults continue to hold onto that magical belief at an unconscious level. Essentially, these people are gambling, assuming the consequences of behavior will show up in others but not in themselves. The smoking adult provides us with a good example of this type of thinking. Another related form of magical thinking is evidenced in the smoker who says, "I know I smoke, but I take extra vitamin C, which helps my body stay in repair, so I am safe." This is a variation of the same theme of "playing the odds."

A typical statement, "I can stop when it causes symptoms," is evidence of an assumption being made by a person who continues to smoke. A person who makes such an assumption fails to grasp the notion that much of the early damage from smoking and related toxic substances is not noticeable to the smoker. By the time symptoms of lung or heart disease appear or a malignancy is detected, the chances of cure are greatly reduced. Education about body physiology and the causes of cancer may help persuade the individual to change.

Compliance with treatment of chronic illness is related to time lines (how long the illness will last) and identification of the causes of symptoms (Redeker, 1988). The side effects of the medication and the symptoms of the disease may become confused. Kloeppel and Henry (1987) list the following factors that can diminish compliance:

1. Denial—Clients who do not see themselves as needing information are not likely to listen to or use advice.
2. Complexity—Non-compliance increases with the complexity of the regimen, and with the amount of life-style interference the client experiences. It appears easier to add a new behavior than to remove a gratifying habit.
3. Comprehension—Clients may not understand the directions. Consumers rely too heavily on their own interpretation of medical information. Many get less than the amount of education they desire.
4. Side effects—Side effects that disrupt the client's life are negatively correlated with compliance. For example, medication for hypertension frequently interferes with a man's ability to maintain a satisfactory erection. Antipsychotic drugs often have a negative effect on an individual's libido. In addition, these drugs frequently cause symptoms of parkinsonism. If the drug regimen is long term, brain damage may make these symptoms permanent.
5. Differing cultural beliefs—Various groups have beliefs about health promotion and illness prevention that may hinder their cooperation.
6. Cost—The greater the cost of the treatment, the fewer the chances of compliance. Some clients may not be able to afford the expense of the desired regimen. A summary of the above phenomena can be found in Figure 13-2.

Promoting affective learning is an important part of intervening in noncompliance. Long-term consequences that may or may not occur are very remote concepts, even to well-educated people. The decision to relinquish a habit, however odious, is very difficult to make. Current events in our country offer encouraging evidence that affective change is possible even through mass media education. In terms of attitudinal change, Naisbitt (1982) noted that Americans have changed their health behaviors monumentally. The change is toward living

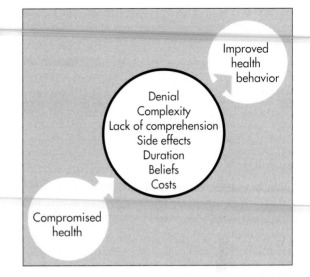

Figure 13-2   Factors that deter compliance include denial, complexity, lack of comprehension, side effects, duration, beliefs, and costs.

more healthfully, and it represents a fundamental shift in the thinking of people. This is evident in grass-root demands for salad bars, smoking-free seating in restaurants and other public places, jogging and bike paths, athletic clothing, and fitness centers. The clients you will be teaching have been influenced by these changes and many have either made life-style changes or are already aware of the need to do so.

Some of your concerns about noncompliance will be solved by factors other than the health education that you provide. For example, public pressure against smoking is mounting and people who smoke are reporting the adverse responses they are getting from nonsmokers. "I find fewer and fewer places where I can smoke undisturbed outside my own home," says one smoker.

The Older Client

Although compliance is a challenge for clients of any age, the older adult has some unique characteristics that make compliance more of a challenge.

For instance, older adults are notorious for failing to comply with medication schedules (Hussey, 1991). The primary problems older adults face are difficulty with remembering, sensory deprivation related to diminished vision and auditory acuity, and slower cognitive and motor processes. In other words the client is going to have trouble hearing what you have to say if you speak too rapidly or softly. Older clients might also have difficulty reading the directions, particularly if the page is too crowded with dense, small type. You may need to find out if the client can read and comprehend written directions. Even if the client says she or he understands the directions, the client may have trouble remembering them. If you keep in mind the strategies we offered in Chapter 7, you can prevent many compliance problems. At this point we will offer some additional strategies for helping older clients to comply. To begin, find out what motivates the older client, or what obstacles she or he experiences that interfere with compliance. Resnick (1991) found that the side effects of medication, nutritional problems, sensory changes, and cognitive disorders may interfere with compliance as well as your teaching.

Ley, Bradshaw, Eaves, and Walker (1973) showed that dividing medical information into labeled categories significantly increased the amount recalled. Information that is labeled receives a special focus in the client's mind. Information connected with a particular concept is remembered better when it is understood. This is particularly important when you teach information that is new to the client. Your challenge is to organize the information so that it is interesting, logical, and sufficiently detailed for the client to associate it with things the client already knows (Slavin, 1992). An additional hint is to highlight the most important points:

Example: "I want you to remember three things to do to protect your skin, especially the skin on your feet: Keep it clean, keep it dry, and wear good shoes.
1. Keep your skin clean.
2. Dry your skin thoroughly, especially between your toes and any other folds of skin.
3. Wear good shoes so your feet have proper support and protection."

The aforementioned directions, given to a 75-year-old, obese, diabetic female, helped her focus on and remember the needed behavioral changes.

Advice presented in concrete, specific statements was substantially more likely to be recalled than the same advice couched in more abstract terms (Ley, Bradshaw, Eaves, & Walker, 1973). "If you eat less meat, you will probably get some relief from your gout," is more concrete than, "Gout seems to be aggravated by an intake of large amounts of purine in your diet."

Skill training *is* possible with the elderly. A client who goes through behavioral rehearsal with feedback and reinforcement is more likely to comply, but the older client may need more time to learn the new skill. The amount of time will depend on the age and physical condition of the individual being taught. The elderly are just as intellectually capable of new learning as anyone else. However, to be effective, you must exercise the additional patience necessary for putting the older client at ease and take your time during the teaching/learning process. As with any change in behavior, clients are more likely to comply and/or succeed if they try out the behavior while you encourage and coach them. An older client had bought a new appliance—a mini food processor—to comply with recommendations to process his food, but he was afraid to use it. The nursing student read the directions and tried running the appliance. She then had the client read the directions step by step while she performed each step. The nursing student then had the client perform each step while she coached. She then asked the client if he wished to try again. This allowed the client to exercise control over the pace of the learning. He could repeat the performance at that time to solidify his learning, or he could wait until the nurse visited again, therefore practicing intermittently.

The importance of client control has also been validated by research (Poon, Fozard, & Popkin,

1978). A feeling of control is correlated with improved blood pressure, adherence to the prescribed regime, understanding, and fewer medication errors. The client's taking control may be aggravating to you, but it is more likely to lead to cooperation and compliance. Such control can be viewed as the client's intuitive knowledge that she or he *must* take control in order to learn whatever is at hand.

Poon and colleagues (1980) looked for correlations between memory difficulties and other symptoms of error proneness. They found that people differ in their vulnerability to minor cognitive failures. Some individuals tend to have liabilities across the board, and different forms of error proneness tend to correlate with each other. Poon also found there is no significant correlation between intelligence, neuroticism, or trait anxiety. Memory taps a dimension not easily assessed by existing psychometrics. However, a higher error rate does correlate with increased vulnerability to stress. Although researchers are not in agreement about the causes and the extent of memory changes, many older individuals and their associates are aware of problems with short-term memory. Fortunately, a number of promising and tested remedies are available to the interested older individual. Using poems, imagery, lists, color coding, and other memory crutches may help. One of the most valuable remedies is association.

Keep in mind that compliance increases with cuing. For example, a client who has a memory aid is more likely to follow the regime prescribed. Specificity also helps. For example, a client is more likely to remember to take a medication with breakfast, lunch, supper, and bedtime tea than she is to remember to take it four times a day. Such specificity needs to be qualified. It is important to ask a particularly thin client about his or her weight.

> *Example:* "I know as we get older our appetite sometimes changes. Tell me, how many times a day do you usually sit down for a bite to eat or a cup of tea?"

Find a way to attach the new health behavior to an established routine. For example, when helping an elderly man set up a regime for faithfully taking his medications at home, the nurse asked him to demonstrate his routine. The nurse noticed that he kept his medication in one little box—the plastic kind in which you get four tomatoes. When he tried to count out his medication for the day, he got mixed up and had trouble handling the individual envelopes another nurse had tried the time before. He also found the little white weekly boxes confusing. Replacing his box with another that was just a little bigger and was divided into front and back with a piece of cardboard helped the man separate the medications he took twice a day from those he took once a day. Putting big black numbers "1X" and "2X" on top of each bottle and on the floor of the box also helped. You can make use of these helpful hints when you are helping an older client learn information, skills, and/or attitudinal changes to promote health. Make use of the research; adapt learning theories and principles to enhance the older client's chances of success.

As with all clients, positive reinforcement is a powerful force for changing behavior. Positive reinforcement, monitoring, home visiting, and tailoring a regimen to the client's daily activities all led to improved compliance (Haynes, Taylor, & Sackett, 1979). Shaping is an important principle for getting clients to comply. Cooperation in a simple low-key activity raises the chances of cooperation in a more demanding activity (Haynes, Taylor, & Sackett, 1979); for example, during colostomy care, ask the client to hold equipment for you, then ask the client to apply the tape, and then invite the client to do the entire procedure while you coach.

Culturally Diverse Clients

Persuading culturally diverse clients to modify their health-related behaviors because such a change is in their best interest is your responsibility as a health educator. This is particularly challenging as you work with ethnic groups that believe their own role in shaping their future health is small. Some Hispanics may believe that life is under the control of God and there is little one can do to control events. You are more likely to be successful with future-oriented cultural groups, such as blacks and Asian Americans.

Many black Americans have a mental orientation toward prevention of health problems. This may facilitate your attempts to teach them preventive health concepts. Blacks may emphasize knowledge of the rules of nature that govern life and may believe that failure to follow the rules may result in illness. Some may believe in moderation of diet, rest, and exercise to help maintain health.

> The body, if protected from extremes of heat and cold, adequately fed, kept clean inside and out, kept limber by work and exercise and properly rested, should remain free of most health problems. There is a special emphasis on monitoring the state of the blood, thought to mirror the state of the system, and on the processes of digestion and elimination. (Snow, 1983, p. 821)

Care must be taken to evaluate the preventive health behaviors in which clients engage. Some practices may not be in the client's best interest from a medical viewpoint. For example, to rid the body of impurities, many blacks overuse laxatives. A culturally sensitive nurse will see an opportunity for education here. Advising the person to stop using laxatives is unlikely to succeed. You raise your chances of success in eliminating an undesirable behavior by introducing a desirable competing behavior, such as increased consumption of bran and dolomite, which are possible aids to regularity that have more nutritional value than laxatives.

What has been labeled noncompliance may really result from inadequate communication. A young Hispanic mother, age 18 and 6 weeks post partum, had developed a yeast infection. The physician prescribed vinegar douches twice a day. The nurse gave the mother directions for preparing the correct mix of vinegar and water. When the nurse revisited the client later in the week, the nurse asked about the vaginal drainage. The client explained that it was about the same but that she just could not continue the treatments anymore. The solution simply tasted too terrible to drink.

Many ethnic groups have extended families and networks for support. If this is the case with your client, it may be important to include such persons in your teaching. If extended family members are going to help care for the client, it is important that they hear the same message. Family members can assist the client in complying with the treatment regimen or making the necessary behavioral changes to live more healthily. You will want to be sensitive to those instances where involvement of family members may not be welcomed by the client. An example of this may be seen across the generations where a younger client may not value the extent of family involvement valued by the parents (Nidorf & Morgan, 1987).

In teaching compliance with drugs, be sure the client takes the correct drug at the correct time and in the correct amount, and through the correct orifice. Fundamental to this is the expectation that the client is even willing to take the drug. Inquire about the herbs that the client may be taking along with Western medications. These must be known so that problems do not arise. For example, ginseng, a commonly used herb among Chinese Americans, is used as a panacea. Ginseng also has a stimulant property, so its use is contraindicated in hypertension (Campbell & Chang, 1981).

Chinese Americans may expect medications to be immediately effective in treating an illness. Such clients may not understand why Western medications, such as that used in the treatment of hypertension, must be taken over a period of time. In Chinese folk treatment, if one herb is ineffective, it is discontinued and another one tried (Campbell & Chang, 1981).

In working with ethnic clients, you should remember that they may be engaging in some traditional health practices along with the nursing and medical interventions they are receiving. By respecting traditional health practices that are helpful or harmless, you will keep the avenues of communication open. Clients will be more likely to comply with medical instructions and expectations if these are compatible with their traditional beliefs and values. Remember, compliance in transcultural interchanges may not be as high as you expect. If the client's belief system is counter to your health message, the resulting level of compliance will be low (Bushy, 1992). Even though the nonverbal behavior of the client may be interpreted by you to mean compliance, it may only be an effort on the client's part to be courteous. Be realistic in your expectations of culturally diverse clients (Charonko, 1992). In the final analysis, it is the client's right to determine his or her own future (Andrews, 1989).

Past literature focused on helping the nurse teach the client how to assume the compliant role (Redman, 1988). However, this view of the nurse's role is rapidly changing. Siegel (1986) and others (Lowery, 1991) pointed out that clients who are not compliant do not always fare worse because of their choices. Clients who attempt to master their illnesses and control their own recovery seem to experience beneficial effects, such as enhanced healing capacity (Siegel, 1986).

Additional Strategies to Help People Comply

In the preceding part of this chapter, we identified some factors that interfere with a client's cooperation with recommended treatments. What else will increase the chances that the client will comply with your recommendations? Compliance improves when clients experience individual appointments, decreased waiting time, and lower costs (Levanthal, 1982). During individual appointments, nurses conducted thorough investigations into clients' perceptions of the cause, symptoms, and the course of the illness. The manner in which you communicate health messages also influences compliance. When you master the art of persuasion, you will enhance the probability of compliance.

Threats are less reliable (Bauman & Keller, 1991). An example of a threat would be to inform the client of the death rate of those who do not comply. The threat of death appears quite remote to most of us, so such a threat may have little meaning. A threat may work when it is put into a framework of concern for the client. For example, a woman who had smoked for years had appeared impervious to the pleas from her family and threats from her medical caregiver. Eventually she developed sores in her mouth that would not heal. Her caregiver declared that the sores were on the verge of becoming cancerous. Then she stopped smoking.

Groups can be very helpful getting people to adopt life-style changes. Some of the strategies these groups use are listed in the box on p. 260. Public commitment also increases the chances that clients will comply. Clients who are willing to state out loud what they will do are more likely to do it. Clients who write and/or sign statements outlining their changes are also more likely to follow through. If you use contracts, keep in mind they should be the end result of consultation and negotiation, not something you dictated and the client signed. Some of the strategies listed in the box can be started in the hospital. In the community health setting you have the opportunity to apply all of the strategies.

Adaptation

Adaptation is the process by which a living system modifies itself to suit a new or changing environment. Adaptation also suggests a change in structure, function, or form that improves the chance of survival for an animal or plant within a given environment (Neufeldt, 1991). The symptoms of disease are efforts on the body's part to adapt to changing conditions. For example, inflammation is the body's adaptation to an irritation, bruising, straining, and/or invasion by pathogens. Obesity is an effort on the body's part to get the fat out of circulation and out of harm's way; storage in adipose tissue is potentially less harmful to the body than its remaining in the circulatory system.

Your task as a health educator is to facilitate the client's adaptation to his or her problem in such a way that she or he moves to a higher level of wellness. If the inflammation were due to a stress injury, such as pitcher's elbow, you would treat it with an ice pack. If the client's obesity is due to inadequate activity and excessive caloric intake, then you would attempt to influence both behaviors. Running might raise the obese person's chances of a stroke or heart attack, but walking a few steps farther each day would eventually encourage his or her body to start

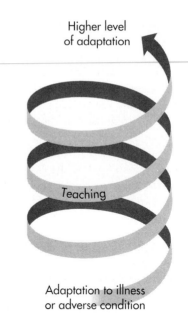

Higher level
of adaptation

Teaching

Adaptation to illness
or adverse condition

Figure 13-3   Teaching facilitates moving toward a
higher level of adaptation.

burning the excess fat. A gradual substitution of one
piece of fruit for one dessert or fatty snack would
also promote a change in the desired direction.

The corollary to teaching clients to adapt their
behaviors to reach higher levels of wellness is for
you as teacher to adapt your teaching to reach
clients. You will raise your chances of success if you
spend the time necessary to focus on clients' motivators, and attempt to engage those motivators in
your plan. See how we have attempted to apply this
principle in our intervention with Mr. Perez below.
Teaching, when it is well-timed and well-aimed, can
lead to a higher level of adaptation as illustrated in
Figure 13-3.

Compliance Considerations
for Lincoln Perez

If Mr. Perez is complying, he will be walking and
doing at least one relaxation technique daily. He
also will be taking his pulse and recording it every
day. When we take his blood pressure, we will have

an additional parameter to assess whether he is getting better or worse.

If Mr. Perez tells us he is not complying, our first response should be to reinforce his honesty and then talk with him about the problem as he sees it. After hearing his story, we will help Mr. Perez identify options that would surmount the problems. As we identify these options, we might preface them with, "Have you thought about . . . ," or "How would . . . work for you?" For illustrative purposes, we are going to create the problems interfering with Mr. Perez's compliance. He tells us he has two sons and a daughter and they are all on different softball teams. His wife works, so it is a major task to coordinate everyone's schedules. When he comes home from work, he does not have time to relax or walk. Some of the options we will pursue with him include getting up earlier to walk, parking his car two blocks farther from his office, and parking his car two blocks farther from any of the construction sites he visits. We asked him what he does for a coffee break and asked if he could do an imagery break with it or instead of it. We asked if he has electric plugs in his office and if he could play a tape before he starts his day. We also asked if he has a favorite prayer he could put in a picture frame and hang facing his desk, so he could see it every time he looks up. By now we hope you have the idea about how we are exploring various options with Mr. Perez.

Summary

Effective client teaching will lead to behavioral change. In one way or another the client must adapt by doing things in a different way, such as letting go of one behavior and taking on new ones. The challenges you will face are influenced by the age and cultural background of your clients and their present health status.

When you become knowledgeable about the principles of learning, behavior modification, cognitive field theories, humanistic education, and information processing theories you are more likely to succeed in selecting strategies appropriate to a specific client or group of clients. We also urge you to keep in mind the power of warmth and caring as motivating forces to help clients change. The bottom line is that clients are in charge of their own behavior and the consequences of their choices (Williams, D'Aguila, & Williams, 1987). You can provide an interesting, stimulating, and timely health message but you cannot enforce compliance. Your role is that of teacher and guide, not health police officer.

COMPLIANCE VS. VALUES

Purposes:

- Acknowledge the dilemma of conflicting values confronting clients who need to change health behaviors
- Propose several strategies to assist clients in changing behavior
- Examine the assumptions and goals behind each strategy

Directions:

1. Divide into four groups.
2. Read about the couple in the situation that follows.
3. In your group, come up with a plan for increasing the client's compliance.
4. Keep your goal in mind as you develop a plan.
5. Be prepared to defend your plan and your rationale for the actions you recommend.

Identify the assumptions and goals behind each strategy.

Situation

You are caring for a 70-year-old man who is 50 pounds overweight. You are trying to help him reduce his blood triglycerides and his blood cholesterol. He retired a few years ago and his wife decided that she would retire with him, particularly from the kitchen. Their primary source of recreation was to go out daily to lunch at the local burger place. In addition to being their only outing for the day, it was also a major social event because they went with another couple. Such a lunch was all they could afford, but they both considered it quite a treat after all these years. Going to this hamburger place was luxurious living for them.

You are well aware that the hamburgers and french fries are high in fat content and that the man's current eating pattern is a threat to his health. The doctor has urged the man to stop going to the local burger place.

COMPLIANCE ACROSS THE AGES AND CULTURES

Purposes:

- Integrate compliance theory with practical clinical situations
- Practice implementing various strategies for improving compliance

Directions:

- The following activities are to be done in the classroom.
- Form groups and choose which assignment(s) your group will prepare.

Group 1 Assignment

1. Put on a show, demonstrating various biologic, psychologic, and sociologic factors that interfere with compliance.
2. Ask the audience to identify the problem.
3. Continue the scene by demonstrating how you might promote compliance.

Group 2 Assignment

1. Have a conversation between yourself and a young mother whose 2-year-old child is going home from the hospital. The child is still sick and crabby. You must help the mother carry out the physician's orders of forcing fluids, clear liquids only.

Group 3 Assignment

1. You are a nurse giving follow-up care to an Asian family that has a new baby. When the young mother says she wants to know about "no babies" you promise to provide her with instruction the next time you meet. What equipment will you bring? You must keep in mind that the family is extremely poor.
2. When you return you find that she has four other women with her. The woman's English is very limited and the other women know even less English than she does. The young mother translates for the other women, and it appears that they are asking you the following questions.
   "What is the operation where they cut you (demonstrates a large vertical abdominal incision) and take everything out, and then you can not walk for a long time?"
   "How many times can you use it (pointing to a condom).
3. Discuss how you would respond to such questions.

Group 4 Assignment

1. Describe the five conditions under which people are likely to take a health action. Give an example(s) that illustrates each of these conditions.
2. Describe the phenomena that do and do not seem to affect client compliance.
3. Name and apply five strategies that have helped clients adopt life-style changes.

References

Andrews, M.M. (1989). Culture and nutrition. In J.S. Boyle & M.M. Andrews, *Transcultural concepts in nursing care* (pp. 742-775). Boston: Scott, Foresman.

Bauman, L.J. & Keller, M.L. (1991). Responses to threat information. *IMAGE Journal of Nursing Scholarship*, 23(1), 13-18.

Bushy, A. (1992). Cultural considerations for primary health care: Where do self-care and folk medicine fit? *Holistic Nursing Practice* 6(3), 10-18.

Campbell, T. & Chang, B. (1981). Health care of the Chinese in America. In G. Henderson & M. Primeaux. *Transcultural health care* (pp. 162-171). Menlo Park, CA: Addison-Wesley.

Charonko, C.V. (1992). Cultural influences in "noncompliant" behavior and decision making, *Holistic Nursing Practice*, 6(3), 73-78.

Froman, R.D., Owen, S.V. & Daisy, C. (1992). Development of a measure of attitudes toward persons with AIDS. *IMAGE: Journal of Nursing Scholarship*, (2), 149-152.

Germain, C.P. (1992). Cultural care: A bridge between sickness, illness, and disease. *Holistic Nursing Practice*. 6(3), 1-9.

Hanlon, J.J. & Pickett, G.E. (1984). Public health: Administration and practice. St. Louis: C.V. Mosby.

Haynes, R.B., Taylor, D.W. & Sackett, D.L. (Eds.). (1979). *Compliance in health care*. Baltimore MD: The Johns Hopkins University Press.

Hentinen, M. & Kyngas, H. (1992). Compliance of young diabetics with health regimens. *Journal of Advanced Nursing*, 17(5), 530.

Hilbert, G.A. (1985). Accuracy of self-reported measures of compliance. *Nursing Research*, September/October (34):319-320.

Hussey, L.C. (1991). Overcoming the clinical barriers of low literacy and medication noncompliance among the elderly. *Journal of Gerontological Nursing*, 17(3), 27-29.

Jane Doe, RN fights to keep HIV status secret. (1989). *American Journal of Nursing*, 89(6), 869.

Kleoppel, J.W. & Henry, D.W. (1987). Teaching patients, families and communities about their medications. In C.E. Smith (Ed.), *Patient education: Nurses in partnership with other health professionals* (pp. 271-296). Orlando, FL: Grune & Stratton.

Leventhal, H. (1982). Wrongheaded ideas about illness. *Psychology Today*. April: 48.

Ley, P., Bradshaw, P.W., Eaves, D. & Walker, C.M. (1973). A method for increasing patients' recall of information presented by doctors. *Psychological Medicine*, 3:217-220.

Lowery, B.J. (1991). Psychological stress, denial and myocardial infarction outcomes. *IMAGE: Journal of Nursing Scholarship*, 23(1), 51-55.

Naisbitt, J. (1982). *Megatrends*. New York: Warner Books.

Neufeldt, V. (1991). *Webster's new world dictionary* (3rd ed.). New York: Webster's New World.

Nidorf, J.F. & Morgan, M.C. (1987). Cross cultural issues in adolescent medicine. *Primary Care*, 14(1), 69-83.

Pidgeon, V. (1989). Compliance with chronic illness regimens: School-aged children and adolescents. *Journal of Pediatric Nursing*, 4(1), 36.

Poon, L.W., Fozard, J.L., Cermack, L.S., Arenberg, D. & Thompson, L.W. (Eds.) (1980). *New Directions in Memory and Aging*—Proceedings of the George A. Talland Memorial Conference. Hillsdale, NJ, Lawrence Erlbaum Associates.

Poon, L.W., Fozard, J.L. & Popkin, S.J. (1978). Optimizing adult development: Ends and means of an applied psychology of aging. *American Psychologist*, 33: 975-989.

Redeker, N.S. (1988). Health beliefs and adherence in chronic illness. *IMAGE: Journal of Nursing Scholarship*, 20(1), 31-35.

Redman, B. (1988). The process of patient education. St. Louis: Mosby.

Resnick, B.M. (1991). Geriatric motivation: Clinically helping the elderly to comply. *Journal of Gerontological Nursing*, 17(5), 17-20.

Reynolds, C. (1992). An administrative program to facilitate culturally appropriate care for the elderly. *Holistic Nursing Practice*. 6(3), 34-42.

Schmidt, L.E., Klover, R.V. & Arfken, C.L. (1992). Compliance with dietary prescriptions in children and adolescents with insulin dependent diabetes mellitus. *Journal of the American Dietetic Association*, 92(5), 567.

Siegel, B.S. (1986). *Love, medicine and miracles*. Harper & Row.

Slavin, R.E. (1992). *Educational psychology: Theory into practice.* Englewood Cliffs NJ: Prentice Hall.

Smith, D.P. & Nix, K.S. (unit eds.) (1991). *Comprehensive child and family nursing skills.* St. Louis: Mosby-Year Book.

Snow, L.F. (1989). Traditional health beliefs and practices among lower class Black Americans. *The Western Journal of Medicine, 139*(6), 820-828.

Streiff, L. D. (1986). Can clients understand our instructions? *IMAGE: The Journal of Nursing Scholarship, 18*(20), 48-52.

Thorne, S.E. & Robinson, C.A. (1989). *Guarded illness: Health care relationships in chronic illness.* IMAGE: The Journal of Nursing Scholarship, 21(3), 153-157.

Williams, A., D'Aguila, R. & Williams, A. (1987). HIV infection in intravenous drug users. *IMAGE: Journal of Nursing Scholarship, 19*(4), 179-183.

Wong, D.L. (1990). *Clinical manual of pediatric nursing.* St. Louis: Mosby.

Evaluating the Teaching Module

The fault is not in using crude
measures but in doing nothing
until perfection comes along.

Mager, 1984.

Objectives

Upon completion of this chapter you will be able to:

- Describe the purpose of measurement and evaluation.
- Discuss four sources of error in evaluation.
- Select measurement techniques best suited for the following objectives: cognitive, psychomotor, and affective.
- Design evaluation techniques to measure a client's achievement of each of the learning objectives in the teaching module.

Key Words

evaluation	rating scales	true-or-false
measurement	check lists	questions
direct measurement	opinion surveys	fill-in-the-blank
indirect measurement	charts and graphs	questions
documentation		multiple-choice
		questions

Introduction

Throughout the text we have looked at the teaching/learning system from the perspective of the suprasystem, selected subsystems, input of theories, principles, and other information, and we have examined the process, using the nursing process model. In this last chapter we concentrate on evaluation—examination of the output of the system, its meaning, and its value as feedback to provide ongoing direction to the teaching/learning system. To evaluate something means to ascertain its value or worth, to examine and judge; appraise, or estimate (Neufeldt, 1991). In nursing you will use the process of evaluation in many contexts. For instance, in nursing practice you will use evaluation to help you decide whether or not you met your goals of nursing care: Does the client function more effectively or feel more comfortable as a result of your intervention? Educators in general consider evaluation to be one of the most sophisticated of the cognitive functions (Bloom, Madaus, & Hastings, 1981). Evaluation is a complex process that combines all other aspects of cognition: knowledge, compre-

—Continued next page

hension, application, analysis, and synthesis. In this chapter we will concentrate on evaluation of the teaching you have done, the teaching module, and the establishment of meaningful measurement methods. If you have written learning objectives clearly and precisely, you will find that your development of evaluation instruments flows relatively smoothly. Throughout the chapter we have included samples of evaluation methods appropriate for measurement in the cognitive, affective, and psychomotor domains. At the close of the chapter, we have included evaluation instruments that would be appropriate for Lincoln Perez, given the objectives we established at the close of Chapter 9.

Purposes of Evaluation

When teaching clients, your main objective is to help them achieve the highest possible level of functioning. As a result of your teaching, you hope clients will assume more responsibility for their health. You also hope they will be better able to promote and maintain their health and prevent further illness (Fawcett, 1989). Evaluation helps you judge how well you facilitated that process. Evaluation also serves as reinforcement and allows for feedback, correction, improvement, and learning.

Success, as mentioned previously, is very reinforcing. When you know you have succeeded at something, you experience a positive emotion that motivates you to repeat the behavior that led to that successful feeling. Evaluation provides you with the opportunity to know whether or not you have succeeded. Frequent feedback and correction help you keep the system effective. Clients are less apt to waste energy in nonproductive trials if they receive feedback in a timely fashion. Evaluation can tell both clients and you if improvement is occurring. This helps clients with motivation and helps you judge whether or not the selected strategy is working. Evaluation also facilitates your learning as a teacher. You learn what works with clients of this type in this situation while clients learn another step in the lesson at hand.

Another purpose of evaluation is documentation. It is vital to your survival as a health educator that you document the importance and effectiveness of your teaching. It is equally important that you document the time teaching takes, and the positive, cost-effective results of your time investment. In addition to the above political and financial factors, you need to be aware of the legal responsibilities of documentation. Nurses' notes are considered weighty in the courts (Bernzweig, 1987). The absence as well as the presence of notes are equally telling. As a professional, you will be legally responsible for evaluations of your clients' biologic, psychologic, social, and cultural responses to your teaching. It is vital that you document your interventions and conclusions. If there are inadequate tools for documenting your interventions and the results, then you can invent devices for capturing the data and corroborating your subsequent judgments based on the data. Such devices will serve the above-mentioned purposes as well as encourage other caregivers to record their relevant actions and observations.

Measurement

To evaluate something, you must set up criteria against which you can compare the results. Measurement means gauging the dimensions, quantity, or capacity of something by comparing it to some kind of a scale (Neufeldt, 1991). Measurement ranges from the more concrete, such as taking a client's pulse, to the more nebulous, such as estimating the client's will to live. No experienced nurse would deny that both phenomena are extremely important; most nurses would agree that the former is much easier to measure than the latter.

Methods of measurement can be ordered along a continuum from direct to indirect as illustrated in Figure 14-1. Measurement involves both observation and recording of behavior whether it is direct or indirect. The most direct measurement takes place in the situation over time. It is dependent on direct observation. You will make such observations at the bedside, in the home and clinic, in the emergency department, and in the presence of machines, such as the electrocardiogram (EKG)

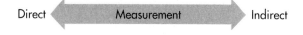

Direct ← Measurement → Indirect

Figure 14-1 Measurement can be ordered along a continuum, from direct to indirect.

monitor, which extends your senses.

More indirect measurements take place when you set up substitute situations or take incomplete samples. When you role play with clients, you will set up substitute situations that are most likely to imitate, or substitute for, the real one. When you give clients paper-and-pencil tests, you are attempting to measure cognitive processes indirectly. No one knows what thinking is or what it looks like. Therefore you must infer from what clients write whether or not they have thought about, retained, and/or gained the knowledge and understanding you hoped they would grasp.

Sources of Error

Error is possible in measurement, and the more indirect the measurement, the more likelihood there is that error may occur. Redman (1988) noted the following common sources of error: indirect measurement, the complexity of behavior, observer bias, and sampling error. Below, we have noted each of those errors and provided examples.

Indirect Measurement   You may get a false picture of how a client would react unless you observe that person in the real situation. The saying, "He talks a good game," indicates that many people know the difference between talking about a situation and actually handling it. Because your time is so limited, you may be tempted to measure objectives by indirect means, such as oral quizzing and paper-and-pencil tests. Keep in mind that these methods are indirect.

Complex Behavior   Behavior, by nature, is very complex. The causes of behavior, especially thought patterns, feelings, and attitudes, are very difficult to identify. Causes are difficult for the observer—as

well as the individual who is exhibiting the behavior—to identify. As a teacher, you may not be able to discover what, if any, effect you had on your clients. Clients may act agreeable just to placate you, or they may choose to not tell you all of the variables involved in their failure to achieve the change you want for them. Indeed, clients may not be aware of all of the factors that might help or hinder their learning.

Observer Bias   You are human, which means you are limited in the amount of stimuli you can notice. You tend to draw conclusions based on your own perceptual base. Winning teachers look for clients' successes and take part of the credit. Losers notice clients' failures and look for someone to blame. One of the advantages of group learning is that the other clients can help balance your perceptions of an individual client. When you team teach, you and your colleagues give balanced views of your clients by sharing your perceptions with each other. All of us are influenced by our culture and other life experiences. We are also influenced by the perceptions of other colleagues. If a colleague tells you a client, a family, and/or a group of clients are particularly difficult to deal with, you are likely to approach these individuals in a guarded manner. Such behavior on your part influences the behavior of those you are approaching.

Sampling   The sample you choose may not be representative of a client's learning. Clients may have learned A, B, and C; but if you measure D, E, and F, you may get a false picture of the clients' abilities and achievements.

The sample of time you choose during which to measure the behavior can also be misleading. You form a different perception of your arthritic client's willingness and ability to do range-of-motion exercises if you test him at 7 A.M. before he is out of bed, than you might if you waited until later in the day, and after he has had time to warm up. It is not possible to observe all of the required behaviors. Therefore your task is to select samples that are as truly representative as possible and relevant to the variables that are the most crucial. In general you can compensate for measurement errors by using a variety of measurement methods.

Measurement Techniques and Tools

Direct Observation of Behavior

Direct observation occurs when you scrutinize the client in person, while the client exhibits mastery of the task at hand. An example is watching a client smoothly navigating on crutches with no axillary pressure and no loss of balance. You also observe directly with mechanical extension of your senses. An example is listening to the client's chest sounds through a stethoscope after a guided session of turning and deep breathing.

Video Cassette Recorders Video cassette recorders (VCRs) are valuable adjuncts to the direct measurement of behavior. Video recordings offer many advantages for unassisted personal observation. One major advantage is their accuracy. The video camera observes and records what happened, rather than your interpretation of what happened. Not only can you study the tape, but also clients can, enabling both of you to get accurate feedback. While being videotaped, clients are freer to focus on internal sensations and their efforts to produce the desired behaviors without the need to be externally self-conscious during the process. The tape can be studied minutely and at length without exhausting clients' or your powers of observation. VCRs have been used with great success in studying various processes, such as the bonding of parents and offspring. VCRs have also proved valuable in sports medicine and rehabilitation. Clients and clinicians can study the tape together, discuss it, try new behaviors, and study the results on a split screen. Videotape provides visual as well as auditory feedback. Because clients can exercise control over the time and pace of self-scrutiny, they can absorb more and evaluate the feedback themselves.

Individuals who are attempting to learn new ways to relate to other human beings, sometimes find it easier to accept feedback from the objective VCR. The VCR presents data from an objective point of view, whereas you can slip into a critical stance and appear judgmental. It is also easier for the client to remain objective; while viewing a screen she or he is less apt to slip into a defensive posture (Keepers & Babcock, 1986). When clients feel defensive, they may hear only part of what is said, or they may distort what they hear.

Families who are puzzled by their communication difficulties can sometimes make sense out of their pattern when they view it from a different perspective. The videotape helps them move out of feeling stuck and defensive. They can be more objective when they sit there watching themselves as spectators. If clients are feeling defensive during one viewing, they can go back later when they are ready to learn.

Rating Scales Rating scales are very useful tools for measuring and recording direct observations of behavior as seen in Figure 14-2, which is designed

✓	1	Rejects client ignores clues
	2	Gives advice, talks about others
	3	With client, reflects
	4	Adds to client's expressions
	5	Adds to client's meaning and feelings

Figure 14-2 Sample rating scale. Because a rating scale is used to measure complex behaviors, levels of competency must be spelled out very carefully.

Name of client: _____

Behaviors	Dates				Comments
1. Selects appropriate equipment.					
2. Identifies action, use, side effects, and dosage range of medication.					

3. Maintains sterility:
   a. Of equipment.
   b. In administration.					

4. Prepares accurate dosage:
   a. Verifies dosage prescribed.
   b. Draws up medication within one minum of a correct dose.					

5. Selects acceptable injection site.					

6. Injects at appropriate angle:
   a. 30-60 degree angle for SQ
   b. 90 degree angle for IM					

7. Aspirates plunger before injecting					
8. Injects medication.					
9. Disposes of needle safely or begins cleansing process correctly.					

Figure 14-3　Sample of a checklist for a complex behavior: giving an injection.

to record the interaction between a caregiver or significant other and the client. Rating scales, such as the Apgar (1953), distinguish between clusters of behaviors. Each cluster is assigned a rank ranging from desirable to undesirable. Rating scales are frequently used in nursing education in the Nursing Arts laboratory.

When you design a rating scale you must use words that are as precise as possible in their meaning. The scale should also be tested with several observers. Ask several colleagues, who are experts in making the necessary observations, to critique the scale to help determine its accuracy. Does the scale describe the behaviors you intend to measure? Colleagues can also help determine its reliability. Each of them should use the scale and then compare results. Note whether individual ratings of the client's behavior are similar.

Because the rating scale is used to measure complex behaviors, levels of competency need to be spelled out very carefully. We recommend that you use no more than three to five levels of discrimination. More than five levels becomes unwieldy. If you feel the need to discriminate among more levels, we suggest that you add another scale because it is likely that too much material is being included in the one scale.

Checklists　Checklists are more precise tools than rating scales because they spell out each of the desired behaviors and provide space for recording the presence or absence of each designated behavior.

Remember to identify every critical element in the desired psychomotor behavior and to exclude non-essentials. For instance when you attempt to measure an Italian or an American mother's bonding to her baby, it is not critical to determine if she sings to her baby or talks to it. Two critical elements would be that she supports the baby's head and attempts to communicate with it in her own style. In Figure 14-3 we have provided a sample checklist of critical requirements for giving an injection. The learning being measured in this figure is psychomotor and a suitable objective is to "Be able to give an injection according to procedure." Appropriate accompanying cognitive objectives follow:

1. Identify action, use, side effects and range of dosage of each medication.
2. Correlate changes in dosage to changes in activity level.
3. Point to 15 acceptable injection sites.
4. Explain three benefits of rotating injection sites.

Figure 14-4 illustrates a sample checklist for evaluating behaviors in a group of children. As illustrated, the specific behaviors you are looking for are clearly identified.

Assistance from your colleagues is also valuable in measuring the accuracy and reliability of a checklist. Colleagues can be enlisted to do trial runs with the checklist to refine the items and the wording. Because the clients do not "pass" until they can do every critical element correctly, you should establish the number of times the clients must exhibit the correct behaviors in order for you to be satisfied that they have mastered the task.

Anecdotal Notes   An anecdotal note is a small vignette that gives a word picture of the client at a particular moment in time. This type of recording is used in psychiatric facilities, because it helps observers detect changes in clients' behaviors over time. It is also valuable to track the circumstances under which changes occur. For example, an adolescent female who was hospitalized for severe behavior problems, was consistently cooperative and easy to relate to in the presence of her therapist.

She was just as consistently obstinate and defiant with the caregivers on the unit. Three questions worthy of pursuit follow:

1. Was the girl obstinate and defiant at home with her family but a delight to outsiders?
2. What are the sexes of the therapist and other caregivers?
3. How are the therapists' transactions with the girl different from that of the staff?

It is crucial for various members of the caregiving unit to use the observations as important data for evaluation and not to automatically jump to the conclusion, "The client always acts just fine for *me*." (The hidden implication is, What are all the rest of you doing wrong?) Anecdotal notes must be recorded consistently over time in order for the caregivers to pick up patterns and changes. Anecdotal notes are usually very interesting and thus more likely to be read than some other methods of recording. Therefore we recommend that you make the notes pertinent to the teaching objectives and that your comments relate to those objectives.

A professional's notes should also be free of color words and bias. Some comments are not very helpful or specific.

> *Example:* "The client is obnoxious and uncooperative."

It would be far more clear to restate such an observation.

> *Example:* "The client refuses to get out of bed until. . . ."
> "When client is approached with the importance of exercises to his recovery, he turns his face to the wall and does not respond."

Such observations may help create a climate of investigation rather than disapproval. If you are curious rather than judgmental, you will be more likely to discover clues that help you create a learning environment more conducive to success. If you can maintain an attitude of curiosity, you are more likely to discover if there is an important disparity between the clients' goals and your goals.

Evaluator: ______________________ Date: __________

Objective: Each child experiments with 3 easy snacks to make at home (Tasty Frosty, Bumps on a Log, and Snappy Apple).

	Snacks								
	Tasty Frosty		Bumps on a Log				Snappy Apple		Comments
Names:	Shakes	Tastes	Chooses celery	Spreads peanut butter on stalk	Adds raisins on top of peanut butter	Tastes	Selects apple slice	Tastes	

Figure 14-4 Sample checklist for evaluating behaviors in a group.

Direct Questioning

Although questioning is a direct transaction between you and the client, it can be used to measure unobservable activity, such as understanding of the principles underlying a particular psychomotor skill. Questioning has several advantages, which include immediate feedback about the level of understanding the client has attained. Questioning also allows you to pick up any gaps or misunderstandings immediately, which, in turn, allows for correction and feedback before the learning episode is completed.

Direct questioning also gives you some clues about the client's learning style and general ability level. The language the client uses to answer the questions offers you important clues to the senses through which the client learns most easily.

> *Example:* "I get it."
> "I see your point."
> "I hear you."

If your client makes one of these statements, you might entertain the hypothesis that the client learns most easily in the kinesthetic or visual or auditory modes, respectively. You can also use questioning to help the client anticipate the future.

> *Example:* "How will you be able to do this when you get home?"
> "What will you do if . . . ?"

There are disadvantages to asking questions. First of all, questioning takes time and energy, and it is less suitable for a large group because you cannot quiz each client. Questions in a discussion group are also complicated by the hazard that they may lead to discussion of tangential topics.

When using questioning, you should avoid expecting clients to read your mind. Remember that people are trained to give teachers and other authority figures exactly what they want to hear. Your question should contain all of the information necessary for the client to understand the context and to decipher what is needed or missing.

Questions that require only a "yes" or "no" are of limited value in evaluation. Usually what you learn from such a question is whether the client is cooperative or rebellious.

> *Example:* "Do you understand these directions?"
> "Do you know the circumstances under which you should call your caregiver right away?"

These questions may allow clients to say "yes" because caregivers look harried, and the clients do not want to be bothersome. Clients usually have more questions than they ask (Kloeppel & Henry, 1987). Clients may also say "yes" to avoid giving the impression that they are stupid. A more effective approach might be the following.

> *Example:* "Now was that in English or Jargonese? Would you explain to me in your own words what these directions say?"
> "Giveaways" should also be avoided: "You know digoxin slows your heart rate, right?"

It is also important to avoid putting the client at risk for giving a socially unacceptable answer. For instance, most young parents would say "yes" if the visiting nurse asked the following question.

> *Example:* "Are you doing everything they told you to do in the hospital for your baby?"

A more tactful approach might be the following.

> *Example:* "When you come home with a new baby it is impossible to recall everything they told you to do. Tell me what you remember and I can help fill in the gaps."
> "All babies are different; is your baby anything like the ones they described in your parenting classes?"
> "Tell me how your baby is like they said she or he would be."
> "Tell me how she or he is different from the babies described in your parenting classes."

Written Measurement

So far we have considered measurements involving direct transactions with clients, in which you have observed the learning directly or asked clients for their perceptions of the learning that took place. A more indirect technique is written measurement. There are some prerequisites to the use of this method. To use a written measurement tool clients must be able to read. This includes attainment of the skill in addition to the ability to see. A well-educated client who is taking medications that cause double vision cannot participate in written measurement nor can clients whose reading glasses are unavailable. Those who are bilingual but read only in another language, or clients who are so weak that they cannot hold the questionnaire, test, or pen would also be inappropriate subjects for written evaluations.

Written tools have some distinct advantages. Most people in our culture are used to reading and writing under many different circumstances. Most clients have been expected to do a considerable amount of writing before they encounter you. Chances are good that you used some reading materials in your teaching. If your clients had self-paced learning modules, they probably had to write some responses in the learning booklet.

One of the main advantages of written measurement is its efficiency in terms of time and energy. One person (not necessarily the teacher) can distribute a written measurement tool to many people at once. The data can be analyzed at the evaluator's convenience and can be easily stored along with the conclusions. As we move into the computer age, written tools are being converted to this new medium of communication. Tomorrow, the client will use a portable answering device and will be able to enter the data directly into the data base. Some nurses may be working on units where this technology is already available.

Test Construction

When the tool is a test or resembles a test, another point you need to consider is the client's perception of taking a test. In addition to noting the client's emotional reaction, you should ask yourself how much test-taking skill the tool requires.

To construct an effective test you must keep many variables in mind. A good test covers all of the relevant material; therefore it should be related to the objectives of the learning module. What do you expect the client to learn? By the time the module is completed, do you hope that the client will be able to recall, recognize, state, select, or choose? If so, what should clients be able to choose? How? How well?

The test should be relevant to the group of clients in terms of life experience and readability. If your clients' reading skills are very limited, you may need to use very simple words and supplement these with pictures. You may need to give the directions out loud. Doing a couple of sample items with clients can help them understand your expectations. Many people can do something if you show them what you mean, show them how, or both. Such behavior is not limited to the illiterate. Think of how many times people put together a piece of machinery, or sew or crochet an item by looking at the pictures? Many people read the directions only as a last resort. Think of how many times you have taken tests without reading the directions. Many people attempt to decipher the directions from the context. These human traits must be acknowledged during the process of giving the client a written test.

A good test uses different types of items, such as true-or-false, matching, multiple-choice and short-answer questions, that provide variety for the client, as well as options for you. True-or-false and fill-in-the-blank questions are good for testing knowledge of facts. Matching is good for testing recall of related concepts. Multiple choice questions are helpful for distinguishing myths from reality, and they measure some levels of problem solving, inference, and generalizations. Short answers are useful for discovering the client's thinking processes. Short answers also provide clues to the use the client is making of the information you attempted to convey. In the box on p. 276, you will find helpful guidelines for writing test questions.

The test should avoid using the exact wording you used during the teaching module, because that measures memory rather than understanding. The use of "giveaway" words should also be avoided. "Never," "always," and "all" are usually false; "generally," "mostly," and "usually" are usually true. If words such as these are used, the test may

Guidelines for Writing Test Questions

1. Group the questions according to type: true or false, matching, multiple choice, fill in the blank, short answer, or essay.

2. State general directions at the beginning of the test: "This test is designed to measure what you know about how to take care of yourself. It will help us plan further teaching." (For clients at a lower reading level say: "Please take this test. The results will tell us what else we need to teach you.")

3. State specific directions before each group of questions.

4. Indicate where to record the answer, and provide a place for clients' answers.

5. Use vocabulary that fits the reading level of the group.

6. Make the directions as clear and as short as possible.

7. Underline and/or bold the directions and special words.

8. Make all multiple choice options similar in length.

9. Put the multiple choice question and answers on the same page.

10. Make all multiple choice options grammatically parallel.

---

measure the test-wise skills of clients, rather than their attainment of the learning objectives. Be specific about what you want to ask.

Each multiple choice question has three parts: the stem, the correct answer, and the distractors. The stem is the main part or the lead-in sentence to which the client must then fit the correct answer. The distractors are the other possible, but incorrect, answers. A good test question is grammatically consistent with all of the possible answers. All answer options should be about the same length. Inconsistencies can give clues to the correct answer. A client can sometimes guess the right answer by looking for the best grammatical fit in matching or multiple-choice questions. Myths and plausible answers are good distractors. If all of the options begin

with the same word or phrase, that should be stated only once at the end of the stem. See the example in the box on the next page. Try to avoid negatively stated items. If you use negative items, be sure to underline the <u>negative</u>. An example of this is test question 2 in the box on the next page.

A table of random numbers will help you arrange answers in a random manner, because it is very easy to slip into a predictable pattern for arranging correct responses. Another way to randomize the sequence of choices in multiple-choice questions is to arrange the possible answers alphabetically.

In a matching question the number of possible answers should be longer than the column of items presented for identification or description. If the list of matching items is exactly the same number as the test items, then the question is testing the client's ability to use logic and the process of elimination rather than testing the client's knowledge.

Fill-in-the-blank questions should contain blanks that are all the same size. If the blanks vary in size, mind reading is encouraged—clients will try to guess what word you had in mind when constructing the test. If you choose to provide a list of the correct words, then it too should contain distractors.

Questions should be grouped according to the type of question. The test taker has to switch mental processes to answer each type. For instance, all true-or-false questions should be together, and all multiple-choice questions should be grouped together. If the test is likely to produce some anxiety, it may help to start it with some easy items. This also will help you measure clients' learning, rather than how the clients think when stressed.

Making directions clear is a very difficult task. A good way to clarify the directions is to do a trial run. Try it out on someone who knows the subject and someone who does not; each have valuable critiques to offer. There may be times when you intend to give clients helps and hints. This would be especially true when a written tool is used to test young children. If the client is to grade him or herself, a key can be included somewhere at the bottom, upside down, or on the back of the page.

1. Which of the following statements is true about parenthood? It is a/an:
   a. Impossible role for most couples.
   b. Demanding but growth enhancing experience.
   c. Essential element of a healthy marriage.
   d. Necessary aspect for a well-rounded, fulfilled life.
2. Effective crutch walking includes all of the following except:
   a. Avoidance of slippery surfaces so that you remain stable.
   b. Keeping the crutch snug in your armpits by leaning on them.
   c. Practicing until you have developed a smooth rhythm.
   d. Placing your most important items in a fanny pack.

Pretests and Posttests

The pretest is useful for assessing the client's current knowledge about the subject to be learned; therefore, use of the pretest assumes that clients have a knowledge base. Pretests are also good for piquing the curiosity of the client. One possible disadvantage of pretests is that they are often perceived as threatening. This threat may be outweighed by the fact that pretests are quite helpful as self-diagnostic devices. As adult clients assume more and more of the responsibility for directing their own learning, you will see more of the pretest, both in written and computer form.

Pretests and posttests must be the same when the posttest is used to determine the gains made as a result of the teaching/learning (Aiken, 1982). The results of both tests are compared to measure the learning. Some large testing services have designed equivalent posttests. This means that although the tests are not exactly alike, they test the same knowledge or skills (Litwack, Linc, & Bower, 1985). The process for developing equivalent tests is lengthy, expensive, and must be done with populations of a significant size. Development of equivalent tests also involves sophisticated statistical manipulations.

Choosing Appropriate Measurement Techniques

How do you evaluate what clients are thinking or what they know? When the objectives have focused on cognitive learning, oral questions and written measurement are usually most appropriate. These methods are indirect because you cannot measure thinking directly.

How can you evaluate changes in clients' attitudes or feelings? You may be able to question them directly if they trust you, because so much of a client's willingness to share is affected by the interpersonal client/teacher relationship. Direct observation is also an excellent technique because you can infer much from the client's behavior. Clients are not always fully aware of or willing to admit their attitudes and feelings. However, a client's behavior may give clues to you if you are an astute observer. Videotapes and anecdotal notes are two good ways to capture the needed data.

Written measurement in the form of an attitude scale or an opinion survey may also be useful. The use of open-ended questions is another way to measure attitudes and feelings. The lack of personal interaction may act as a facilitator or a deterrent to self-disclosure. Many factors influence a person's willingness to admit attitudinal change or lack of change.

How can you decide whether or not clients can perform a skill at a satisfactory level? Direct observation is the main method for evaluating the attainment of psychomotor skills. If performance is the subject of evaluation, the videotape is an excellent tool. Checklists and rating scales are also useful because they enable you to remain objective with a previously constructed and well-thought-out list as in Figure 14-3. Checklists also reduce the likelihood that crucial elements of the desired performance will be neglected.

Evaluation of Lesson Plan for Lincoln Perez

We are now ready to evaluate the learning of Mr. Perez. We focused on his learning about relaxation

Sample Test Questions

Sample True-or-False Questions

Directions: Circle **T** if the statement is true. Circle **F** if any part of the statement is false.

T   F   1. A daily program of exercise and relaxation will improve the efficiency of your body.

T   F   2. You can tell when your blood pressure is up.

T   F   3. If you exercise and rest, you do not need to take blood pressure medicine.

Sample Multiple-Choice Question

Directions: Put an **X** in front of the one best answer.

1. Regular exercise and relaxation are most likely to:

_____ a. Have little effect on your life.

_____ b. Reduce your blood pressure.

_____ c. Make blood pressure medicine unnecessary.

_____ d. Build up muscle mass and endurance.

Sample Short-Answer and Fill-In Questions

Directions: Fill in the blanks to make this statement correct. The missing words are listed at the bottom.

1. Although _____ and _____ are good activities to make a regular part of your _____ routine, they will not _____ the need for medication. They will help you to control _____ , and they may help you _____ your blood _____ as well as your pulse _____ .

Possible missing words:

daily	pressure	relaxation	exercise
style of life	eliminate	rate	stress
reduce			

2. List as many benefits of relaxation that you can.

a.

b.

c.

d.

e.

Sample Attitude Scale

Directions: Place an **X** in the column that most closely describes your feelings toward each of the statements. Be as honest as you can; this is for *you*.

Statement	Agree	Neutral	Disagree
1. I am too busy to exercise.			
2. I am too tense to relax.			
3. I can tell when my blood pressure is up.			
4. I am worried about stroke or heart disease.			
5. Everyone must die of something sometime.			
6. Exercise can have a positive effect on my life.			
7. I can relax in front of the television.			
8. There is a difference between deep relaxation and sitting in front of the television.			

as a method of stress reduction. If he has succeeded in the objectives, he will be able to select three benefits of relaxation from a list; agree to experiment with walking and various relaxation techniques; and lower his pulse rate by five beats per minute. Before we can expect him to measure and record his pulse rate, we must make sure he can locate his pulse and count it correctly. We will use our own measurement of his pulse to evaluate his accuracy. Lowering his pulse rate is indicative of the effectiveness of exercise and relaxation. Our long-term goal is reduction of blood pressure.

Cognitive Objective

Our first objective was cognitive: Select three benefits of relaxation from a list. This objective can be measured in a variety of ways. Mr. Perez can verbally expound on the benefits of relaxation to you or you can give him a brief paper-and-pencil test. If you chose the latter format, your questions can be true-or-false, multiple-choice, short-answers, or fill-in-the-blank types. See the box at the top of p. 278 for sample test questions.

Affective Objective

The affective objective for Lincoln Perez can be evaluated several ways. The short-term measure is to have him fill out an attitude scale as seen in the box at the bottom of p. 278. The long-term measure is whether or not he sticks to a regular exercise and relaxation schedule. To measure this we have made up charts to record his pulse and blood pressure. If he is indeed changing his life-style to include regular exercise and relaxation, it will be evident in these vital signs. The ability to take his own pulse is a psychomotor skill, so the charts will measure his success in two domains at once.

Psychomotor Objective

To measure Mr. Perez's ability to take his pulse correctly, we have developed a checklist (see the box at the top of the previous column), a place for him to record his results, and a place for us to record our results. He will be considered successful when his count approximates ours. We will have him perform this procedure once initially to see whether he acts familiar with the procedure. If he does, and if his total is correct, we will test him once. If he does not, then we will repeat the procedure until he is accurate and acts comfortable with the procedure. The criteria will be that his total is within three beats of the pulse rate obtained by the nurse. If he is already used to 10 seconds multiplied by 6 and measures accurately, we will accept his method.

The charts we have developed will measure pulse and blood pressure over time. Mr. Perez will keep the pulse chart himself on a daily basis (see Figure 14-5). We will also chart his blood pressure, which will be measured each time he returns to the clinic for weekly checkups (see Figure 14-6). The horizontal axis on both charts is time. The vertical axis is pulse rate on one chart (Figure 14-5) and systolic and diastolic values on the other chart (Figure 14-6).

Teacher Evaluation

Hopefully every evaluation is a learning opportunity for both the client and you. Some important questions to ask include: How well did my performance facilitate the client's learning? Was my content clearly related to the objectives? Did I share the information in language that my clients could un-

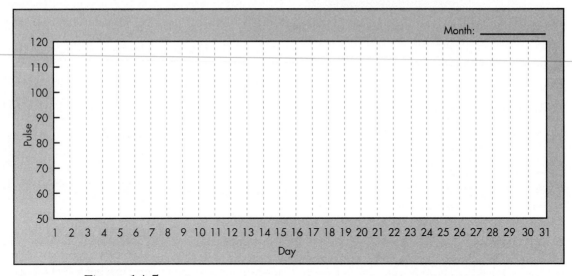

Figure 14-5 Pulse rate can be monitored over time on a chart such as this one.

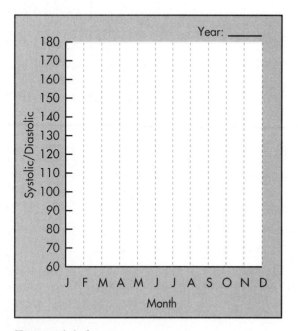

Figure 14-6 Blood pressure values can be readily monitored on a chart such as this one.

derstand? Were my strategies appropriate to these clients in this situation? Had I practiced using the strategies and equipment sufficiently to be able to use them in a smooth manner? Did the materials I chose make the learning more enjoyable and more likely to be retained? Did I assess my audience accurately? Did I gather sufficient baseline data? Did I make the assumption that adults start with a large knowledge base (for good or bad) and that children have some knowledge base? Did I seek feedback during the teaching process? Did I notice whether or not I was succeeding, or did I notice a need, lag, snag, and change my approach accordingly?

Was my teaching cost-effective? Was my teaching lengthy enough to be thorough? Did I make the best use of the time and materials available? Did I use materials that had been used before successfully? Were the materials commercially prepared or

Figure 14-7 Opposite page. This teacher evaluation form covers objectives, content, strategies, teaching aids, and teaching performance. Space is allowed for additional comments.

Teacher Evaluation Form

Key:
0 = not applicable
1 = definitely below average
2 = slightly below average
3 = average
4 = slightly above average
5 = definitely above average

Speaker: _____

Evaluator: _____

                                                                    0 1 2 3 4 5

Objectives — Were the objectives:

Clearly presented to the clients?...

Evident throughout the presentation?....................................

Content — Was the content:

Clearly explained?...

Accurate?...

Clearly explained?...

At the right vocabulary level?..

Appropriate to the audience's background?..........................

Strategies — Were the strategies:

Appropriate for the content?...

Appropriate for the audience?...

Teaching aids — Were the materials:

Appropriate to the context?..

Appropriate to the objectives?..

At the client's level of comprehension?..............................

Pleasing to the eye?...

Visible (contrast, size & location)?.....................................

Used in a practiced manner?..

Performance — Did the teacher:

Dress appropriately to the client's & topic?........................

Maintain eye contact with the audience?............................

Speak in a clear audible voice?...

Use a pace appropriate to the audience?...........................

Stay attuned to the audience?..

Give recognition for contributions?....................................

Allow time for questions?...

Seek feedback periodically?...

Show preparation by smooth performance?.........................

Comments:

From Babcock/Miller: *Client Education: Theory and Practice* Copyright 1994, Mosby.

homemade? How well were the materials received? How could I tell? Did the clients laugh? Did clients' faces light up with comprehension? Did clients come up and study the materials after the presentation?

Did I collect data to evaluate each of my objectives? Were my evaluation tools appropriate for my objectives? Did I provide opportunity for clients to tell me what they thought of my presentation style? Did I build in a mechanism that would invite clients' suggestions for future presentations? These questions are summarized in the teacher evaluation form shown in Figure 14-7.

Summary

In this chapter we addressed the final phase of the nursing process within the teaching/learning system. We reviewed the importance of evaluation and stressed the need for documentation. We identified evaluation as an essential component of teaching/learning through which you determine the effectiveness of your efforts. Evaluation becomes feedback into the teaching/learning system that allows you to self-correct so that you can continually improve as a teacher. We included examples of each type of evaluation measurement and showed how they might be applied to the teaching/learning of Lincoln Perez. You will find more examples in the appendix along with directions for producing and evaluating a teaching module.

It takes a lot of courage and humility to actively seek feedback from clients. It may be helpful for you to recall comforting or encouraging phrases, such as "Be patient. God's not through with me yet," or "I can grow and learn, and that's exciting."

INTERPRETING PATTERNS

Purposes:

- Practice noting a pattern
- Relate a pattern to its possible meaning in terms of client learning

Directions:

- Study the following patterns of satisfactory (S) and unsatisfactory (U) performance. They represent repetitions of a particular performance over a period of time for three different clients.

- Discuss with one another what the various patterns might mean.
- Discuss the implications for the nurse/teacher evaluating the client who exhibits each of the patterns.

Key: U = Unsatisfactory S = Satisfactory

Pattern of Client I
U U S U S U S S S S

Pattern of Client II
S S S U S S S S S S

Pattern of Client III:
S U S U S U U S U S

FIND THE FLAWS

Purposes:

- Make an inference about the purpose of this test
- Apply guidelines for proper test construction

Directions:

- Find all of the flaws in this test.
- State your rationale for your opinions.
- Rewrite the test to improve form, to clarify questions, and to maintain the purpose of the test.
- Share your perception of the test's purpose with your peers.
- State your rationale for your conclusion.

Hospital of St. Anywhere—Critical Care Unit

Directions:

- Circle the statements you feel to be true:

1. The damage in a heart attack is due to:
   a. Too much fat in the blood.
   b. Too much blood in the heart chambers.
   c. Too little blood to the heart muscles.
   d. No heart damage; only damage is a clot in a blood vessel.
2. The pain involved in a heart attack is from:
   a. Heart irritability.
   b. Too little oxygen to the heart muscle.
   c. Too little blood to the heart chambers.
   d. Damaged heart muscle.

3. The damage to the heart muscle from a heart attack is:
   a. Similar to a deep cut.
   b. Similar to a muscle sprain.
   c. Similar to a bruise.
4. The healing of the heart following an attack is:
   a. Never really complete, there is always a scar that is subsequently weaker than the natural heart muscle.
   b. Totally complete, leaving no trace or damage.
   c. Leaves a scar.

Directions:

- Mark **T** for true; **F** for false.

____ 5. After a heart attack a client will not return to his or her previous level of physical capacity.

____ 6. After a heart attack one's sex life always has to be reduced (in future years).

____ 7. It was my last meal that led to my heart attack.

____ 8. Even an occasional cocktail is bad for your heart.

____ 9. High blood cholesterol signals a proneness to heart attack.

____ 10. About medication:
   a. You should not become dependent on them as a "crutch."
   b. It may help to carry nitroglycerine tablets in your pocket.
   c. Once you leave the hospital, medications you are given in the hospital are not to be changed in the future by your doctor.

E X E R C I S E   I I I

EVALUATION PHRASES

Purposes:

- Practice giving compliments
- Break the habit of giving negative criticism
- Specify positive concrete suggestions

Directions:

- Divide into small groups.
- Look at the criticisms listed below. They point out common errors that detract from teaching effectiveness.
- Find ways to restate the criticisms in positive terms. Do not give generalities such as "be more clear." Do give concrete, specific recommendations. For example, you could tell a client to organize your speech in an outline; make a handout that lists all of the causes together," or "Make a handout."

- Discuss your recommendations with the rest of the group.

Criticisms

1. Your voice trailed off.
2. Your poster was hard to read.
3. Your vocabulary was too technical.
4. You said "um" a lot.
5. You fidgeted with your rings and cards.
6. You tried to teach too much without asking questions.
7. You did not involve the audience until the end.
8. You were very confusing.
9. You jumped around from one subject to another.
10. You went too fast.
11. You looked at your notes too much and read them.

FINAL SPEECH

Purpose:

- Practice assertive criticism
- Integrate and consolidate learning

Directions:

- Prepare a final speech of evaluation.

- Address the following:

1. This is what I am going to do with what I learned in this course.
2. This is my advice for the instructor on what to keep, delete, and add.

References

Aiken, L.R., Jr. (1982). *Psychological testing and assessment* (4th ed.). Boston: Allyn & Bacon.

Apgar, V. (1953). A proposal for a new method of evaluation of the newborn infant. *Anesthesia, 32:* 260.

Bernzweig, E.P. (1987). *The nurse's liability for malpractice* (4th ed.). New York: McGraw-Hill.

Bloom, B.S., Madaus, G.F. & Hastings, J.T. (1981). *Evaluation to improve learning.* New York: McGraw-Hill.

Fawcett, J. (1989). *Analysis and evaluation of conceptual models of nursing* (2nd ed.). Philadelphia: F.A. Davis.

Keepers, T.D. & Babcock, D.E. (1986). *Raising kids O.K.* (2nd). Menlo Park CA: Menalto Press.

Kloeppel, J.S. & Henry, D.W. (1987). Teaching patients, families and communities about their medications. In C.E. Smith (Ed.), *Patient education, nurses in partnership with other health professionals* (pp. 271-296). Orlando FL: Grune & Stratton.

Litwack, L., Linc, L. & Bower, D. (1985). *Evaluation in nursing: Principles and practice.* New York: National League for Nursing.

Mager, R.F. (1984). Preparing Instructional Objectives (3rd ed.). Belmont CA: Pitman Learning.

Neufeldt, V. (Ed.). (1991). *Webster's New World Dictionary* (3rd ed.). Cleveland: Webster's New World.

Redman, M.K. (1988). *The process of patient education* (6th ed.). St. Louis: Mosby.

APPENDIXES

Reader Learning Profile

Purposes:

- Assess the subject's current level of teaching experience
- Facilitate the planning of meaningful activities
- Collect data for study of class participants

Directions:

- Please copy these pages, fill them out, and hand them in.

Name _____

Date & Time of Class _____

Other Commitments This Term

1. Employment (numbers of hours weekly) ____
2. Other courses (number of hours) _____
3. Family (number in household) _____
4. Community activities _____

5. Other languages spoken besides Standard English _____
6. Anticipated concerns _____

Previous Experiences Related to This Course

1. Nursing courses in which I gave class presentations include:

2. Work or other teaching experiences (Check all that apply):
   - ____ a. Led small group discussion
   - ____ b. Wrote behavioral objectives
   - ____ c. Wrote course description
   - ____ d. Wrote lesson plans
   - ____ e. Lectured to a small group ____ large group

_____ f. Gave a demonstration to a small group _____ large group

_____ g. Gave individualized planned instruction

_____ h. Participated in team teaching

_____ i. Led a game or exercise and postgame discussion

_____ j. Role played

_____ k. Wrote an illustrated pamphlet

_____ l. Performed in front of a video camera

_____ m. Other (describe) _____

3. I have used (Check all that apply):

_____ a. Tape recorder

_____ b. Video camera, recorder

_____ c. 16 mm movie projector

_____ d. Audiocassette tape and filmstrip projector

_____ e. Audiocassette tape and slide carousel

_____ f. Opaque projector

_____ g. Overhead projector

_____ h. Microphone

_____ i. Computer assisted instruction

_____ j. Other (specify)

4. (Check one) I believe I know
_____ a lot, _____ a moderate amount,
_____ very little about client teaching.

5. Expectations of this course:

a. Concerns, apprehensions, fears:

b. Things I expect to be doing, based on what I have heard or read about this course:

c. Things I particularly want to do, discuss, or need to know:

6. Learning style or needs (Use extra paper if necessary):

a. Teacher behaviors that:
(1) Facilitate my learning are:

(2) Inhibit my learning are:

b. To help myself learn, I:

c. To facilitate my participation and success in this course, you should also know:

Jigsaw

Purposes:

- Experience a cooperative learning endeavor
- Lower anxiety through progressive desensitization
- Practice teaching in small steps
- Learn by teaching others
- Experiment with various teaching strategies

Directions:

1. Choose one to three objectives from the list of behavioral objectives that are found at the beginning of each chapter.
2. Your job is to help your classmates achieve these objectives.
3. The instructor should identify those objectives that are not suitable for peer teaching and therefore should **not** be chosen for this exercise.
4. Plan to address the objective you choose on the day that it is to be covered in the class schedule.
5. To prepare, read the material in the chapter related to your chosen objective, and then teach the content to your peers.
6. Use whatever strategies and materials you need to promote cognitive, affective, and psychomotor learning of the objectives you selected. You are **not** expected to drain your time, budget, and energy preparing handouts for all of your peers during these activities, because they already have the material in their own texts.
7. Because these are practice sessions you will not be graded on your performance. The point is to get feedback and helpful suggestions from your peers and the teacher.

Written Outline of the Teaching Module

Purpose:

This activity is to help you integrate all of the knowledge, skills, and attitudes you have gained during your study of this book. This activity will take you through the process of assessing clients; analyzing their learning needs; and planning, implementing and evaluating the teaching module. The document you will create can be used as a model for all of your future teaching activities. This model will not be the best or most complete model, but it is theoretically sound and helpful for beginners. Hundreds of nursing students have found the model helpful and practical for use in clinical practice.

The following instructions will be helpful no matter where you present your teaching module because they will provide you with anticipatory set and serve as advance organizers. The instructions contain all of the learning experiences—in a brief, outline form—that we discussed in detail throughout the text.

Directions:

The first page of your teaching module should contain general instructions. These instructions should be written so that a colleague can flip through the module, read the first paragraph and decide whether or not she or he can use it. Preparing the instructions will give you experience developing an advance organizer.

In the opening paragraph(s), explain what the module is about, who the intended audience is, how the module should be presented, the length of time

it usually takes to present the material, and what kind of surroundings are most conducive or crucial to the learning. You should also identify where audiovisual materials can be obtained and how much anyone teaching this module can expect to pay to rent, buy, or borrow the materials.

Description of the Participants

In this description, include all essential variables that are important for assessing your potential clients. Assess:

1. Biologic, psychologic, sociologic, and cultural characteristics.
2. Clients' perceptions of their own health status and their present health behaviors—reported or observed.
3. Psychosocial adaptation to health problems.
4. Ability to meet basic needs, such as rest, elimination of bodily waste, comfort, and nutrition.
5. Expectations of health care providers.
6. Ability to communicate.
7. Motivation or emotional readiness to learn.
8. Developmental and experiential readiness.

As you describe your clients, become aware of the connection between their characteristics and the design of your module. If you see people with glasses and hearing aids, you will need to strengthen your voice. If the clients are children, you should incorporate physical activities and song. If clients are culturally different, you will need to educate yourself on what beliefs they hold. If they are of limited education, you will need to simplify your vocabulary. The above examples are offered only as reminders, and they are meant to inspire you and not to limit your options.

Describe your own biologic, psychologic, social, and cultural characteristics as they pertain to the preparation of your teaching module.

Describe how the similarities and differences between you and your clients might affect your potential relationship. You are to plan how you will approach your clients to minimize barriers and to enhance positives. If you are white and will be talking to a nonwhite racial group, you can predict that clients will perceive your color before they notice anything else. They may hold stereotypes about you as you might of them. If you have a New York accent, you probably talk at a fast pace. If you are talking to clients who are Midwesterners, you need to take into account that they are likely to react to both your clipped, speedy delivery and your New York "city slicker," accent. It is also important to remember that you were probably exposed to different social and cultural influences than they were.

It is possible to soften the above-mentioned developmental, racial, social, cultural, and ethnic barriers. Being aware that the barriers are present is a first step.

Teaching Principles

Identify two principles of learning and of teaching that are specific to your module, and briefly describe how you have applied those principles in your teaching plans. The use of these principles should be evident to the instructor when she or he sees you use the module.

Lesson Plan

Many good structures for lesson plans have been designed. However, in the typical hospital and clinic setting, lesson plans often consist of an outline of the content "to be covered." Although the outline of content is a necessary part of the lesson plan, it is deficient if used alone. This part of the teaching module is devoted to placing the outline of content in a more complete structure entitled the lesson plan. The lesson plan consists of three columns in which the objectives, the content, and the strategies are arranged, one across from the other, so that you can see your aim, your content, and your strategies in one glance.

1. State the behavioral objectives in the first column. These objectives should reflect client outcomes. In other words, by the time the module is completed clients should be able to demonstrate that they have acquired new knowledge, can perform a new skill, or have changed their attitude. The more clearly you state these objectives, the easier they will be to evaluate.

2. The second column of the lesson plan contains an outline of the content you intend to impart. This outline is similar to many of the topical outlines you will find on many hospital units.

3. The third column specifies the strategies you plan to use, questions you plan to ask, the materials you will gather or prepare, the audiovisual aids, and specific directions you plan to give. You are expected to develop and use teaching aids that are appropriate for the audience, the topic, you, and the situation. If you choose to use a commercially prepared video, film, or slide show, it should take up less than one third of the time allotted for the lesson. A sample lesson plan regarding Mr. Lincoln Perez can be found in Chapters 10, 11, and 12.

Evaluation

The evaluation section of the written module should be thoroughly developed as if there were no time constraints or exigencies that could occur.

For each objective you state, you must have a way of measuring whether or not that objective was met. It is part of your responsibility to design tools to measure the objectives you choose. Chapter 14 contains samples of measuring tools for Mr. Perez's objectives as well as other samples.

The tools should suit the domains you choose. If the objectives are cognitive outcomes, the evaluation tool should test increased knowledge. If a change in attitude is to be accomplished, then the evaluation tool will measure an attitude change. If the outcome is acquisition of a psychomotor skill, then the tool must specify each of the desired steps involved in the successful performance of the skill.

The evaluation measures should include standards of performance. A key that contains the desired responses should be included along with a standard that you have decided will constitute a satisfactory, passing performance. If clients are learning to do home dialysis, a much stricter measure of performance is necessary than for clients who are learning to apply diapers.

If the test is a self-scoring test, then a key that is either upside down, in a corner, or on the back should be provided on the page.

The readability level of written tests should be appropriate for the clients. For example, if little children or adults with limited reading skills will be cognitively tested, the tool may consist of pictures that should be circled and/or colored.

Format

Your module should conform to the same high-quality standards as an English composition. Therefore you should type the module neatly; present it in a cover so that the title is visible; number all the pages, including the appendixes; use standard English and correct spelling; and use proper bibliographic form for references.

If applicable, the appendix should contain directions, sketches of posters, handouts, evaluation tools, keys, phone numbers, and addresses of resources.

Samples of Nursing Diagnoses and Related Teaching

Acute Care Situation: Lin Wu

Mr. Lin Wu is a 56-year-old Chinese client who was admitted last night to cardiac intensive care with an acute myocardial infarction. This morning you find him diaphoretic, restless, weak, nauseous, anxious, and cyanotic. After administering appropriate measures to relieve his anxiety and circulatory distress, you realize you need to review with him and his family the importance of reporting pain. You suspect that his culture encourages, "Do not complain." You realize you are trying to get him to go against his programming to save his own life. What are you going to do?

Nursing Diagnosis:

- Cardiac output, decreased, high risk for

Related To (R/T):

- Failure to report symptoms
- Failure to push call button
- Failure to alert staff to symptoms
- Insufficient knowledge of importance of reporting symptoms
- Deeply ingrained cultural inhibition against complaining

As Evidenced By (AEB):

weakness   cyanosis
nausea   diaphoresis
frowning   dyspnea
distressed facial
  features

Expected Outcomes:

1. Client will report the next episode of chest pain by alerting the nurse or pushing the call button.
2. Client will verbalize the relationship between signs and symptoms and decreased cardiac blood flow by the next shift change.

Interventions:

1. Explore your hunch that complaining is culturally inhibited by talking with the client or family.
2. Ask the client what information he has already received regarding signs and symptoms.
3. Role play with the client or family by pushing the call button and showing them how the nurse responds.
4. Reinforce any efforts to cooperate.

Discussion:

In this situation, it is important to recognize the teachable moment and the size of the lesson to be taught. Under these circumstances, you will focus only on essential concepts. Clearly this situation limits what the client is able to absorb at this point in time. Right now the most important issue is getting Mr. Wu to cooperate in ensuring his own survival. It is imperative for the client to report his symptoms, especially his pain, to you. Other concepts and skills can be taught later. Role playing is important for two reasons. First, role playing will allow you to see if the client understood your message. Second, role playing will get the client to practice a behavior that is culturally alien and will allow you to reinforce his efforts.

Acute Care Situation: Rosa Swiftwind

Mrs. Rosa Swiftwind was diagnosed with diabetes 6 months ago. She is 34, obese, and of Hispanic and Native American heritage. Mrs. Swiftwind has returned to the hospital 6 times since initial diagnosis. The last time she was admitted in ketoacidosis; this time she is in insulin shock. When asked, Mrs. Swiftwind claims to know all about her disease and its treatment.

Nursing Diagnosis:

- Altered Health Maintenance
- Noncompliance

Related To:

- Failure to regulate glucose, insulin, exercise, rest, and/or balance

As Evidenced By:

- Repeated hospitalizations for ketoacidosis and insulin shock

Expected Outcomes

1. Client agrees to daily phone consultations with the nurse specialist for diabetics.
2. Client differentiates between hyperglycemia and hypoglycemia.
3. Client verbalizes appropriate emergency measures to take when experiencing symptoms of either condition.
4. Client balances diet and exercise with insulin intake.
5. Nutritionist develops culturally appropriate exchange list.
6. Client agrees to daily monitoring of glucose levels.
7. Client reduces her weight by 10 pounds in 3 months.
8. Client verbalizes the relationship between genetics and vulnerability to diabetes mellitus.
9. Client verbalizes the relationship between good diabetes management and health.
10. Client reduces the episodes of ketoacidosis or insulin shock by half within the next 6 months.

Interventions:

1. Assess the client's knowledge base about diabetes mellitus.
2. Explore the client's perception of the cause of the multiple hospitalizations and identify her central problems with controlling the disease.
3. Work with the client on prioritizing health goals.
4. Prepare lesson plans that address the client's health education needs as she identifies them.

Discussion:

It is apparent that more is going on in this situation than a straightforward need for knowledge. You may need to collaborate with the public health nurse, who can visit the client's home, or your Native American or Hispanic cultural expert to give you ideas on what might be interfering with this woman's ability to cope with her medical diagnosis. You may also need to consult with folk healers to come up with a workable plan of management. Retelling the client knowledge that has already been presented to her will not solve the problem. You will get frustrated by repeating yourself and she will feel demeaned if you have to tell her something twice. Another possibility is that the barrier between the two of you is so large that she will not benefit from hearing the health education message from you again. The client's learning needs may be affective rather than cognitive. It is best for you to identify what is really going on and then address her learning needs at that level.

Acute Care Situation: Fred Roe

Mr. Fred Roe is a 70-year-old, white male admitted for prostate surgery. The anesthesiologist instructed Mr. Roe to stop smoking before surgery. However, you will be satisfied if you can get him to stop for a week.

Nursing Diagnosis:

- Gas exchange, impaired, high risk for

Related To:

- Chronic smoking, 55-year duration
- Surgical assault

As Evidenced By:

- Heavy infiltration of tar in lungs
- Shortness of breath
- Chronic cough
- Cyanosis in nail beds and nose

Expected Outcomes:

1. Client verbalizes the relationship between coughing and smoking.
2. Client verbalizes the relationship between smoking, coughing, and postsurgical, incisional pain.
3. Client stops smoking for 2 days prior to surgery and 1 week following surgery.

Interventions:

1. Assess client's previous efforts to stop smoking.
2. Explore client's motivation for a maximally comfortable, postsurgical experience.
3. Propose a contract that will get the client to stop smoking 2 days before surgery and 1 week after surgery.
4. Ask the anesthesiologist about the compatibility of a nicotine patch and anesthesia.

Discussion:

We realize that smoking cessation is in the client's best interest but that it is probably not realistic given how many years he has been smoking. Mr. Roe is well aware of the need to stop smoking, and you believe it will not help the situation for him to hear reasons one more time from you. However, it may be possible to find an immediate motivator in the present situation. You ask Mr. Roe if he will agree to stop smoking for a week, which would mean fewer coughing episodes and less incisional pain. You can not promise Mr. Roe freedom from pain but you offer it as a possibility for controlling and improving his own comfort level. After this week, he might be ready to continue smoking cessation. At that point, you could help him plan, one day at a time, a contract for not smoking. In the meantime both of you have shared a positive learning experience, and, if he agrees to the contract, he will have a more comfortable postsurgical experience.

Acute Care/Home Care Situation: Dotty Wall

Miss Dotty Wall is a 10-year-old, white female who has been diagnosed with osteomyelitis. She is in the hospital to receive aggressive, intravenous, antibiotic treatment. Your job is to prepare her and her mother for self-care of the catheter at home, administration of antibiotics, maintenance of a clean insertion site, clamping off the catheter, administration of medications by learning to remove air before injection, and maintenance of a patent catheter.

Nursing Diagnosis:

- Skin integrity, impaired, high risk for
- Anxiety and fear

Related To:

- Central venous catheter
- Insufficient knowledge of catheter care

As Evidenced By:

- Frowning, anxious facial expressions
- Confessed ignorance of catheter care

Expected Outcomes:

1. Client describes the route of the catheter in the body.
2. Client expresses confidence in her ability to assist her mother with catheter care within one week of insertion.
3. Client assists mother with catheter care without contamination while following the established protocol.
4. Client assists mother with established protocol for IV antibiotic administration twice daily without contamination.
5. Client keeps catheter securely bandaged in between IV treatments.
6. Client keeps catheter clean and dry during bathing.
7. Client verbalizes signs and symptoms of incipient infection, side effects of antibiotics, and allergic reactions.

Interventions:

1. Assess client's previous experiences with changing dressings, administering medication by syringe, and incisional care.
2. Explain the anatomy and physiology components of the procedure.
3. Demonstrate full protocols for catheter care, IV antibiotic administration, and incision care.
4. Invite and reinforce step-by-step participation by the mother and client in the procedures.
5. Explain the signs and symptoms of incipient infection, side effects of antibiotics, and allergic reactions.

Discussion:

This situation is a good example of the value of audiovisual aids, objects and models, reinforcement, demonstration and return demonstration. Using the real things as well as pictures and charts, will facilitate teaching the mother and child the necessary skills. You should watch facial expressions for signs of comprehension, overload, or both. Choose activities that are likely to promote immediate success. Encourage the mother and client to participate at their own pace. Build gradually by giving them things to hold before giving them things to do. For example, have them handle the bandage and then apply it. Assure them they do not have to do the entire procedure until they are ready.

Explain your collaborative relationship with the home health nurse who will pick up where you have left off. Assure them that the home health nurse will be with them the first time any of the protocols are performed at home. Send home a videotape of the procedure that they have already watched in the hospital.

Checklist for Community Teaching

The following checklist is provided to help you organize the teaching you will do away from your ordinary work area. This teaching might take place in a clinic, church, home, senior citizen community center, or school. You should use this checklist as a starting point in the creation of your own list.

Hints

Arrive early to:

- Locate bathroom.
- Replan in case something changes.
- Set up all of your equipment.
- Provide for any last-minute inspirations.
- Have an alternative plan in case electrical appliances fail.
- Locate light switches in case you want to dim the lights.
- Have a plan for getting others to help with activities.

Materials List

Teaching module
Posters
Poster holder
Transparent tape
Masking tape
Scissors
Transparencies and pens/blank flip-chart paper
Handouts
Evaluation tool(s)
Extra paper
Cards for last-minute signs
Appliances if necessary
Microphone if your voice is soft or space is large
Long (30-foot) cord, 3-way plug, and converter plug

Chalk and eraser
Pencils and eraser
Facial tissue
Cup of water
Cough drops or lemon drops
Self-adhesive notes
Refreshments if topic is nutrition
Tape recorder if using music
Tapes of music or other appropriate matter
Eye- and lip-enhancers (makeup) to improve visibility of features

Children and Play

Things to Remember about Play

1. For children, play is the equivalent of adults' work and can be equally productive. Play is self-education—it provides practice in physical, lingual, social, and emotional activities. We should not "sell it short".
2. Observe play because it gives us good clues as to the child's feelings, needs, growth, and development.
3. Be observant. Watch for fatigue.
4. Avoid play that increases tension.
5. Give the child one activity at a time.
6. Give children freedom of expression, but set necessary limits.
7. Give simple directions.
8. Remember that the attention span is short, especially for younger children. Be helpful and permissive in activity changes.
9. Be sure to arrange things so that the child in bed is comfortable and can reach things she or he wants.

Requirements for Hospital Toys

1. Ensure that the toys are easily cleanable and able to withstand frequent cleaning, or cheap enough to be discarded.
2. Toys should be sturdy and durable; hospital toys get more continuous use than home toys.
3. Toys should be easy to play with. Sick children often want toys a little below their normal developmental level.
4. Appropriate toys have few small parts to be lost.
5. For young children, the toy should have no parts small enough to be swallowed.

Special Cases

1. Diabetes—Avoid giving these children sharp toys and tools that could scratch them and lead to infections.
2. Brain tumor—Avoid playing bending games because they may cause dizziness.
3. Nephrosis—Avoid close eye work because these children have difficulty seeing.
4. Asthma—Avoid fuzzy materials. Do water sports.
5. Casts—Avoid small objects that may get pushed under the child's cast, and wet materials that may make the cast lining soggy.
6. Postoperative—Avoid any game that will put strain on the suture line.
7. Oxygen—Avoid toys that have been oiled or mechanical toys that put out sparks.
8. Cardiac or respiratory conditions—Avoid fatigue.
9. Small children—Avoid play materials that contain poisons, such as paints or paste, which may be eaten when your back is turned. Avoid toys that have small parts that might be swallowed, put in ears, or put up nostrils.

10. Ear surgery—Avoid bending games to prevent dizziness.
11. Hemophilia—Avoid sharp toys and rough play.

Infancy

General Information

1. Toys should be free of removable parts and sharp or pointed edges.
2. Yarn and fuzzy stuffed dolls should be avoided.
3. The paint on toys should not be the type that washes off.
4. Eyes on stuffed animals should be painted on—no removable buttons or pins.
5. Pull-string toys should be avoided in the hospital situation because the child may wrap the string around his or her neck.

Infancy (birth to 2 years)

Characterized by sensory exploration, development of motor control, and beginning of speech.

Birth to 3 Months

Characterized by sucking, looking, and listening
Attraction to bright dangling objects—mobiles, simple patterns
Likes a bright piece of cloth over the crib
Plays with a ring rattle—brightly colored plastic rings on one larger ring
Interested in small silver dumbbell rattles
Enjoys rubber, squeaking toy

3 to 9 Months

Characterized by touching objects
Enjoys a cradle gym
Likes rubber blocks with bells inside
Needs a sturdy rattle
Uses teething beads
Interested in a water ball
Likes looking into a large mirror (4 to 6 months peak)

6 to 12 Months

Characterized by banging, inserting, poking, twisting, squeezing, dropping, shaking, biting, throwing
Enjoys a recliner swing
Uses a spoon and cup
Likes nested measuring cups

9 to 12 Months

Characterized by stacking, in and out, pouring out, fitting, opening and closing, pressing levers, pushing balls and cars
Needs a playpen
Enjoys hard rubber blocks—good for biting
Likes square or round block stacks—colorful blocks fitted on a large peg
Plays with a ball
Likes water toys
Uses brightly colored, heavy, plastic cereal bowls or nested cups

12 to 18 Months

Characterized by action
Uses a jumper chair
Likes a walker—low enough so that child has whole foot on ground
Plays with pull and push toys
Enjoys sweeping sets with broom and mop
Likes balls
Plays with blocks—small, brightly colored
Likes opening and closing simple boxes
Plays with a color cone—brightly colored rings of graduated sizes that fit one on top of the other
Enjoys water toys
Likes cloth, soft animals and dolls—no removable parts, eyes should be painted or embroidered, no buttons or sharp points, lightweight
Likes turning pages of books—should be cloth and heavy cardboard with familiar objects and bright colors

18 to 24 Months

Ready to climb stairs
Likes swinging

Rides a rocking horse
Enjoys using a push cart
Plays with a large ball
Likes a—hammer and peg toy
Enjoys pull toys—peg wagon, small cart
Likes pots and pans with covers

Finds a pocketbook interesting
Likes soft, cloth animals
Wears wrist bells
Listens to a music box
Plays with small (2-inch), colored blocks

Preschool

Characterized by physical activity, an ability to do things for oneself, pretending, and using working parts

	2 to 3 years	4 to 5 years
1. For development of strength and skill	Push and pull toys Large colored wooden beads for stringing together Wagon Wheelbarrow Toy car to ride Three-wheeled scooter Sandbox and sandbox toys	Lock box Ten-in game Balls
2. For developing creativity with constructive toys	Sandbox Large hollow blocks or boxes Blunt scissors and colored paper Large pegboard and pegs Tinker toys Hammer and large nail set Picture puzzles Nest of blocks	Blunt scissors Smaller beads to string Simple tool chest Felt-o-grams Picture puzzles (10-25 pieces) Hammer and small nail set Paper to cut Simple construction sets
3. For dramatic and initiative play (peak at age 5)	Doll carriage Broom and sweeper Dump truck Simple train Toy animals Small autos for dolls	Garden tools Housekeeping toys Fire engine Garages and gas station Toy telephones
4. For social development	Dolls Beds, chairs, table, etc. Balls Blocks Wagons	First board games Simple computer programs that test colors, numbers, and sounds Sandbox Fishpond games Toy village Tea table, chairs, dishes

5. For artistic development	Large crayons	Large paints and crayons
	Modeling clay	Modeling clay
	Drum	Finger painting material
	Jingle bells	Plasticin

School Age (6 to 10 years)

Characterized by desire to learn simple skills, imitative and dramatic play games, and group activities

1. For development of strength and skill

Gymnastic equipment—increasingly complex
Ring toss game
Archery with rubber-tipped arrows
Jump rope
Kites

Beanbag
Toys to spin
Marbles
Races

2. Constructive play for creativity

Metal and wood construction sets:
motorized parts, complex gears
Picture puzzles (12 pieces or more)
Modeling wax
Felt-o-grams
Soap-bubble sets

Wire puzzles
Paper craft materials
Constructive blocks
Word processors

3. Adventurous play

Circus sets
Play stories
Cash registers
Families or small dolls
Costumes, lots of accessories

Puppets and marionettes
Boats
Dolls and paper dolls
Doll trunk
Video games

4. For social development

Games (such as purchase, dominoes, bingo,
Junior Scrabble)
National costume dolls
Ring toss
Role playing with elaborate costumes and makeup

Checkers
Tiddlywinks

5. For artistic development

Painting sets
Swing sets
Bead looms
Rhythm instruments
Design or pattern toys

Weaving sets
Modeling clay, wax
Mosaics
Crayons, paints, markers

6. Hobbies and special interests

Map puzzles
~~Blackboard and crayons~~
Printing sets
Magnet sets
Collective books, birds, and animals
Conceptual models: body, world, stars, science kits, clocks and watches, calculators, and storybooks

Dominoes
Puzzle clock
Counting games
Blueprint outfits
Stamp albums

Preadolescence (girls, 10 to 13; boys, 10 to 14)

Characterized by interest in teamwork and athletics, competitions, skill development, and dexterity

1. For constructive and creative play

Construction kits—airplane, birdhouse, boat
Games—Monopoly, ping-pong, tennis, etc.
Card games
Video and tape player, blanks to make own tapes

Picture puzzles
Advanced creator sets
Science fiction
Computers, word processors

Early Adolescence (14 to 17)

Characterized by interest in games of intellectual competition, hobbies, motor skills, group recreational activities involving both sexes

1. For intellectual and physical development

Tennis racquet
Baseball and football equipment
Workbench and tools
Board and card games
Typing
Compass
Telescopes
Collections
Woodburning
Ceramics
Video equipment

Target games
Jigsaw puzzles
Camp equipment
Chemistry sets
Reading
Electric motors
Microscopes
Needlework
Leatherwork
Science fiction
Complex computer games
Electronic/music equipment

Sources of Audiovisual Materials

Introduction

When you are looking for audiovisual aids, consider your phone book as the first place to start. Look under your state and local health departments. You can also look under voluntary health organizations, such as the American Cancer Society, the Kidney Foundation, the American Heart Association, the American Stroke Association, and any other diseases related to your teaching needs. Planned Parenthood is one organization that maintains local offices and clinics throughout the country. The National Dairy Council may have a local office and actual teaching packages for various age groups on the subject of nutrition. Teacher stores are loaded with teaching materials and ideas. Art stores sell copyright-free cartoons and other materials for posters and transparencies. Librarians can be very helpful in telling you what the library has to offer. Many libraries, both public and college, have audiovisual departments. They can also help you locate addresses for other resources. Colleges and universities—particularly those with nursing, teacher education, and medical departments—may be helpful, too. Other sources of information are pharmaceutical companies. Additional resources follow.

Aging

American Foundation for the Blind (AFB)
15 W. 16th Street
New York, NY 10011
(212) 620–2000

AFB Products Catalog
100 Enterprize Place
Dover, DE 19901
(800) 829–0500

American Association of Retired Persons (AARP)
601 E Street N.W.
Washington, D.C. 20049
(202) 434–2277

National Eye Care Project
P.O. Box 429098
San Francisco, CA 94142-9098
(800) 222–3937
(assist the disadvantaged elderly locally)

National Council on Aging
409 Third Street S.W., Suite 200
Washington, D.C. 20024
(800) 424–9046

International Hearing Society
20361 Middlebelt Road
Livonia, MI 48152
(800) 521–5247 (Hearing Aid Help Line)

Self Help for Hard of Hearing People, Inc.
7800 Wisconsin Ave.
Bethesda, MD 20814
(301) 657–2248

Consumer Interests

U.S. Consumer Product Safety Commission
Office of the Secretary
Washington, D.C. 20207
(800) 638–2772

Consumer Information Catalog
P.O. Box 100
Pueblo, CO 81002

Disease-Oriented Organizations

American Cancer Society
1599 Clifton Road N.E.
Atlanta, GA 30329
(404) 320–3333

American Diabetes Association
National Service Center
1660 Duke Street
Alexandria, VA 22313
(703) 549–1500

American Heart Association
7320 Greenville Ave.
Dallas, TX 75231
(214) 373–6300

Epilepsy Foundation of America
4351 Garden City Drive
Landover, MD 20785
(800) 332–1000

CDC National AIDS Clearinghouse
P.O. Box 6003
Rockville, MD 20849-6003
(800) 458–5231

National Cancer Institute
9000 Rockville Pike

Bethesda, MD 20892
(800) 4–CANCER

National Association for Sickle Cell Disease, Inc.
3345 Wilshire Blvd. Suite 1106
Los Angeles, CA 90010-1880
(800) 421–8453

National Hemophilia Foundation
110 Green St., Room 406
New York, NY 10012
(212) 219–8180

National High Blood Pressure Education Program Information Center
P.O. Box 30105
Bethesda, MD 20824-0105
(301) 951–3260

National Jewish Center for Immunology and Respiratory Medicine
1400 Jackson
Denver, CO 80206
(800) 222–LUNG (Lungline)

National Kidney Foundation
30 East 33rd Street
New York, NY 10016
(800) 622–9010

National Multiple Sclerosis Society
205 E. 42nd Street
New York, NY 10017
(800) 532–7667

National Stroke Association
300 East Hampden Avenue, Suite 240
Englewood, CO 80110-2654
(303) 762–9922

General Health Information

American Association of Sex Educators, Counselors, Therapists
35 N. Michigan Ave.
Suite 1717
Chicago, IL 60611-4066
(312) 644–0828

American College Health Association
P.O. Box 28937
Baltimore, MD 21240-8937
(410) 859-1500

American Dental Association
211 E. Chicago Avenue
Chicago, IL 60611
(800) 621-8099

Channing L. Bete Co., Inc.
200 State Road
South Deerfield, MA 01373
(800) 628-7733

National Health Information Center
Office of Disease Prevention and Health
Promotion
P.O. Box 1133
Washington, D.C. 20013-1133
(800) 336-4797

National Institutes of Health
9000 Rockville Pike
Bethesda, MD 20205
(301) 496-4000

Office of Minority Health Resource Center
P.O. Box 37337
Washington, D.C. 20013-7337
(800) 444-6472

Maternal and Child Health

La Leche League International
9616 Minneapolis Avenue
P.O. Box 1209
Franklin Park, IL 60131
(800) 525-3243

March of Dimes Birth Defects Foundation
1275 Mamaroneck Ave.
White Plains, NY 10605
(914) 428-7100

National SIDS Foundation
10500 Little Patuxent Parkway, Suite 420
Columbia, MD 21044
(800) 221-SIDS

Mental Health

National Institutes of Mental Health
Public Inquiries Section
5600 Fishers Lane, Room 15C-05
Rockville, MD 20857
(301) 443-4515

National Mental Health Association
Information Center
1021 Prince Street
Arlington, VA 22314
(703) 684-7722

National Clearinghouse for Alcohol and Drug
Information
P.O. Box 2345
Rockville, MD 20852
(301) 468-2600

Nutrition and Nutritional Problems

National Dairy Council (Dairy and Nutrition
Council)
O'Hare International Center
10255 W. Higgins Road, Suite 900
Rosemont, IL 60017-5616
(708) 803-2000

Smoking and Tobacco

Adventist Information Ministry
Berrien Springs, MI 49104-0970
(800) 253-3000
(smoking cessation)

American Lung Association
1740 Broadway
New York, NY 10019
(212) 315-8700

American Cancer Society
(see selected disease-oriented organizations)

National Cancer Institute
(see selected disease-oriented organizations)

National Institutes of Health
9000 Rockville Pike
Bethesda, MD 20205
(301) 496-4000

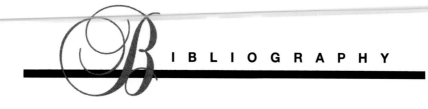
Aiken, L.R., Jr. (1982). *Psychological testing and assessment* (4th ed.). Boston: Allyn & Bacon.

Ailinger, R.L. (1982). Hypertension knowledge in a Hispanic community. *Nursing Research, 31*(4), 207-210.

Alford, D.M. (1982). Tips for teaching older adults. *Nursing Life,* September/October: 60-64

Allport, G. (1955). *Becoming a person.* New Haven: Yale University Press

American Association of Retired Persons. (1987). *A profile of older Americans.* Washington DC: Author.

American Heart Association. (1991). *1991 heart and stroke facts.* Dallas: Author.

American Hospital Association (1972). *A patient's bill of rights.* Chicago: Author.

American Nurses Association. (1991). *Nursing's agenda for health care reform,* (PR-12-91). Author.

Anand, K.J.S. & Hickey, P.R. (1992). Halothane-morphine compared with high-dose sufentanil for anesthesia and postoperative analgesia in neonatal cardiac surgery. *New England Journal of Medicine, 326*(1), 1-9.

Anderson, G.C. (1989). Skin to skin: Kangaroo care in western Europe. *American Journal of Nursing, 89*(5), 662-666.

Andersen, J. & Briggs, L. (1988). Nursing diagnosis: A study of quality and supportive evidence. *IMAGE: Journal of Nursing Scholarship. 20*(3), 141-4.

Andraesen, N.C. (1984). *The broken brain.* New York: Harper & Row.

Andresen, G.P. (1989). A fresh look at assessing the elderly. *RN,* June, 28-39.

Andrews, M.M. (1989). Culture and nutrition. In J.S. Boyle & M.M. Andrews, *Transcultural concepts in nursing care* (pp. 333-355). Boston: Scott, Foresman.

Apgar, V. (1953). A proposal for a new method of evaluation of the newborn infant. *Anesthesia, 32:* 260.

Babcock, D. & Zak-Dance, C. (1981). Developing skills as a public speaker. *American Operating Room Nurses Journal, 33*(5), 994-1000.

Baca, J.E. (1978). Some health beliefs of the Spanish speaking. In R.A. Martinez, (Ed.). *Hispanic culture and health care* (pp. 92-98). St. Louis: Mosby.

Backer, B., Frost, A. & Mason, D. (1985). High tech-high touch it's high time for nursing. *Nursing & Health Care, 6*(5), 263-266.

Bahrick, H.P. (1989). The laboratory and ecology: Supplementary sources of data for memory research.

In L.W. Poon, D.C. Rubin, & B.A. Wilson (Eds.), *Everyday cognition in adulthood and late life* (pp. 73-83). Cambridge: Cambridge University Press.

Bainbridge, L. & Quintanilla (Eds.). (1989). *Developing skills with information technology.* New York: Wiley.

Bandman, E.L. & Bandman, B. (1988). *Critical thinking in nursing.* Norwalk: Appleton & Lange.

Bates, B. (1991). *A guide of physical examination and history taking* (5th ed.). Philadelphia: Lippincott.

Bauer, K.G. (1980). *Improving the chances for health: Lifestyle changes and health evaluation.* San Francisco: National Center for Health Education.

Bauman, L.J. & Keller, M.L. (1991). Responses to threat information. *IMAGE: Journal of Nursing Scholarship, 23*(1), 13-18.

Beden, H. & Carrea, N. (Winter, 1988). The effects of andragogical teacher training on adult student attendance and evaluation of their teachers. *Adult Education Quarterly, 38*(2), 75-87.

Bellock, N.B. & Breslow, L. (1972). Relationship of physical health status to health practices. *Preventive Medicine, 1,* 409-421.

Benson, H. (1980). *The mind-body effect.* New York: Simon & Schuster.

Berne, A.S., Dato, C., Mason, D.J., & Rafferty, M. (1990). A nursing model for addressing the health needs of homeless families. *IMAGE: Journal of Nursing Scholarship, 22*(1), 8-13.

Bernzweig, E.P. (1987). *The nurse's liability for malpractice* (4th ed.). New York: McGraw-Hill.

Bigge, M. (1982). *Learning theories for teachers* (4th ed.). New York: Harper & Row.

Bingham, A. & Bargar, J. (1985). Children of alcoholic families. *Journal of Psychosocial Nursing, 23,* 13-15.

Bingham, R. (Writer, Director). (1987) *The sexual brain* [Videorecording]. Princeton NJ: Films for the Humanities & Sciences.

Bloom, B.S., Englehart, M.B., Furst, E.J., Hill, W.H. & Krathwohl, D.R. (eds.) (1956). *The classification of educational goals. Handbook I: Cognitive domain.* New York: McKay.

Bloom, B.S., Madaus, G.F. & Hastings, J.T. (1981). *Evaluation to improve learning.* New York: McGraw-Hill.

Bolles, E.B. (1988). *Remembering and forgetting: An inquiry into the nature of memory.* New York: Walker & Company.

Boyle, J.S. (1989). Alterations in lifestyle: Transcultural concepts in chronic illness. In J.S. Boyle & M.M. Andrews, *Transcultural concepts in nursing care* (pp. 223-241). Boston: Scott, Foresman.

Boyle, J.S. & Andrews, M.M. (1989). Transcultural perspectives in the nursing process. In J.S. Boyle & M.M. Andrews, *Transcultural concepts in nursing care* (pp. 67-92). Boston: Scott, Foresman.

Brookfield, S.D. (1991). *Developing critical thinkers.* San Francisco: Jossey-Bass.

Brophy, C.J. & Mitchell, M.E. (1989). Children with chronic illness: A structured strategic family approach. *Journal of Psychotherapy and the Family, 6*(34), 129.

Browne, M.N. & Keeley, S.M. (1986). *Asking the right questions: A guide to critical thinking* (2nd ed.). Englewood Cliffs NJ: Prentice-Hall.

Brundage, D.H. (1980). *Adult learning principles and their application to program planning.* Ontario: The Ministry of Education.

Brunner, E., Wilder, D.K., Kirchner, D. & Newberry, Jr. J. (1959). *Adult education,* Chicago: Adult Education Association.

Brunt, B. & Scott, N. (1986). Factors to consider in the development of self instructional materials. *Journal of Continuing Education in Nursing, 17*(3), 87-93.

Bushy, A. (1992). Cultural considerations for primary health care: Where do self-care and folk medicine fit? *Holistic Nursing Practice 6*(3), 10-18.

Cain, E. (1988). *Fulfilled Parents.* Brighton, CO: Nanel Unlimited.

Califano, J.A., Jr. (1986). *America's health care revolution.* New York: Random House.

Campbell, T. & Chang, B. (1981). Health care of the Chinese in America. In G. Henderson & M. Primeaux, (eds). *Transcultural health care* (pp. 162-171). Menlo Park CA: Addison-Wesley.

Capers, C.F. (1992). Teaching cultural content: A nursing education imperative. *Holistic Nursing Practice, 6*(3), 19-28.

Carmack, B.J. (1992). Balancing engagement/detachment in AIDS-related multiple losses. *IMAGE: Journal of Nursing Scholarship, 24*(1), 9-14.

Carnegie, D. (1980). *The quick and easy way to effective speaking*, 2nd ed. New York: Dale Carnegie & Associates.

Carnegie, D. (1980). *How to win friends and influence people*. New York: Dale Carnegie & Associates.

Chalick, T. & Smith, L. (1992). Nursing at the grass roots. *Nursing & Health Care*, 13(5), 242-246.

Chang, K. (1991). Chinese Americans. In J.N. Giger & R.E. Davidhizar, *Transcultural nursing assessment and intervention* (pp. 359-377). St. Louis: Mosby.

Carnes, L.S. & Moore, P.S. (1992). Meeting patients' spiritual needs: The Jewish perspective. *Holistic Nursing Practice*, 6(3), 64-72.

Charonko, C.V. (1992). Cultural influences in "noncompliant" behavior and decision making, *Holistic Nursing Practice*, 6(3), 73-78.

Cherry, B. & Giger, J.N. (1991). Black Americans. In J.N. Giger & R.E. Davidhizar, *Transcultural nursing assessment and intervention* (pp. 147-182). St. Louis: Mosby.

Choi, M.W. (1985). Preamble to a new paradigm for women's health care. *Image: The Journal of Nursing Scholarship*, 17(1), 14-16.

Charness, N. (1989). Age and expertise: Responding to Talland's challenge. In L.W. Poon, D.C. Rubin, & B.A. Wilson (Eds.), *Everyday cognition in adulthood and late life* (pp. 437-456). Cambridge: Cambridge University Press.

Claxton, C.S. & Murrell, P.H. (1987). *Learning styles: Implications for improving education practices*. ASHE-ERIC Higher Education Report No. 4. Washington DC: Association for the Study of Higher Education.

Colorado State Board of Nursing. (1991). *Colorado nurse practice act*. Denver, CO: Author.

Coppens, N. (1990). Parental responses to children in unsafe situations. *Pediatric Nursing*, 16(6), 571-574.

Corell, J. (1984). Ethnicity and cancer prevention in a tri-ethnic urban community. *Journal of the National Medical Association*, 76(10), 1013-1019.

Cowling, W.R. & Campbell, V.G. (1986). Health concerns of aging men. *The Nursing Clinics of North America*, March. Philadelphia: W.B. Saunders.

Crovitz, H.F. (1989). Memory retraining: Everyday needs and future prospects. In L.W. Poon, D.C. Rubin, & B.A. Wilson (Eds.), *Everyday cognition in adulthood and late life* (pp. 681-691). Cambridge: Cambridge University Press.

Crowe, C. (1986). Innovations in family and community health. *Family and Community Health*, 9(1), 82-85.

Curran, D. (1985). *Stress and the healthy family*. Minneapolis: Winston.

Davis, C.M. (1981). Affective education for the health professions. *Physical Therapy*, 6(11), 1587-1593.

Davis, H. & Hurwitz, M.B. (Eds.). (1977). *Operant-Pavlovian interactions*. Hillsdale, NJ: Erlbaum.

Davis, L.N. (1974). *Planning, conducting and evaluating workshops*. Austin, TX: Learning Concepts.

Dellarosa, D. (1988). A history of thinking. In R.J. Sternberg & E.E. Smith (Eds.), *The psychology of human thought* (pp. 1-18). New York: Cambridge University Press.

Detection and diagnosis of breast cancer. (1984). In *The breast cancer digest* (2nd ed.). (NIH Publication No. 84-1691). Bethesda: National Cancer Institute.

deTornyay, R. & Thompson, M.A. (1982). *Strategies for teaching nursing*. New York: John Wiley & Sons.

Dewey, J. (1938). *Experience and education*. New York: Macmillan.

Dewey, J. (1922). *Human nature and conduct*. New York: Holt, Rinehart & Winston.

Disch, J.M. (June, 1989). *Are we fostering excellence in practice?* Paper presented at the Nursing Education 89: The Conference for Nursing Faculty. Philadelphia: Medical College of Pennsylvania, Continuing Nursing Education.

Doak, C.C., Doak, L.G. & Root, J.D.H. (1985). *Teaching patients with low literacy skills*. Philadelphia PA: Lippincott.

Dobson, K.S. (ed.) (1988). *Handbook of cognitive-behavioral therapies*. New York: Gilford Press.

Donar, M.E. (1988). Community care: Pediatric home mechanical ventilation. *Holistic Nursing Practice*, 2(2), 68-80.

Donnelley, G.F. (1988). Imaginative play and the physically disabled child. *Holistic Nursing Practice*, 2(2), 81-88.

Dossey, B.M., Keegan, L., Gouzetta, D. & Kolkmeier, L.G. (1988). *Holistic nursing: A handbook for practice*. Rockville, MD: Aspen Publishers.

Ebersole, P. & Hess, P. (1990). *Toward healthy aging: Human needs and nursing response* (3rd ed.). St. Louis: Mosby.

Ennis, R.H. (1985). A logical basis for measuring critical thinking skills. *Educational Leadership, 43*, 44-48.

Erickson, E.H. (1963). *Childhood and society* (2nd ed.). New York: W.W. Norton.

Erikson, E.H. (1968). *Identity: Youth and crisis.* New York: W.W. Norton.

Ersek, M. (1992). *Examining the process and dilemmas of reality negotiation.* IMAGE: *Journal of Nursing Scholarship, 24*(1), 1925.

Evaneshko, V. (1984). Ethnic and cultural considerations. In Steffl, B.M. (ed.). *Handbook of gerontological nursing.* New York: Van Nostrand Reinhold.

Fawcett, J. (1989). *Analysis and evaluation of conceptual models of nursing* (2nd ed.). Philadelphia: F.A. Davis.

Fein, R. (1992). Health care reform: Is it time for our medicine? *Modern Maturity, 35*(4), 22-35.

Feinblum, S. (1989). Pinning down the psychosocial dimensions of AIDS. *Nursing & Health Care, 7*, 255-257.

Fernald, A. & Kuhl, P. (1987). Acoustic determinants of infant preference for motherese speech. *Infant Behavioral Development,* 10:279-293.

Fishel, R. (1988). *Time for joy: Daily affirmations.* Deerfield Beach FL: Health Communications.

Fisher, N.L. (1992). Ethnocultural approaches to genetics. *The Pediatric Clinics of North America, 39*(1), 55.

Flaskerud, J.H. (1989). Transcultural concepts in mental health nursing. In J.S. Boyle & M.M. Andrews, *Transcultural concepts in nursing care* (pp. 243-269). Boston: Scott, Foresman.

Flavell, J.H. (1985). *Cognitive development.* (2nd ed.). Englewood Cliffs NJ: Prentice-Hall.

Flavell, J.H., Green, F.L. & Flavell, E.R. (1986). *Development of knowledge about the appearance-reality distinction.* Chicago: Society for Research in Child Development.

Folks, D.G., Freeman, A.M., Sokol, R.S. & Thurstin, A.H. (1988). Denial: Predictor of outcome following coronary bypass surgery. *International Journal of Psychiatry in Medicine, 18,* 57-66.

Foster, G.M. (1981). Relationships between Spanish and Spanish-American folk medicine. In G.

Henderson & M. Primeaux, (Eds.), *Transcultural health care* (pp. 115-135). Menlo Park CA: Addison-Wesley.

Frey, M.S. & Denyes, M.J. (1989). Health and illness self care in adolescents with IDDM: A test of orem's theory. *Advances in Nursing Science, 12*(1), 67-75.

Freedman, A., Kaplan, H. & Sadock, B. (Eds.). (1975). *Comprehensive textbook of psychiatry* (2nd ed.). Baltimore: Williams & Wilkins.

Froman, R.D., Owen, S.V. & Daisy, C. (1992). Development of a measure of attitudes toward persons with AIDS. IMAGE: *Journal of Nursing Scholarship, 24*(2), 149-152.

Fry, E. (1968). A readability formula that saves time. *Journal of Reading, 11,* 513-516, 575-577.

Fulghum, R. (1988). *All I really need to know I learned in kindergarten.* New York: Ivy Books.

Gage, N.L. & Berliner, D.C. (1992). *Educational psychology* (5th ed.). Boston: Houghton Mifflin.

Garcia-Coll, C.T.G., Halpern, L.F., Vohr, B.R., Seifer, R., & Oh, W. (1992). Stability and correlates of change of early temperament in preterm and full term infants. *Infant Behavior and Development, 15*(2), 137.

Gawlinski, A. and Jensen, G.A. (1991). The complications of cardiovascular aging. *American Journal of Nursing, 91*(11), 26-30.

Germain, C.P. (1992). Cultural care: A bridge between sickness, illness, and disease. *Holistic Nursing Practice, 6*(3), 1-9.

Giardano, D.A. & Dusek, D.E. (1988). *Changing health behaviors.* Scottsdale AZ: Gorsuch Scarisbrick, Publishers.

Ginsburg, H. & Opper, S. (1979). *Piaget's theory of intellectual development* (2nd ed.). Englewood Cliffs NJ: Prentice Hall.

Gold, A.R. (July 30, 1989). The struggle to make do without health insurance. *New York Times.*

Gortner, S.R., Dirks, J. & Wolfe, M.M. (1992). Elders after CABG. *American Journal of Nursing, 92*(8), 44-49.

Gose, K. & Levi, G. (1988). *Dealing with memory changes as you grow older.* Toronto: Bantam Books.

Groer, M.W., and Shekleton, M.E. (1989). *Basic pathophysiology* (3rd ed.). St. Louis: Mosby.

Gronlund, N.E. (1985). *Stating behavioral objectives for classroom instruction* (3rd ed.). New York: Macmillan.

Gronlund, N.E. (1978). *Stating behavioral objectives for classroom instruction.* (2nd ed.). New York: Macmillan.

Guthrie, E.R. (1935). *The psychology of learning.* New York: Harper & Row.

Hall, C. & Lindzey, G. (1957). *Theories of personality.* New York: John Wiley & Sons.

Halpern, D.F. (1984). *Thought and knowledge.* Hillsdale NJ: Lawrence Erlbaum Associates.

Hamilton, E.M., Whitney, E.N. & Sizer, F.S. (1991). Nutrition concepts and controversies. St. Paul MN: West.

Hanley, C.E. (1991). Navajo Indians. In J.N. Giger and R.E. Davidhizar, *Transcultural nursing assessment and intervention* (pp. 215-238). St. Louis: Mosby.

Hanlon, J.J. & Pickett, G.E. (1984). *Public health: Administration and practice.* St. Louis: Mosby.

Harrow, A.J. (1972). *A taxonomy of the psychomotor domain: A guide for developing behavioral objectives.* New York: David McKay.

Harter, S. & Chao, C. (1992). The role of competence in children's creation of imaginary friends. *Merrill-Palmer Quarterly,* 38(3), 350.

Hassanein, S.A. (1991). On the shortage of registered nurses: An economic analysis of the RN market. *Nursing & Health Care,* 12(3), 152-156.

Hautman, M.A. (1979). Folk health and illness beliefs. *The Nurse Practitioner: The American Journal of Primary Health Care,* 4(4), 23-34.

Hawken, P.L. (1990). NLN's national health strategy: A plan for reform. *National League for Nursing Public Policy Bulletin,* Fall 1990, 3-4.

Haynes, R.B., Taylor, D.W. & Sackett, D.L. (Eds.). (1979). *Compliance in health care.* Baltimore MD: The Johns Hopkins University Press.

Heckler, M. (1985). *Report of the secretary's task force on black and minority health,* U.S. Dept of Health and Human Services, 1985.

Heidgerken, L. (1965). *Teaching and learning in schools of nursing: Principles and methods.* Philadelphia: Lippincott.

Hendreson, G. & Primeaux, M. (1981). The importance of folk medicine. In G. Henderson & M. Primeaux, (Eds.). *Transcultural health care* (pp. 59-77). Menlo Park CA: Addison-Wesley.

Hentinen, M. & Kyngas, H. (1992). Compliance of young diabetics with health regimens. *Journal of Advanced Nursing,* 17(5), 530.

Herberg, P. (1989). Theoretical foundations of transcultural nursing. In J.S. Boyle & M.M. Andrews, *Transcultural concepts in nursing care* (pp. 3-65). Boston: Scott, Foresman.

Hickey, S.S. (1986). Enabling hope. *Cancer Nursing,* 9(30), 133-137.

Hilbert, G.A. (1985). Accuracy of self-reported measures of compliance, *Nursing Research.* September/October (34), 319-320.

Hilgard, E. & Bower, G. (1966). *Theories of learning* (3rd ed.). New York: Meredith.

Hoffer, E. (1973). *Reflections on the human condition.* New York: Harper & Row.

Houldin, A.D., & Lev, E., Prystowsky, M.B., Redei, E. & Lowrey, B.J., (1991). Psychoneuroimmunology; A review of literature. *Holistic Nursing Practice,* 5(4), 10-21.

Houle, C.O. (1961). *The inquiring mind.* Madison: University of Wisconsin Press.

Houle, C.O. (1980). *Continuing learning in the professions.* San Francisco: Jossey-Bass.

Huey, F. (1988). How nurses would change U.S. health care. *American Journal of Nursing,* 88(11), 1482-1493.

Hughes, D., Johnson, K., Simons, J., & Rosenbaum, S. (1986). *Maternal and child health data book.* Washington DC: Children's Defense Fund.

Hussey, L.C. (1991). Overcoming the clinical barriers of low literacy and medication noncompliance among the elderly. *Journal of Gerontological Nursing,* 17(3), 27-29.

Ingalls, A.J. (1991). *Maternal and child health nursing.* St. Louis: Mosby.

Irwin, T. (1985). *Nicomachean ethics.* Indianapolis: Hackett.

Jane Doe, RN fights to keep HIV status secret. (1989). *American Journal of Nursing,* 89(6), 869.

Johnson, J.S. & Newport, E.L. (1989). Critical period effects on second language learning: The influence of maturational state on the acquisition of English as a second language. *Cognitive Psychology,* 21: 60-99.

Johnson, P.A. (1990). National health insurance program: A nursing perspective. *Nursing & Health Care,* 11(8), 416.

Jordan, W.C. (1979). The roots and practice of voodoo medicine in America. *Urban Health,* 8(10), 38-48.

Kaluger, G. & Kaluger, M.F. (1984). *Human development: The span of life* (3rd ed.). St. Louis: Mosby.

Kandel, E.R. & Hawkins, R.D. (1992). The biological basis of learning and individuality. *Scientific American,* 267(3), 79-86.

Keepers, T.D. & Babcock, D.E. (1986). *Raising kids o.k. Human growth and development throughout the life span* (2nd ed.). Menlo Park CA: Menalto Press.

Kemp, J.E. & Dayton, D.K. (1985). *Planning and producing instructional media* (5th ed.). New York: Harper & Row.

Kim, M.J., McFarland, G.C., & McLane, A.M. (1989). *Pocket guide to nursing diagnoses.* (3rd ed.). St. Louis: Mosby.

King, E.C. (1984). *Affective education in nursing.* Rockville MD: Aspen Systems.

Kippenbrock, T.A. (1991). Wish I'd been there: A sense of nursing history. *Nursing & Health Care,* 12(4), 208-212.

Kleoppel, J.W. & Henry, D.W. (1987). Teaching patients, families and communities about their medications. In C.E. Smith (Ed.), *Patient education: Nurses in partnership with other health professionals* (pp. 271-296). Orlando FL: Grune & Stratton.

Knowles, M. (1990). *The adult learner: A neglected species.* (4th ed.). Houston: Gulf.

Koehler, W. (1958). Gestalt psychology today. *American Psychologist,* 14, 727-734.

Koffka, K. (1935). *Principles of gestalt psychology.* New York: Harcourt, Brace & World.

Krathwohl, D.R., Bloom, B.S. & Masia, B.B. (1964). *Taxonomy of educational objectives: The classification of educational goals. Handbook II: The affective domain.* New York: David McKay.

Krierger, D. (1990). Therapeutic touch: Two decades of research, teaching and clinical practice. *Imprint,* 37(3), 83, 86-88.

Kub, J.P. (1986). Ethnicity: An important factor for nurses to consider in caring for hypertensive individuals. *Western Journal of Nursing Research,* 18(4): 445-456.

Kuipers, J. (1991). Mexican Americans. In J.N. Giger & R.E. Davidhizar, *Transcultural nursing assessment and intervention* (pp. 185-212). St. Louis: Mosby.

Kurlowicz, L.H., (1990). Violence in the emergency room. *American Journal of Nursing,* 90(9), 34-39.

Lazlo, E. (1972). *The Systems View of the World.* New York: Braziller.

Leigh, R.D. (1930). Comments on education as a lifelong process. *Journal of Adult Education,* 2(2), 123.

Leininger, M. (Ed.). (1988). *Care: The essence of nursing and health,* Detroit: Wayne State University Press.

Leininger, M. (1978). *Transcultural nursing: Concepts, theories, and practices.* New York: John Wiley & Sons.

Leininger, M. (1970). *Nursing and anthropology: Two worlds to blend.* New York: John Wiley & Sons.

Lerner, H. & Bryne, M.W., (1991). Helping nursing students communicate with high risk families. *Nursing & Health Care,* 12(2), 98-101.

Lesmes, G.R. & Donofrio, K.H. (1992). Passive smoking: The medical and economic issues. *The American Journal of Medicine,* 93(1), 385.

Leventhal, H. (1982). Wrongheaded ideas about illness. *Psychology Today.* April: 48.

Levine, S.L. (1989). *Promoting adult growth in schools: The promise of professional development.* Boston: Allyn and Bacon.

Lewin, K. (1955). *A dynamic theory of personality.* New York: McGraw Hill.

Ley, P., Bradshaw, P.W., Eaves, D. & Walker, C.M. (1973). A method for increasing patients' recall of information presented by doctors. *Psychological Medicine,* 3:217-220.

Lindeman, E.C. (1926). *The meaning of adult education.* New York: New Republic.

Little, C. (1992). Health for all by the year 2000; Where is it now? *Nursing & Health Care,* 13(4), 198-204.

Litwack, L., Linc, L. & Bower, D. (1985). *Evaluation in nursing: Principles and practice.* New York: National League for Nursing.

Lowery, B.J. (1991). Psychological stress, denial and myocardial infarction outcomes. *IMAGE: Journal of Nursing Scholarship,* 23(1), 51-55.

Ludman, E.K. & Newman, J.M. (1984). Yin and Yang in the health-related food practices of three Chinese groups. *Journal of Nutrition Education,* 16(1), 3-5.

MacGregor, S.N., Keith, L.G., Chasnoff, I.J., Rosner, M.A., Chisum, G.M., Shaw, P. & Minogue, J.P.

(1987). Cocaine use during pregnancy: Adverse perinatal outcome. *American Journal of Obstetrics and Gynecology, 157:*686-690.

Maduro, R. (1983). Curanderismo and Latino views of disease and curing. *Western Journal of Medicine,* 139(6), 868-874.

Mager, R.F. (1984). *Preparing instructional objectives.* Belmont CA: Lake.

Margalit, M. (1990). *Effective technology integration for disabled children: The family perspective.* New York: Springer.

Marzano, R.J., Brandt, R.S., Hughes, C.S., Jones, B.F., Presseisen, B.Z., Rankin, S.C. & Suhor, C. (1988). *Dimensions of thinking: A framework for curriculum and instruction.* Alexandria: Association for Supervision and Curriculum Development.

Maslow, A.H. (1954). *Motivation and personality.* New York: Harper & Row.

Matteson, M.A. & McConnell, E.S. (1988). *Gerontological Nursing: Concepts and Practice.* Philadelphia: W.B. Saunders.

McAvoy, B.R. & Raza, R. (1991). Can health education increase uptake of cervical smear testing among Asian women? *British Medical Journal,* 302(6780), 833-836.

McCroskey, R. & Kasten, R. (1982). Temporal factors and the aging auditory system. *Ear Hear, 3,* 124-127.

McElmurry, B.J. & LiBrizzi, S.J. (1986). The health of older women. *The Nursing Clinics of North America,* March, Philadelphia: W.B. Saunders.

McFarland, G.K. & McFarlane, E.A. (1989). *Nursing diagnosis and intervention: Planning for patient care.* St. Louis: Mosby.

McHatton, M. (1985). A theory for timely teaching. *American Journal of Nursing, 85*(7), 798-800.

McKenna, M.A. (1989). Transcultural perspectives in the nursing care of the elderly. In J.S. Boyle & M.M. Andrews, *Transcultural concepts in nursing care.* Boston: Scott, Foresman.

Meltzoff, A.N. & Moore, M.K. (1989). Imitation in newborn infants: Exploring the range of gestures imitated and the underlying mechanisms. *Developmental Psychology, 25*(6), 954-962.

Meyer, C. (1992). Bedside computer charting: Inching toward tomorrow. *American Journal of Nursing, 92*(4), 38-44.

Miller, C.A. (1990). *Nursing Care of Older Adults.* Glenview IL: Scott, Foresman/Little, Brown Higher Education.

Miller, M.A. (1989). Social, economic, and political forces affecting the future of occupational health nursing. *Journal of the American Association of Occupational Health Nurses, 37*(9), 361-366.

Miller, M.A. & Malcolm, N.S. (1990). Critical thinking in the nursing curriculum. *Nursing and Health Care, 11*(2), 67-73.

Miller, M.K. & Stokes, C.S. (1978). Health status, health resources and consolidated structural parameters: Implications for public health care policy. *Journal of Health and Social Behavior,* 19(3), 263-278.

Minnesota Educational Computing Corporation. (1990). *Writing and publishing in multimedia computer file version 1.0.* St. Paul: Author.

Moraldo, P.J. (1992). Trends to watch for in '92: Health highest on American agenda. *Executive wire,* New York: National League for Nursing.

Murillo-Rohde, I. (1981). Hispanic American patient care. In G. Henderson & M. Primeaux, (Eds.). *Transcultural health care* (pp. 224-238). Menlo Park CA: Addison-Wesley.

Nahemow, L., McCluskey-Fawcett, K. & McGhee, P. (1986). *Humor and aging.* London: Academic Press.

Naisbitt, J. & Aburdene, P. (1990). *Megatrends 2000.* New York: William Morrow and Company, Inc.

Naisbitt, J. (1982). *Megatrends.* New York: Warner Books.

National Commission to prevent Infant Mortality (1988). *Indirect costs of infant mortality and low birth weight.* Washington DC: The commission.

National League of Nursing Education: Standard curriculum for schools of nursing (1918). Baltimore MD: The Waverly Press.

National League of Nursing Education: A curriculum guide for schools of nursing (1937). New York: The League.

Neufeldt, V. (Ed.), (1991). *Webster's new world dictionary* (3rd ed.). Cleveland: Webster's New World.

Newbern, V.B. (1992). Sharing the memories: The value of reminiscence as a research tool. *Journal of Gerontological Nursing.* 18(5), 13-18.

Nidorf, J.F., & Morgan, M.C. (1987). Cross cultural issues in adolescent medicine. *Primary care*, 14(1), 69-83.

Nightingale, F. (1859). *Notes on nursing.* New York: Appleton-Century-Crofts.

Office of the Surgeon General. (1979). *Healthy people: The surgeon general's report on health promotion and disease prevention; background papers* (DHEW Publication No. 79-55071A). Washington DC: U.S. Government Printing Office.

Office of the Surgeon General. (1990). *Healthy people 2000* (DHHS Publication PHS No. 91-50213). Washington DC: U.S. Government Printing Office.

Okun, B.F. (1987). *Effective helping: Interviewing and counseling techniques* (3rd ed.). Pacific Grove CA: Brooks/Cole.

Pascucci, M.A. (1992). Measuring incentives to health promotion in older adults. *Journal of Gerontological Nursing.* 18(30), 16-23.

Paul, R. (1990). *Critical thinking: What every person needs to survive in a rapidly changing world.* Rohnert Park CA: Center for Critical Thinking and Moral Critique.

Pender, J.J. (1987). *Health promotion in nursing practice.* Norwalk CN: Appleton-Century Crofts.

Perlmutter, L.C. & Monty, R.A. (1989). Motivation and aging. In L.W. Poon, D.C. Rubin, & B.A. Wilson (Eds.), *Everyday cognition in adulthood and late life* (pp. 373-393). Cambridge: Cambridge University Press.

Piaget, J. (1972). Intellectual evolution from adolescence to adulthood. *Human Development,* 15, 1-12.

Pidgeon, V. (1989). Compliance with chronic illness regimens: School-aged children and adolescents. *Journal of Pediatric Nursing,* 4(1), 36.

Pohl, M.L. (1981). *The teaching function of the nurse practitioner.* Dubuque IA: Wm. C. Brown.

Poon, L.W., Rubin, D.C., & Wilson, B.A. (eds.). (1989). *Everyday cognition in adulthood and late life.* Cambridge: Cambridge University Press.

Poon, L.W., Fozard, J.L., Cermack, L.S., Arenberg, D. & Thompson, L.W. (eds.) (1980). *New Directions in Memory and Aging—Proceedings of the George A. Talland Memorial Conference.* Hillsdale NJ: Lawrence Erlbaum Associates.

Poon, L.W., Fozard, J.L. & Popkin, S.J. (1978). Optimizing adult development: Ends and means of an applied psychology of aging. *American psychologist,* 33: 975-989.

Poulson, C.L., Kymissis, E. & Reeve, K.F. (1991). Generalized vocal imitation in infants. *Journal of Experimental Child Psychology,* 51(2), 267.

Practical applications of research. (1981). *Newsletter of Phi Delta Kappa's center on evaluation, development and research.* Bloomington IN: 3(4), 1-4.

Prescott, P.A., Phillips, C.Y., Ryan, J.W. & Thompson, K.O. (Spring, 1991). Changing how nurses spend their time. *IMAGE: Journal of Nursing Scholarship,* 23(1), 23-27.

Primeaux, M. & Henderson, G. (1981). American Indian patient care. In G. Henderson & M. Primeaux, (Eds.). *Transcultural health care* (pp. 239-254). Menlo Park CA: Addison-Wesley.

Putnam, G.L., Brannon, B. & Yanagisako, K.L. (1982). Multimedia public/professional skin cancer education in a multiethnic setting. *Issues in cancer screening and communications.* New York: Alan R. Liss.

Putsch, R.W. (1985). Cross-cultural communication: The special case of interpreters in health care. *Journal of the American Medical Association,* 24, 3344-3348.

Rawl, S.M. (1992). Perspectives on Nursing Care of Chinese Americans. *Journal of Holistic Nursing,* 10(1), 6-17.

Redeker, N.S. (1988). Health beliefs and adherence in chronic illness. *IMAGE: Journal of Nursing Scholarship,* 20(1), 31-35.

Redman, M.K. (1988). *The process of patient education* (6th ed.). St. Louis: Mosby.

Reinisch, J.M., Rosenblum, L.A. & Rubin, D.B. (1991). Sex differences in developmental milestones during the first year of life. *Journal of Psychology and Human Sexuality,* 4(2), 19.

Resnick, B.M. (1991). Geriatric motivation: Clinically helping the elderly to comply. *Journal of Gerontological Nursing,* 17(5), 17-20.

Reynolds, C. (1992). An administrative program to facilitate culturally appropriate care for the elderly. *Holistic Nursing Practice,* 6(3), 34-42.

Rodin, J. (1986). Aging and health: Effects of the sense of control. *Science,* 233, 1271-1276.

Rogers, C. (1969). *Freedom to learn*. Columbus: Charles E. Merrill.

Rogers, C.R. (1961). *On becoming a person*. Boston: Houghton-Mifflin.

Rogers, C.R. (1951). *Client-centered therapy*. Boston: Houghton-Mifflin.

Rollin, B. (1976). *First, you cry*. Philadelphia: Lippincott.

Russell, J.E. (1938). Insights about adult learning. *Journal of Adult Education*, 10(4), 385-386.

Sachs, J.S. & Johnson, M. (1976). Language development in a child of deaf parents. In *Baby talk and infant speech*, W. von Raffler Ergel & Y. le Brun (Eds.), Amsterdam: Swets and Zeitilinger.

Saudino, K.J. & Eaton, W.O. (1991). Infant temperament and genetics: An objective twin study of motor activity level. *Child Development*, 62(5), 1167.

Saylor, C. (1990). Reflection and professional education: Art, science, and competency. *Nurse Educator*, 15(2), 8-11.

Schmidt, L.E., Klover, R.V. & Arfken, C.L. (1992). Compliance with dietary prescriptions in children and adolescents with insulin dependent diabetes mellitus. *Journal of the American Dietetic Association*, 92(5) 567.

Schuster, C.S. & Ashburn, S.S. (1986). *The process of human development a holistic life-span approach* (2nd ed.). Boston: Little, Brown.

Seidel, H.M., Ball, J.W., Dains, J.E., & Benedict, G.W. (1991). *Mosby's guide to physical examination* (2nd ed.). St. Louis: Mosby.

Selder, F. (1989). Life transition theory: The resolution of uncertainty. *Nursing and Health Care*, 10(8), 437-451.

Selkoe, D.J. (1992). Aging brain, aging mind. *Scientific American*, 267(3), 135-142.

S.F. pay jumps 13%, starting now at $43,000. (1991). *American Journal of Nursing*, 91(8), 11.

Shabetai, R. (1983). Cardiomyopathy. How far have we come in 25 years, how far yet to go? *Journal of the American College of Cardiology*, 1, 252.

Shaffer, J. (1978). *Humanistic psychology*. Englewood Cliffs NJ: Prentice-Hall.

Siegel, B. (1986). *Love, medicine and miracles*. New York: Harper & Row.

Slavin, R.E. (1988). *Educational psychology: Theory into practice* (2nd ed.). Englewood Cliffs NJ: Prentice-Hall.

Slavin, R.E. (1991). *Educational psychology: Theory into practice* (3rd ed.). Boston: Allyn & Bacon.

Simpson, E.J. (1972). The classification of educational objectives in the psychomotor domain. In *Contributions of behavioral science to instructional technology: The psychomotor domain*. Mt. Rainier MD: Gryphon.

Smith, D.P. & Nix, K.S. (Eds). (1991). *Comprehensive child and family nursing skills*. St. Louis: Mosby.

Smith, G.R. (1989). Community of caring. *Geriatric Nursing*, 10(5), 248.

Smith, J.A. (1976). The role of the black clergy as allied health care professionals in working with black patients. In Luckraft, D. (Ed.) *Black Awareness: Implications for black patient care*. New York: The American Journal of Nursing.

Smith, M.J., Goodman, J.A. & Ramsey, N.L. (1987). *Child and family: Concepts of nursing practice* (2nd ed.). New York: McGraw-Hill.

Snow, L.F. (1981). Folk medical beliefs and their implications for the care of patients: A review based on studies among black Americans. In G. Henderson & M. Primeaux, (Eds.). *Transcultural health care* (pp. 78-101). Menlo Park CA: Addison-Wesley.

Snow, L. (1983). Traditional health beliefs and practices among lower class black Americans. *The Western Journal of Medicine*, 139(6): 820-828.

Somers, A.R. (Ed.). (1976). *Promoting health, consumer education and national policy: Part III summary and recommendations*. Germantown MD: Aspen Systems Corporation.

Sprague, J. & Stuart, D. (1992). *The speaker's handbook* (3rd ed.). Orlando FL: Harcourt Brace Janovich.

Springer, S.P. & Deutsch, G. (1981). *Left brain, right brain*. New York: W.H. Freeman.

Stein, Z. & Kline, J. (1983). Smoking, alcohol and reproduction. *American Journal of Public Health*, 73:1154-1156.

Steinke, E.E. (1988). Older adults knowledge and attitudes about sexuality and aging. *IMAGE: Journal of Nursing Scholarship*. 20(2), 93-95.

Stevens, M.S. (1987). Which adolescents breeze through surgery? *American Journal of Nursing*, 87(12), 1564-1565.

Streiff, L.D. (1986). Can clients understand our instructions? *IMAGE: Journal of Nursing Scholarship,* 18(20), 48-52.

Suchman, E.A. (1965). Stages of illness and medical care. *Journal of Health and Human Behavior,* 6, 114-128.

Sullivan, K.R. (1990). Maternal implications of cocaine use during pregnancy. *Journal of Perinatal Neonatal Nursing,* 3(4), 12-25.

Thomas, D.N. (1981). Black American patient care. In G. Henderson & M. Primeaux, (Eds.). *Transcultural health care* (pp. 209-223). Menlo Park CA: Addison-Wesley.

Thompson, J.M., McFarland, G.K., Hirsch, J.E., Tucker, S.M., & Bowers, A.C. (1989). *Mosby's manual of clinical nursing,* St. Louis MO: Mosby.

Thorndike, E.L. (1928). *Adult learning.* New York: Macmillan.

Thorne, S.E. & Robinson, C.A. (1989). Guarded illness: Health care relationships in chronic illness. *IMAGE: The Journal of Nursing Scholarship,* 21(3), 153-157.

Tiedt, P.L. & Tiedt, I.M. (1990). *Multicultural teaching.* Boston: Allyn & Bacon.

Toffler, A. (1980). *The third wave.* New York: William Morrow.

Tough, A. (1979). *The adult's learning projects.* Ontario: Institute for Studies in Education.

Tough, A. (1982). *Intentional changes: A fresh approach to helping people change,* Chicago: Follett.

Tripp-Reimer, T., Brink, P.J., Saunders, J.M. (1984). Cultural assessment: Context and process. *Nursing outlook,* 32, 78-82.

U.S. Census Bureau. (1991). *Statistical abstract of the United States: 1991* (111th ed.), Washington DC: Author.

U.S. Senate Special Committee on aging in conjunction with the American Association of Retired Persons. (1989). *Aging America: Trends and projections,* Washington DC: Authors.

Vander Zanden, J.W. (1981). *Human Development* (2nd ed.). New York: Knopf.

von Bertalanffy, L.C. (1968). *General system theory: Foundations, development and applications.* New York: George Braziller.

Watson, G. & Glaser, E. (1964). *Critical thinking appraisal manual.* New York: Harcourt, Brace & World.

Weinrich, S.P., Boyde, M. & Nussbaum, J. (1989). Continuing education: Adapting strategies to teach the elderly. *Journal of Gerontological Nursing,* 15(11), 17-21.

West, R.L. (1989). Planning practical memory training for the aged. In L.W. Poon, D.C. Rubin, & B.A. Wilson (Eds.), *Everyday cognition in adulthood and late life* (pp. 573-591). Cambridge: Cambridge University Press.

Wheeler, R.C., Marcus, A.C., Cullen, J.W., & Konugres, E. (1983). Baseline chronic disease risk factors in a racially heterogeneous elementary school population: The "know your body" program, Los Angeles, *Preventive medicine,* 12, 569-587.

Willitt, J.B. (1988). Sticks and stones may break my bones . . . Reasoning about illness causality and body functioning in children who have a chronic illness. *Pediatrics,* 88(3), 608.

Wilson, B.A. (1989). Designing memory-therapy programs. In L.W. Poon, D.C. Rubin, & B.A. Wilson (eds.), *Everyday cognition in adulthood and late life* (pp. 615-637). Cambridge: Cambridge University Press.

Winslow, E.H. (1985). Cardiovascular consequences of bed rest. *Heart & Lung,* 14, 236.

Witt, B.S. (1991). The homeless shelter: An ideal clinical setting for RN/BSN Students. *Nursing and Health Care,* 12(6), 304-307.

Wong, D.L. (1990). *Clinical manual of pediatric nursing.* St. Louis: Mosby.

Yesavage, J.S., Lapp, D., & Sheikh, J.I. (1989). In L.W. Poon, D.C. Rubin, & B.A. Wilson (Eds.), *Everyday cognition in adulthood and late life* (pp. 598-611). Cambridge: Cambridge University Press.

Yesavage, J.A., Rose, T.L., & Bower, G.G. (1983). Interactive imaging and judgments improve face-name learning in the elderly. *Journal of Gerontology,* 29, 197-203.

Zakaluk, B.L. & Samuels, S.J. (Eds.). (1988). *Readability: its past, present and future.* Newark, DL: International, Reading Association.

Zerwekh, J.V. (1992). Public health nursing legacy. *Nursing and Health Care,* 13(2), 84-91.

Zimmerman, B.J. (1990). Self-regulated learning and academic achievement: An overview. *Educational Psychologist,* 25(1), 3-17.

INDEX

American College Health
Association, address and
phone number of, 305
American Dental Association,
address and phone
number of, 305
American Diabetes Association,
address and phone
number of, 305
American Foundation for the Blind,
address and phone
number of, 304
American Heart Association,
address and phone
number of, 305
American Lung Association,
address and phone
number of, 306
Analogue model, teaching with,
208
Analysis
cognitive domain and, 168
health teaching and, 5-6
Andragogy, 94-99
Anecdote, use of, 238-239
Angal, Andral, Association for
Humanistic Psychology
founded by, 41
Anger
motivation for learning through,
61
teaching through use of, 61
in young child, teaching and, 76
Anxiety
about memory loss, in older
adult, 112
lecture preparation and, 187
parental, 73
speech, dealing with, 187-188
Apgar scale, 271
Appearance, lecture affected by,
186, 187
Applicability, learning affected by,
47
Application, cognitive domain and,
168
Aristotle, learning theory and, 34
Arousal
learning affected by, 47, 56-57
memory affected by, 114
Art-O-Graph, teaching with, 214
Arteriosclerosis, aging as cause of,
105

Asian American(s)
attitude toward aging of, 115
compliance to health education
and, 257
definition of, 128
folk medicine and, 140-142
holistic health paradigm and,
137
hot and cold imbalance and,
138
importance of family to, 149
nonverbal communication and,
146
nutrition patterns of, 150-152
verbal communication style of,
145
Assessment
communication difficulties and,
61-62
of culturally diverse clients,
124-159
data from
analysis of, 162-179
general considerations about,
164
dynamics of, 56-57
fundamentals of, 54-67
health teaching and, 5
process of, 55
psychosocial, education level of
client and, 60
of readability of teaching
materials, exercise for, 227
Assimilation, learning and, 40
Association, learning through use
of, 46
Association for Humanistic
Psychology, 41
Atherosclerosis, aging as cause of,
105
Attention
learning affected by, 47
memory affected by, 114
teaching/learning process and,
113
Attentiveness, teaching success
and, 239
Attitude scale, sample of, 278
Attitude(s)
adjustment of, appropriate
teaching strategy for, 198
affective domain of learning and,
24

measurement of, 277
perception affected by, 56
teacher, successful teaching and,
232-233
teaching learning process
affected by, in older adult,
105
Audience
consideration of, in lecture
preparation, 183
participation of, use of
chalkboard for, 215-216
Audiocassette tape
advantages and disadvantages of,
224t-225t
filmstrip accompanied by, 211
instruction of young child with,
76
teaching with, 211-212
Audiovisual materials, sources of,
304-306
Audiovisual materials, use of, with
lecture, 184
Authenticity, teaching success and,
239-240
Awareness, affective domain and,
169

B

B vitamin, memory and, 119
Balance, holistic health paradigm
and, 136
Behavior
adult, health education and, 254
change in, compliance to health
education and, 250
complex, measurement of, 269
definition of, 37
reinforcement of, 240-244
respondent, learning and, 35
Behavior modification, learning
theory and, 36
Behavior theory
child development and, 71
learning and, 34-38
propositions of, 35-36
Behavioral objectives, writing of,
exercise for, 177-178
Behaviorism, learning and, 35-38
Beliefs
affective domain of learning and,
24
cultural diversity and, 129

Bias, observer, measurement and, 269
Black American(s)
    attitude toward aging of, 115
    communication challenges and, 146
    compliance to health education and, 258
    folk medicine and, 140-142
    holistic health paradigm and, 137
    hypertension in, 152
    importance of family to, 149
    magico-religious health paradigm and, 132
    nutrition patterns of, 150-151
Black English, communication and, 144-145
Blood flow, changes in, aging as cause of, 105
Body humors, holistic health paradigm and, 138
Body integrity, fear of loss of, in preschool child, 78
Bone, absorption of, aging as cause of, 105
Boundary, definition of, in health teaching system, 7
Brain, information processing in, 44
Bronchitis, older adult health problem because of, 110
Brujeria, illness associated with, in magico-religious health paradigm, 132
Bulletin board, use of, 218

C

CAI; *see* Computer assisted instruction
Calcification, arterial, aging as cause of, 105
Cancer
    magico-religious health paradigm and, 132
    older adult health problem because of, 110
Cardiovascular disease, older adult health problem because of, 110
Cardiovascular system, changes in, aging as cause of, 105
Caretaker, of young child, teaching of, 76

Cartesian dualism, definition of, 135
Cartoon
    advantages and disadvantages of, 224t-225t
    teaching and use of, 217-218
Cassette recorder, operation of, 211-212
Caucasian American(s), holistic health paradigm and, 137
CDC National AIDS Clearinghouse, address and phone number of, 305
Chaining, behavior influenced by, 242-243
Chalkboard
    advantages and disadvantages of, 224t-225t
    guidelines for use of, 215-216
    teaching with, 214-215
Channing L. Bete Co., Inc., address and phone number of, 306
Characterization, affective domain and, 169-170
Checklist, measurement with, 271-272
Chicano, definition of, 127
Child; *see also* Adolescent; Infant
    assessment of, exercises for, 87
    behavioral theories and development of, 71
    as client for health education, 252-254
    health education for, 8
    health of, sources of audiovisual materials on, 306
    information processing by, 72
    play and, 299-303
    preschool, 77-79
        cognitive characteristics of, 78
        language development in, 78
        play and, 301
        psychosocial characteristics of, 77-78
    psychologic environment of, 70
    school-age, 79-82
        cognitive characteristics of, 80-81
        language characteristics of, 81

psychosocial characteristics of, 80
teaching of, 81-82
school-age, play and, 302
sexual development of, 72
stress and development of, 72-73
teaching to, 68-89
temperament of, 72
toddler, 74-77
    cognitive development in, 75
    language development in, 75-76
    psychosocial characteristics of, 74
    teaching of, 76-77
Child development, stages of, nursing implications for, 85t-86t
Chinese American(s)
    compliance to health education and, 258
    folk medicine and, 140, 141
    nonverbal communication and, 146
    verbal communication style of, 145
Christianity, holistic health paradigm and, 140
Chronic illness; *see* Illness, chronic
Church, Black American cultural tradition and, 141
Cigarette smoking
    health education about, client compliance and, 255
    sources of audiovisual materials on, 306
Cigarette smoking, health education and, 9
Client; *see also* Adolescent; Adult; Child
    adaptation of, to health problem, 259-260
    compliance of, 248-265
    convalescing, teaching to, 58-59
    cultural assessment of, 143
    cultural differences between nurse and, 154-155
    culturally diverse
        assessment of, 124-159
        compliance to health education and, 257-259
        teaching to, 126-129

Focus
  of discussion, 190-191
  maintenance of, in teaching, 239
Focusing, learning affected by, 45
Folk illness, 133t-135t
Folk medicine, 140-143
Folk practitioner, 140-143
Food, holistic health paradigm and,
    138
Forgetfulness; *see* Memory, loss of
  causes of, in older adult, 106
Frames, programmed instruction
    and, 194
Fry's graph, readability measured
    with, 221, 222f

G

Gallstones, older adult health
    problem because of, 110
Gastrointestinal system, problems
    in, older adult and, 110
Gender, sensitivity to, 239
Genuineness, teaching success and,
    239-240
Gestalt frame of reference, 25
Gestalt psychology, 38-41
Gestalt theory, child development
    and, 71
Gesture(s), lecture and, 186
Glare, sensitivity to, aging and, 107
God, magico-religious health
    paradigm and, 132
Goldstein, Kurt, Association for
    Humanistic Psychology
    founded by, 41
Grade(s), behavioral response to,
    243-244
Group activity, teaching through
    use of, 196
Guilt, development of preschool
    child and, 77
Guthrie, Edwin, learning theory
    and, 35

H

Harmony, holistic health paradigm
    and, 136, 138-140
Health
  belief systems about, 129-140,
    139t
  learning affected by, 48
Health care, current trends in,
    11-12

Health education
  approaches to, for culturally
    diverse clients, 155-156
  intergenerational conflict and,
    153-154
  knowledge about cultures and,
    143-153
  limiting factors of, 13
  motivation and, 9
  research and development of, 10
  special problems in, 153-155
  target groups for, 8
  theory development in, 34
Health information, sources of
    audiovisual materials on,
    305-306
Health teaching; *see also* Teaching
  context of, 7-10
  history of, 7-8
  limiting factors of, 13
  research and development of, 10
  target groups for, 8
Health teaching system, nurse's role
    in, 2-17
Healthy People, 8-9
Healthy People 2000, 9, 10
Hearing
  changes in, aging as cause of,
    108-109
  impaired, communication with
    client with, 62
  Heart, changes in, aging as cause
    of, 105
Heart disease, older adult health
    problem because of, 110
Hechiceria, illness associated with,
    in magico-religious health
    paradigm, 132
Height, loss of, aging as cause of,
    105
Herbal specialist, folk medicine
    and, 141
Herbs, holistic health paradigm
    and, 138
Hex, illness associated with, in
    magico-religious health
    paradigm, 132
Hierarchy of needs, 41
High blood, definition of, 151
Hispanic American(s)
  attitude toward aging of, 115
  compliance to health education
    and, 257

folk medicine and, 140-142
holistic health paradigm and,
    137
hot and cold imbalance and,
    138
importance of family to, 149
magico-religious health paradigm
    and, 130
nutrition patterns of, 150-151
verbal communication style of,
    144
Hoodoo, illness associated with, in
    magico-religious health
    paradigm, 132
Hot and cold forces, holistic health
    paradigm and, 137-138
Houle, C.O., adult learning theory
    and, 92, 93
Human development
  environmental influences on, 70
  systems theory and, 70-71
Human growth movement, nursing
    and, 10
Human potential movement, 41
Humanism
  learning theory and, 41-42
  theories about child
    development and, 72
Humor, use of, in teaching, 239
Hygiene, personal, instruction
    about, 81
Hypertension
  health education for client with,
    152-153
  older adult health problem
    because of, 110
Hypertrophy, aging as cause of, 105

I

Illness
  belief systems about, 129-140,
    139t
  chronic, teaching to client with,
    58
  definition of, 130
  folk, 133t-135t
  holistic health paradigm and,
    138
  levels of client compliance to
    health education and, 254
  severity, teaching/learning
    process affected by, 61
  symptoms of, instruction about,
    81

Illustration
    on posters and pamphlets,
        216-217
    use of, 238-239
Imitation
    child development and use of,
        71
    learning through use of, 46
Immune system suppression, ill
        health in elderly client
        associated with, 109
Immunization, programs for, history
        of, 7-8
Implementation
    health teaching and, 6
    of teaching strategies, 230-247
Individual, definition of, 5
Infant; *see also* Child
    development of, 70
    family of, instruction of, 73
    information processing in, 72
    language development in, 74
    play and, 300-301
    psychosocial characteristics of,
        73
    sensorimotor development in,
        73-74
Information processing, 42-44
    thinking defined as, 25
Initiative, development of, in
        preschool child, 77
Input
    as component of learning, 22
    in teaching/learning system, 5
Instruction
    group, instruction to adolescents
        with, 84
    programmed, examples of, 44
Integrity, older adult psychosocial
        development and, 104
Interest, teaching/learning process
        and, 113
International Hearing Society,
        address and phone
        number of, 305
Interpreters, use of, in health
        situations, 147-148
Iris, changes in, aging as cause of,
        106
Iron, memory and, 119

J

Journal of Adult Education, 92

K

Kangaroo Care, 72
Kellogg Foundation, health
        education research by, 10
Knowledge
    cognitive domain and, 167
    definition of, 26
Knowles, M.
    adult learing theory and, 94
    adult learning theory and, 92, 98
Koehler, W., learning theory
        developed by, 38
Koffka, K., learning theory
        developed by, 38
Kroy machine, transparencies made
        with, 212

L

La Leche League International,
        address and phone
        number of, 306
Lactase, deficiency of, in ethnic
        groups, 150-151
Lactose, intolerance to, in ethnic
        groups, 150-151
Language
    acquisition of, child
        development and, 73
    adolescent vocabulary and,
        83-84
    as barrier, in communication
        with elderly client, 116
    cultural diversity and, 144
    development of
        in infant and child, 74
        in preschool child, 78
        in school-age child, 81
        in toddler, 75-76
    figurative, readability of teaching
        materials and, 221
    impaired, communication with
        client with, 62
Latino; *see* Mexican American(s);
        see also Hispanic
        American(s)
Law of Contiguous Conditioning,
        35
Law of Effect, learning and, 35
Learner, learning-oriented, 93-94
Learning
    activity-oriented, 93
    affective
        humanistic psychology and,
        42

measurement of, 279
    promotion of, 255
affective domain and, 24
behavioral change and, 37
behavioral theories of, 34-38
    compliance to health
        education and, 252-253
in childhood, 68-89
cognitive
    humanistic psychology and,
        42
    measurement of, 277, 279
definition of, 22
domains of, 22-24
    learning objectives and, 166-
        167
gestalt view of, 38
goal-oriented, 92-93
information processing and,
    42-44
motivation for, 56
multicultural, exercise for, 157
operant, 35
orientation to, 97
    by adult learner, 92-93
    exercises for, 100
principles of, 45-48
psychomotor, measurement of,
    279
reader profile for, 288-289
readiness for, 56-57, 96-97
reinforcement of, 238
self-paced, computer assisted
    instruction for, 218
theories and principles of, 32-51
    historical perspective of, 34
    thinking and, 25-26
transactional nature of, 70-71
Learning, objectives of; *see* Learning
    objectives
Learning environment, teaching
        success and, 233
Learning objectives
    affective domain and, 168-169
    clear definition of, 235
    cognitive domain and, 167-168
    components of, 166-167
    criteria for, 166
    establishment of, 164-165
    historical context of, 167
    psychomotor domain and,
        170-172
    purpose of, 166
    taxonomy of, 167
    writing of, exercise for, 177-178

Sexually transmitted disease, instruction about, to adolescents, 84
Shaman, folk medicine and, 140-142
Side effects, drug, compliance to health education affected by, 255
Silence, need for, in question and answer situation, 237
Sin, illness attributed to, 140
Skill building, appropriate teaching strategy for, 198
Skill(s)
    development of, health education and, 9
    measurement of, 277
    training for, older adult client and, 256
Skin, changes in, aging as cause of, 105
Skinner, B.F., learning theory and, 35
Skinner box, 35
Slide-audiocassette, teaching with, 210
Slides
    advantages and disadvantages of, 224t-225t
    teaching and use of, 210-211
Smallpox, eradication of, 8
Smoking; see Cigarette smoking
Social isolation, ill health in elderly client associated with, 109
Socioeconomic characteristics, consideration of, in lecture preparation, 183
Sorcery, illness explained by, in Hispanic culture, 130
Spiritualist, folk medicine and, 140-142
Standard English, communication and, 145
Stanford Heart Disease Program, 10
Statistics, lecture supplemented with, 185
Stereotyping, definition of, 129
Stimulus persistence, aging associated with, 108
Stimulus-response theory, learning and, 34-38
Stress, compliance to health education affected by, 257

Substance abuse, instruction about, to adolescents, 84
Subsystem, definition of, in health teaching system, 7
Success, behavioral response to, 240
Suprasystem, definition of, 6
Symbol, teaching and use of, 208-210
Synthesis, cognitive domain and, 168
System
    coexisting, 7
    definition of, 4
Systems theory
    definition of, 4-5
    human development explained through, 70-71
    thinking and, 25

T

Taboo, illness explained by, in Hispanic culture, 130
Tape recorder, operation of, 211-212
Task Force on Black and Minority Health, 155
Task Force on Consumer Health Education, 9
Taxonomy
    definition of, 167
    of learning objectives, 167
Teacher
    evaluation of, 279-282
    relationship of, with client, 63
    as subsystem in teaching/learning system, 63
Teaching; see also Health teaching
    of adolescent, 84
    audiovisual materials and, 206-207
    behavioral change and, 37
    of caretakers of infant, 74
    clinical, 5
    community, checklist for, 298
    to culturally diverse clients, 126-129
    demonstration as method for, 192-194
    discussion as method for, 188-192
    evaluation of, 266-285
    formal, 182

general health, older adult client and, 110
gestalt psychology in, 40
group activity as method for, 196
informal, 182
materials for; see Teaching materials
modeling as method for, 194
module of
    evaluation of, 293
    written outline for, 291-293
    nursing diagnosis and, 294-297
as nursing function, 12-13
of preschool child, 78-79
principles of, 232-238
programmed instruction as method for, 194-195
quality, exercise for, 245
role playing as method for, 196-197
of school-age child, 81-82
simulated environment as method for, 195-196
strategies for, 180-203
    advantages and disadvantages of, 201t
    exercise for selection of, 202
    implementation of, 230-247
    selection of, 198-199
team, use of posters and, 217
team approach to, 197-198
    advantages and disadvantages of, 201t
theory-based, 34
of toddler, 74-77
types of, 182
Teaching/learning process
    chronic disease and, 109-111
    communication and, 147
    description of, 4-7
    educational level of client and, 60
    environment of, 63-65
    evaluation of, 266-285
    physiologic changes due to aging and, 104-110
    settings of, 65
    sociologic factors and, 59-60
Teaching/learning system
    description of, 4-7
    purpose of, 4